2005
YEAR BOOK OF
UROLOGY®

The 2005 Year Book Series

Year Book of Allergy, Asthma, and Clinical Immunology™: Drs Rosenwasser, Boguniewicz, Milgrom, Routes, and Weber

Year Book of Anesthesiology and Pain Management™: Drs Chestnut, Abram, Black, Gravlee, Mathru, Lee, and Roizen

Year Book of Cardiology®: Drs Gersh, Cheitlin, Graham, Kaplan, Sundt, and Waldo

Year Book of Critical Care Medicine®: Drs Dellinger, Parrillo, Balk, Bekes, Dorman, and Dries

Year Book of Dentistry®: Drs Zakariasen, Horswell, McIntyre, Scott, and Zakariasen Victoroff

Year Book of Dermatology and Dermatologic Surgery™: Drs Thiers and Lang

Year Book of Diagnostic Radiology®: Drs Osborn, Birdwell, Dalinka, Gardiner, Levy, Maynard, Oestreich, and Rosado de Christenson

Year Book of Emergency Medicine®: Drs Burdick, Cydulka, Hamilton, Handly, Quintana, and Werner

Year Book of Endocrinology®: Drs Mazzaferri, Bessesen, Howard, Kannan, Kennedy, Leahy, Meikle, Molitch, Rogol, and Rubin

Year Book of Family Practice®: Drs Bowman, Apgar, Bouchard, Dexter, Miser, Neill, and Scherger

Year Book of Gastroenterology™: Drs Lichtenstein, Burke, Dempsey, Drebin, Ginsberg, Katzka, Kochman, Morris, Nunes, Shah, and Stein

Year Book of Hand Surgery and Upper Limb Surgery®: Drs Berger and Ladd

Year Book of Medicine®: Drs Barkin, Frishman, Klahr, Loehrer, Mazzaferri, Phillips, Pillinger, and Snydman

Year Book of Neonatal and Perinatal Medicine®: Drs Fanaroff, Maisels, and Stevenson

Year Book of Neurology and Neurosurgery®: Drs Gibbs and Verma

Year Book of Nuclear Medicine®: Drs Coleman, Blaufox, Royal, Strauss, and Zubal

Year Book of Obstetrics, Gynecology, and Women's Health®: Dr Shulman

Year Book of Oncology®: Drs Loehrer, Arceci, Glatstein, Gordon, Hanna, Morrow, and Thigpen

Year Book of Ophthalmology®: Drs Rapuano, Cohen, Eagle, Grossman, Hammersmith, Myers, Nelson, Penne, Sergott, Shields, Tipperman, and Vander

Year Book of Orthopedics®: Drs Morrey, Beauchamp, Peterson, Swiontkowski, Trigg, and Yaszemski

Year Book of Otolaryngology-Head and Neck Surgery®: Drs Paparella, Otto, and Keefe

Year Book of Pathology and Laboratory Medicine®: Drs Raab, Grzybicki, Bejarano, Bissell, and Stanley

Year Book of Pediatrics®: Dr Stockman

Year Book of Plastic and Aesthetic Surgery™: Drs Miller, Bartlett, Garner, McKinney, Ruberg, Salisbury, and Smith

Year Book of Psychiatry and Applied Mental Health®: Drs Talbott, Ballenger, Buckley, Frances, Jensen, and Markowitz

Year Book of Pulmonary Disease®: Drs Phillips, Barker, Dunlap, Lewis, Maurer, and Willsie

Year Book of Rheumatology, Arthritis, and Musculoskeletal Disease™: Drs Panush, Hadler, Hellmann, Hochberg, Lahita, and Seibold

Year Book of Sports Medicine®: Drs Shephard, Alexander, Cantu, Feldman, McCrory, Nieman, Rowland, Sanborn, and Shrier

Year Book of Surgery®: Drs Copeland, Bland, Cerfolio, Daly, Eberlein, Fahey, Mozingo, Pruett, and Seeger

Year Book of Urology®: Drs Andriole and Coplen

Year Book of Vascular Surgery®: Dr Moneta

2005

The Year Book of UROLOGY®

Editors

Gerald L. Andriole, Jr, MD

Professor and Chief of Urology, Washington University School of Medicine; Chief of Urology, Barnes-Jewish Hospital, St Louis, Missouri

Douglas E. Coplen, MD

Associate Professor of Surgery (Urology), Washington University School of Medicine; Director of Pediatric Urology, St Louis Children's Hospital, St Louis, Missouri

ELSEVIER
MOSBY

ELSEVIER
MOSBY

Vice President, Continuity Publishing: Timothy M. Griswold
Publishing Director, Continuity: J. Heather Cullen
Developmental Editor: Dana M. Lamparello
Senior Manager, Continuity Production: Idelle L. Winer
Senior Issue Manager: Jason Gonulsen
Illustrations and Permissions Coordinator: Dawn Vohsen

2005 EDITION

Printed in the United States of America
Composition by Thomas Technology Solutions, Inc.
Printing/binding by Sheridan Books, Inc.

Editorial Office:
Elsevier
Suite 1800
1600 John F. Kennedy Blvd
Philadelphia, PA 19103-2899

International Standard Serial Number: 0084–4071
International Standard Book Number: 0-323-02119-0

Contributors

Sam B. Bhayani, MD
Assistant Professor of Urology, Surgery, Washington University School of Medicine, St Louis, Missouri

Adam S. Kibel, MD
Associate Professor of Urologic Surgery, Washington University School of Medicine, St Louis, Missouri

Venkatesh Krishnamurthi, MD
Director, Kidney/Pancreas Transplant, Cleveland Clinic Foundation, Cleveland, Ohio

Cathy K. Naughton, MD
Assistant Professor of Urologic Surgery, Director of Male Infertility and Microsurgery, Washington University School of Medicine, Barnes-Jewish Hospital, St Louis, Missouri

David K. Ornstein, MD
Assistant Professor, University of California, Irvine, University of California Irvine Medical Center, Orange, California

Claus G. Roehrborn, MD
Professor and Chairman, Department of Urology, University of Texas Southwestern Medical Center; Professor and Chair, University of Texas Southwestern, Parkland, Dallas, Texas

Eric S. Rovner, MD
Associate Professor of Urology, Medical University of South Carolina; Attending Physician, Medical University Hospital, Charleston, South Carolina

John T. Wei, MD, MSc
Associate Professor of Urology, University of Michigan, Ann Arbor, Michigan

Table of Contents

Journals Represented xi

Introduction xiii

1. **Clinical Research** 1

2. **Medical Education** 5

3. **Practice Management** 9

4. **Imaging** 15

5. **Endourology and Stone Disease** 19

6. **Laparoscopy** 27

7. **Transplantation** 43

8. **Female Urology** 55
   - Incontinence and Voiding Dysfunction 55
   - Tension Free Vaginal Tape/Transobturator Tape 69
   - Sling/Pelvic Prolapse 78
   - Sexual Function 83

9. **Urinary Tract Infection** 85

10. **Sexually Transmitted Disease** 87

11. **Benign Prostatic Hyperplasia** 89
    - Epidemiology 89
    - Diagnostics 93
    - Medical Treatment 104
    - Surgical Treatment 110

12. **Male Incontinence** 123

13. **Renal Tumors** 125

14. **Urothelial Cancer** 145

15. **Prostate Cancer** 161
    - Epidemiology/Outcomes 161
    - Screening/Diagnosis 175
    - Radical Prostatectomy 189
    - Radiation Therapy 195
    - Systemic Chemotherapy 199
    - Advanced Disease—Imaging and Treatment 203

16. Scrotum 213
17. Infertility 215
18. Sexual Function 229
19. Urethral Reconstruction 235
20. Pediatric Urinary Tract Infection 237
21. Vesicoureteral Reflux 243
22. Voiding Dysfunction 247
23. Neurogenic Bladder 251
24. Antenatal Hydronephrosis 255
25. Neurogenic Reconstruction 261
26. Urinary Reconstruction 265
27. Hypospadias 269
28. Genital Ambiguity 277
29. Cryptorchidism 279
30. Varicocele 283
31. Pediatric Oncology 285
SUBJECT INDEX 287
AUTHOR INDEX 301

Journals Represented

Journals represented in this YEAR BOOK are listed below.

Academic Emergency Medicine
Acta Obstetricia et Gynecologica Scandinavica
Acta Paediatrica
American Journal of Epidemiology
American Journal of Obstetrics and Gynecology
Annals of Internal Medicine
Archives of Pediatrics and Adolescent Medicine
British Journal of Urology International
British Medical Journal
Cancer
Cancer Research
Clinical Cancer Research
European Urology
Human Reproduction
Journal of Clinical Endocrinology and Metabolism
Journal of Clinical Oncology
Journal of Pediatrics
Journal of Ultrasound in Medicine
Journal of Urology
Journal of the American College of Surgeons
Journal of the American Medical Association
Journal of the American Society of Nephrology
Journal of the National Cancer Institute
Kidney International
Lancet
Mayo Clinic Proceedings
Medical Care
Medical Decision Making
Neurology and Urodynamics
New England Journal of Medicine
Pediatrics
Prenatal Diagnosis
Proceedings of the National Academy of Sciences
Psychiatric Services
Science
Surgery
Transplantation
Urology

STANDARD ABBREVIATIONS

The following terms are abbreviated in this edition: acquired immunodeficiency syndrome (AIDS), cardiopulmonary resuscitation (CPR), central nervous system (CNS), cerebrospinal fluid (CSF), computed tomography (CT), deoxyribonucleic acid (DNA), electrocardiography (ECG), health maintenance organization (HMO), human immunodeficiency virus (HIV), intensive care unit (ICU), intramuscular (IM), intravenous (IV), magnetic resonance (MR) imaging (MRI), ribonucleic acid (RNA), ultrasound (US), and ultraviolet (UV).

NOTE

The YEAR BOOK OF UROLOGY is a literature survey service providing abstracts of articles published in the professional literature. Every effort is made to assure the accuracy of the information presented in these pages. Neither the editors nor the publisher of the YEAR BOOK OF UROLOGY can be responsible for errors in the original materials. The editors' comments are their own opinions. Mention of specific products within this publication does not constitute endorsement.

To facilitate the use of the YEAR BOOK OF UROLOGY as a reference tool, all illustrations and tables included in this publication are now identified as they appear in the original article. This change is meant to help the reader recognize that any illustration or table appearing in the YEAR BOOK OF UROLOGY may be only one of many in the original article. For this reason, figure and table numbers will often appear to be out of sequence within the YEAR BOOK OF UROLOGY.

Introduction

The 2005 Year Book of Urology has been assembled from more than 3000 articles selected from worldwide peer-reviewed publications. It represents an attempt to summarize some of the best and most important contributions this year to the specialty of urology.

Evidence-Based Medicine and Clinical Research

There is increasing awareness that urology needs to develop methodology and measures for both quality of care and quality of life. The first 2 chapters address these issues in medical education and clinical research.

Laparoscopy

Laparoscopy continues to evolve with an emphasis on increasing complex ablative and reconstructive procedures. Abstracts 6–1 through 6–3 discuss laparoscopic prostatectomy costs and outcomes. Laparoscopic nephrectomy is now an acceptable standard, and the laparoscopic approach to partial nephrectomy is more widely accepted as surgeons become more adept at intracorporeal suturing (Abstracts 6–9 and 6–10). The role of ablative therapy in small renal masses needs further evaluation (Abstract 6–11). Complications of laparoscopic surgery are discussed in the last 4 abstracts in this section.

Transplantation

Recent studies show excellent rejection-free graft survival with early withdrawal of prednisone. A variety of approaches to reduce donor-specific antibody now enable ABO incompatible and cross-match incompatible transplantation.

Female Urology

Nine abstracts discuss treatment and outcomes of the suburethral tapes. The efficacy of botulinum toxin in the management of overactive bladder and urinary tract dysfunction is detailed in 4 abstracts.

Urinary Infections

Purified antibodies can prevent bacterial adherence and ascending infection.

Benign Prostatic Hyperplasia and Male Incontinence

The appropriate management of benign prostatic hyperplasia includes an understanding of the natural history (Abstracts 11–1 and 11–2), evaluation of outcomes with medical therapy (Abstracts 11–12 through 11–16), and the appropriate utility of newer minimally invasive therapies. While the artificial urinary sphincter is the gold standard for postprostatectomy incontinence, the male urethral sling may have a limited role (Abstracts 12–1 and 12–2).

Renal Tumors

Treatment of advanced renal cell cancer has not improved over the past several years. Antiangiogenesis therapies may not be curative but could improve long-term survival (Abstracts 13–16 and 13–17).

Bladder Cancer

Urethral recurrence after cystectomy and neobladder is uncommon, but the management can be challenging (Abstracts 14–11 through 14–13).

Prostate Cancer

The abstracted articles cover a wide range of topics including prediction of outcomes before and after surgical treatment, controversies in screening and diagnosis, and a section on new chemotherapy with a survival benefit in prostatic adenocarcinoma. The reader is encouraged to look at this excellent section that focuses on one of the most important parts of most urologic practices. Controversy persists with regard to prostate cancer detection and treatment.

Pediatrics

A new technique of injection of dextran polymer for correction of vesicoureteral reflux has increased the success rate (Abstract 21–2). Transitional cell carcinoma is being reported after bladder augmentation, and children with this carcinoma will need to be screened in adulthood (Abstract 25–1). Oxybutynin has now been formally evaluated in children with neurogenic bladder (Abstract 23–1). The importance of the relationship between the magnitude of antenatal renal dilation and postnatal outcomes is better defined (Abstracts 24–1 through 24–4). Tubularized incised plate hypospadias repairs give good results (Abstracts 27–1 and 27–2), but preputial flaps have similar success and may be preferable in some children (Abstract 27–3). Gender reassignment remains controversial and may not be problematic in a 46XY patient with testosterone exposure (Abstract 28–1).

Douglas E. Coplen, MD

Gerald L. Andriole, Jr, MD

1 Clinical Research

Pretest Probability Estimates: A Pitfall to the Clinical Utility of Evidence-based Medicine?

Phelps MA, Levitt MA (Alameda County Med Ctr-Highland Campus, Oakland, Calif)

Acad Emerg Med 11:692-694, 2004 1–1

Introduction.—The Bayesian application of likelihood ratios has been incorporated into the model of evidence-based medicine (EBM). In this approach, a provider's clinical suspicion (or pretest probability) of a given disease in a particular patient is used to generate an individualized posttest probability of disease. As yet, however, there is minimum scientific validation for the clinical application of this approach. To evaluate the ability of this approach to yield consistent posttest disease estimates, a cross-sectional cohort study was designed.

Methods.—The study, conducted at an urban county teaching hospital, included as participants a sample of emergency and internal medicine residents and faculty and midlevel practitioners from the emergency department (ED). The initial step in the approach, clinicians' estimates of pretest probability, was assessed for variability. Those who participated read 4 clinical vignettes representing patients seen in the ED with a possible clinical disease: acute myocardial infarction (AMI), pulmonary embolus, deep vein thrombosis (DVT), and urinary tract infection. Clinicians had history and physical examination findings available, but not the results of laboratory or imaging studies.

Results.—The 56 residents and physicians and 5 emergency physician assistants who took part in the study were asked to estimate the likelihood of the suggested diagnosis as a percentage (0%-100%). Mean pretest probability estimates ranged from 42% to 77%. The smallest difference in pretest probability magnitude for a single vignette was 70% (in DVT); the largest was 95% (for AMI).

Conclusion.—A finding of wide variability in clinicians' pretest probability estimates of disease, even in cases with identical information, raises concerns about EBM based on Bayes' theorem. Such extensive variations may yield inconsistent posttest disease estimates.

► A fundamental tenet of modern medicine is to use medical evidence taken from the literature to guide decision making. A common approach is known as the Bayesian method in which the likelihood of a condition is estimated before the use of a diagnostic test. This pretest estimate is then incorporated with the sensitivity and specificity of a given test to determine the posttest likelihood of having a specific condition. This paradigm applies well in scenarios in which screening tests are performed, such as prostate specific antigen (PSA) screening. In this study, the authors found that the pretest probability estimates by clinicians working in an ED vary tremendously even when given a uniform set of vignettes. Although on the surface this may seem problematic, this degree of variance likely exists whether or not the Bayesian prediction approaches are used. Despite these findings, it is likely that implementation of decision aids such as nomograms for prostate cancer screening will decrease posttest variability. Additional research should focus on how the variability in pretest probability estimates actually affects treatment decisions, eg, the number of patients undergoing prostate biopsy as a result of PSA-based screening.

J. T. Wei, MD, MSc

Impact of FUTON and NAA Bias on Visibility of Research

Murali NS, Murali HR, Auethavekiat P, et al (Mayo Clinic College of Medicine, Rochester, Minn)

Mayo Clin Proc 79:1001-1006, 2004 1–2

Introduction.—Evidence-based medicine (EBM) continues to gain acceptance among health care professionals and to be incorporated into the curriculum of medical schools in the United States. The growth of EBM has been facilitated by the Internet, and most physicians access MEDLINE because it is free, easy to access, and familiar. But scientific articles on MEDLINE/PubMed appear as FUTON (full text on the net), abstracts only, or NAA (no abstract available), with a low percentage available as FUTON. To determine whether the ability to obtain journals as FUTON affects their impact factor, the availability of journals as FUTON on MEDLINE or free FUTON on the Web was examined for the fields of cardiology, nephrology, and rheumatology/immunology.

Methods.—A comprehensive search sought to identify all journals in English related to these specialties, using MEDLINE, PubMed, and EMBASE databases as well as online publishers and several search engines. Excluded were journals published after 1999 and those that discontinued publication between 1998 and 2000. Of 324 journals identified, 159 journals were in existence in both the pre- and post-Internet (1992 and 2001) era. The change in impact factor for these journals was calculated by dividing the number of citations in the current year by the source items published in that journal during the previous 2 years.

Results.—Of the 324 journals, 38.3% were FUTON, 42.6% had abstracts only, and 19.1% had NAA. Mean impact factors were 3.24, 164, and 0.14, respectively. In the subgroup of 159 journals, 19 were available as free FUTON, 132 had free abstracts only, and 8 had NAA. Analysis of the change in impact factor from pre- and post-Internet eras showed no statistically significant difference among groups, but there was a trend for a greater impact for FUTON journals versus those with free abstracts only. More than 90% of the free FUTON journals were not available until 1 year after publication.

Conclusion.—The online availability of medical literature as FUTON or NAA may determine a journal's impact factor. Relevant non-FUTON articles may not reach a wide audience, thereby limiting their potential influence.

► The impact factor is a standardized measure of how frequently a journal article is cited during a particular year of time. It is calculated by determining the number of citations of articles from a journal divided by the total number of articles or proceedings published by that journal during the same period. These data have been published by the Institute for Scientific Information (ISI) since 1975 and are widely quoted. Although the impact factor is explicitly used to rank journals, they also have a direct effect on the choice of journals that are targeted for submission by investigators. In many medical schools they may also have an effect on academic promotion, in that promotion committees often rate the value of the publication according to the impact factor of the journal in which the original publications are published.

This study evaluated how the availability of articles and journals online affects the impact factor. In their cross-sectional analysis, it is clear that journals with full text online have higher impact factors; however, considering that it is possible that higher impact journals may be more likely to provide full text online. The investigators then limited their analysis to the 159 journals that were available before and after the Internet era. Although there was only a marginal statistical significance, there was a trend for a higher impact factor among journals that provided full text online. In fact, in their analysis of subspecialty journals, they clearly demonstrated that full text online journals for cardiology to be associated with a significantly higher impact factor for that specialty. The authors concluded that providing FUTON is likely to have an effect on the impact rating of a journal.

In the present day Internet-based era of medicine, there is a tendency to use the Internet to search for medical information when caring for patients. Consequently, physicians will read articles that are readily available online and therefore available at the bedside. The caveat is that journals that do not provide full text online run the risk of having their publications read less widely and submission of articles to journals that provide full text online are likely to result in greater dissemination of research findings.

J. T. Wei, MD, MSc

2 Medical Education

Trends in Urology Graduate Medical Education: A Brief Update From the Urology Residency Review Committee

Miller DC, and Members of the Residency Review Committee for Urology (Columbia-Presbyterian Med Ctr, New York)

J Urol 172:1062-1064, 2004 2–1

Introduction.—During the past 2 decades, various accreditation and demographic forces have led to modifications in both the number and duration of training programs in urology. There is a growing apprehension among many urologists that these changes may fail to meet the needs of a growing elderly population. Longitudinal data from the Accreditation Council for Graduate Medical Education were reviewed and analyzed for trends in urology training programs. In addition, several publications related to general and urologic graduate medical education were reviewed.

Findings.—The total number of urology residency training programs has decreased by more than 20% since 1982, when there were 153 accredited programs. Many community hospital–based programs were discontinued, often because resources were insufficient to meet more comprehensive program requirements established by the Accreditation Council for Graduate Medical Education. By 1992 there were only 125 accredited urology training programs, a number that has remained relatively stable (119 programs in 2002). And these programs (all but 1 in 2003) have shifted from requiring 3 years of clinical urology to a 4-year program. But in most cases, duration of preurologic general surgical training was reduced from 2 years to 1 year. This reduction was a response to the federal government's policy of reimbursing sponsoring institutions for a maximum of 5 years of postgraduate education in urology. The number of first-year urology residents showed a similar pattern of decline and stabilization. Nevertheless, the total number of urologists in training was greater in 2002 and 2003 than in any year since 1994.

Conclusion.—An examination of recent trends in urologic graduate medical education shows a decline in the number of training programs since 1982, but more recent stabilization. The total number of urologists in training is now increasing, and the specialty appears to be maintaining its focus on graduating a consistent number of high-quality urologic surgeons.

► In 1996 the AUA conducted a Gallup Survey that found nearly half of all practicing urologists believed that there were too many other urologists within 30 minutes of their practice. By and large, the remaining urologists thought that the number of other urologists was just about right. Only 18% of practices were seeking additional urologists for their practice that year. As the proportion of elderly patients in the US population increases, the number of patients requiring urologic care will no doubt increase. The work by Dr Miller and the Residency Review Committee summarize the evolution of training programs during the 1990s. Overall, they found that the number of urologists being trained today is nearly the same as earlier in the decade. Given the increasing elderly population, the Residency Review Committee will need to reconsider manpower requirements to determine whether more urology training slots should now be offered.

In addition, most urology programs have now shortened the general surgery preliminary years and are providing more time in clinical urology training. At the same time, there are fewer programs that support nested research time during residency. Although it has never been proven, it has always been assumed that nested research time will increase trainee interest in subspecialty fellowships and academic research. It remains to be seen whether this trend will affect the propensity of trainees to enter an academic career. This is another area that the Residency Review Committee should monitor closely, as it will ultimately affect the viability of our specialty.

J. T. Wei, MD, MSc

Development of Validated Instrument to Measure Medical Student Learning in Clinical Urology: A Step Toward Evidence Based Education

Kerfoot BP, Baker H, Volkan K, et al (Brigham and Women's Hosp, Boston; California State Univ Channel Islands, Camarillo)

J Urol 172:282-285, 2004 2–2

Introduction.—Published reports designed to assess and improve medical student learning in urology have been limited by the lack of an assessment tool. Thus, previous investigations have examined students' perceptions of learning rather than the actual level of urologic learning. A validated measure of medical student learning in urology was developed to meet this need.

Methods.—As the focus of test development, 4 core topics in clinical urology were selected: prostate cancer, screening with prostate specific antigen, benign prostatic hyperplasia, and erectile dysfunction. Detailed curricula created for each topic were designed to establish the minimum level of knowledge that a medical student should have before graduation. Four medical educators established validity of the curriculum content, and multiple choice questions were developed. The reliability of a preliminary 32-item instrument was tested by administering it to third-year surgery students. Findings were used to create a 28-item instrument.

Results.—Reliability of the 28-item test was 0.76; 1-week test-retest reliability was 0.72. All experts in the field of urology performed well, achieving mean scores significantly higher than the mean student posttest scores (24.9 vs 17.8, respectively). Scores improved with increasing years of training.

Conclusion.—The validated instrument presented here allows medical student learning in urology to be measured, a significant step toward evidence-based education in urology.

► Assessment of medical student training with regard to urologic content is essential to ensure that our graduates are qualified to manage basic urologic problems, regardless of their ultimate specialty or practice. To date, this has largely been ignored by most medical schools and testing has been relegated to the standardized medical board examination that includes relatively few items on urology. These investigators have developed content and test items in a rigorous fashion similar to what is used by other testing groups. Moreover, they have provided validation of their urology curriculum by administration of their tests among urology residents and faculty. They demonstrate that with increasing years of training that test scores improve and that these test scores improve after urology rotations. A limitation of the work is that only 4 specialty topic areas are currently covered. Although this body of research is an important step forward, it is likely impractical for all urology student rotations and medical schools to reproduce this effort. It will remain to be seen in subsequent years if this moves forward to other medical schools.

J. T. Wei, MD, MSc

3 Practice Management

The Value of Your Time: Evaluation of Effects of Changes in Medicare Reimbursement Rates on the Practice of Urology

Lotan Y, Cadeddu JA, Roehrborn CG, et al (Univ of Texas, Dallas)

J Urol 172:1958-1962, 2004 3–1

Introduction.—The standardization of reimbursement for physician services under the Medicare program, designed to decrease overall national health care costs, resulted in relative losses to surgical income. Data from a previously published national survey of urologists were examined to determine the net hourly reimbursement effect of Medicare reforms on income generated from operative and nonoperative services.

Methods.—The 1993 survey randomly sampled 115 urologists. Information sought was related to physician time and work required before, during, and after the most frequently performed urologic services. Three common evaluation and management (E&M) services, 2 outpatient procedures, and 9 inpatient procedures were examined. To determine whether reported times have changed significantly, mean operative times during the last year at the study institution were estimated by averaging the mean times of those surgeons who regularly perform the procedures.

Results.—Over the 3 years used for comparative purposes (1995, 1999, and 2004), there was a steady increase in reimbursement for outpatient services and a decrease in reimbursement for surgical procedures. Reimbursement for outpatient cystoscopy and for transrectal US biopsy of the prostate increased significantly, a result of reimbursement for overhead in 1999. For E&M codes, 2004 reimbursement rates per hour represent a mean increase of 51% since 1995. Hourly rates for surgical procedures, however, have decreased 28.5%. Seven of 9 surgical procedures lost between 25.5% and 32% in reimbursement over the period. The highest reimbursement in 2004 was for office cystoscopy and transrectal US biopsy of the prostate. Except for shock wave lithotripsy, however, hourly reimbursement rates differed little between common surgical procedures and E&M services.

Conclusion.—Rapid changes in the field of urology have had considerable financial impact. Urologists perform fewer operations for fewer diseases, and reimbursement rates for surgery continue to decrease. Some practitioners may discontinue tests or procedures because of decreased reimbursement.

► This study is a gem for those interested in learning how the practice of urology is fairing today. The investigators used a previously published practice survey and calculated the hourly reimbursement for a variety of office visits, office-based procedures, and common inpatient operations. Their chief findings document plainly that there has been significant economic pressures to decrease inpatient surgeries in favor of outpatient-based care. In 7 of the 9 inpatient procedures evaluated, there was at least a 25% decrease in reimbursement between 1995 and 2004. Moreover, the study documented the dramatic increase in outpatient office-based reimbursements. Although all urologists should strive to provide the best possible care for their patients, each must eventually face the economic reality of maintaining solvency in an increasingly expensive medical environment. The changes in urologic practice that follow reimbursement changes are undeniable.

Third-party payers who dictate reimbursement and have ratcheted down inpatient reimbursements over the past decade have done so for 1 reason only: as a cost-saving measure. However, they may have unknowingly done so at a price. Studies have consistently shown that urologists are now offering fewer services that are poorly reimbursed and do not cover the cost of delivering quality care. The lack of services in smaller communities will no doubt impact patient care in the long run.

What is even more notable about the changes in reimbursement is that it is often not dictated by thoughtful cost-effective analyses but rather by lobbyist. If office-based procedures turn out in the long run to be less effective than inpatient operations, then these price pressures are at odds with the delivery of quality care. More research examining the effects of price pressures on practice is clearly needed.

J. T. Wei, MD, MSc

Hospital Costs Associated With Surgical Complications: A Report From the Private-Sector National Surgical Quality Improvement Program

Dimick JB, Chen SL, Taheri PA, et al (Dartmouth Med School, Hanover, NH; Univ of Michigan, Ann Arbor; Brigham and Women's Hosp, Boston; et al)

J Am Coll Surg 199:531-537, 2004 3–2

Background.—The National Surgical Quality Improvement Project (NSQIP) has reduced morbidity rates in Veterans Affairs Hospitals. As the NSQIP methods move to private-sector hospitals, funding responsibilities will shift to the medical center. The objective of the current study was to calculate hospital costs associated with postoperative complications, because reducing morbidity may offset the costs of using the NSQIP.

Study Design.—Patient data were obtained from a single private-sector center involved in the NSQIP from 2001 to 2002 (n = 1,008). Cost data were derived from the hospital's internal cost-accounting database (TSI;

Transitions Systems Inc). Total hospital costs associated with both minor complications and major complications were calculated. Multiple linear regression was used to determine the cost of each type of complication after adjusting for patient characteristics.

Results.—Rates of minor complications (6.3%, 64 events) and major complications (6.6%, 67 events) were similar. Median hospital costs were lowest for patients without complications (4,487 dollars) compared with those with minor (14,094 dollars) and major complications (28,356 dollars) ($p<0.001$). After adjusting for differences in patient characteristics, major complications were associated with an increase of 11,626 dollars (95% CI, 9,419 dollars to 13,832 dollars; $p<0.001$). Minor complications were not associated with increased costs in the adjusted analysis.

Conclusions.—Given the substantial costs associated with major postoperative complications, reducing morbidity may provide sufficient cost savings to offset the resources needed to participate in the private-sector expansion of the NSQIP.

► The risk of incurring surgical complications is accepted by all surgeons. It is discussed with patients preoperatively and documented in the informed consent process. What is often not well documented are the additional costs associated with such complications. In this cost accounting study, the investigators utilized the data collected as part of the NSQIP to estimate the incremental cost of surgical complications. Complications were classified as absent, minor, or major, but following adjustment for potentially confounding factors, only major complications were significantly associated with greater costs (an average of $11,626 more per case with a major surgical complication).

This study is valuable for several reasons. First, it illustrates the power of using NSQIP as a quality assessment infrastructure. The NSQIP has also been shown to be valuable in the identification of factors associated with the quality of care both in the Veterans Health system and in the private sector. Implementation of the NSQIP infrastructure in the Veterans Health system has already resulted in remarkable decrement in morbidity. This study at a single private institution documents the incremental costs attributable to various major and minor complications. The caveat to their findings is likely also true; that is, minimizing complications will result in cost savings. While this may seem intuitive, this study provides documentation of the potential economic benefits of improving the quality of care.

J. T. Wei, MD, MSc

Changes in Prognosis After the First Postoperative Complication

Silber JH, Rosenbaum PR, Trudeau ME, et al (Children's Hosp of Philadelphia; Univ of Pennsylvania, Philadelphia; Leonard Davis Inst of Health Economics, Philadelphia; et al)

Med Care 43:122-131, 2005 3–3

Introduction.—Postoperative complications occur at relatively high rates in Medicare-aged patients, yet no previous study has quantified the increase in the chances of dying that follows an initial postoperative complication in this population. Knowledge of how specific types of complications affect prognosis could help to determine subsequent treatment plans for individual patients and would provide researchers with valuable data.

Methods.—The case-control Surgical Outcomes Study used Medicare claims data to identify subjects and chart abstracts to provide clinical details. A total of 681 randomly selected cases from Pennsylvania included patients age 65 to 85 years who underwent surgical procedures in the years 1995 through 1996 and who died within 60 days of admission. Controls underwent similar procedures and were individually matched to cases, but did not die within 60 days of admission. Models sought to estimate the odds of dying after any 1 of 24 first postoperative complications (defined as the first occurring after discharge from the recovery room).

Results.—Cases and controls were similar in mean age, race, gender distribution, percentage admitted from the emergency department, medical history variables, and types of surgery. Compared with patients without complications, those with complications had a 3.4-fold increased odds of dying within 60 days. If the first complication was respiratory compromise, there was a 7.2-fold increase in the odds of dying. Similarly high increases in the odds of dying were observed with first complications of pneumonia (5-fold) and congestive heart failure (5.1-fold). First complications of hypertension and those of hematologic nature were associated with lower increases of risk than other studied events (1.3 and 1.1, respectively).

Conclusion.—The development of a postoperative complication is an important event that changes prognosis and should prompt an immediate re-evaluation of the patient's care. In this Medicare population, the average increase in the odds of death associated with a first complication was 3-fold. Estimates provided may be used to determine the relative severity of a range of first or early complications.

▶ Through experience and training, surgeons learn to recognize the increased risk of poor outcomes associated with premorbid conditions such as heart or pulmonary disease. It follows then that, as the hospital course evolves, a patient's hazard of dying likely also changes depending on the postoperative events but this has not been previously demonstrated. This is the precise question that Silber et al address in this first of its kind article. In this case-control study, the investigators identified patients who died within 60 days of surgery from a sample of Pennsylvania Medicare patients and matched them by using administrative data to control patients who did not die within 60 days.

Explicit chart abstraction was then undertaken for each case and additional comorbid conditions identified. Moreover, detailed information regarding actual complications that occurred postoperatively was recorded. In their analyses, the presence of any postoperative complication increased 3.4-fold among patients with complications compared with those without complications. High leverage complications included major cardiac events, strokes and deep vein thromboses (each increased the odds of death within 60 days of admission by at least 10-fold). The authors concluded that occurrence of complications, even those that at face value may seem mild, carry an increased risk of mortality.

Appropriate preoperative counseling of patients involves an appreciation of which patients are likely to experience a poor outcome. This is often incorporated into the discussion by surgeons as a fixed risk but in reality the risk of a poor outcome such as death should more appropriately be viewed as a "hazard." Hazard of any event such as death is a statistic that varies with the patient condition. The concept of hazard is illustrated by an individual who walks to work from his home. At home, his hazard of death may be quite low, then he exits his home and walks along the sidewalk, where the hazard may be increased, particularly when he crosses the street where he may be hit by an automobile. Finally, when he enters his office, this hazard will likely decrease once again to a lower level. This illustrates the situational nature behind the principle of hazard. In a similar manner, patients in the hospital after surgery have a "hazard" that changes with their health status and the occurrence of a postoperative complication has now been demonstrated to clearly increase that "hazard." This new information should be used by surgeons to counsel patients and families when complications occur. Moreover, the ranking of complications with regard to risk of mortality can further help guide their expectations. Although this study is clearly significant, further research should be undertaken to validate these findings in a urologic sample.

J. T. Wei, MD, MSc

4 Imaging

Helical Computed Tomography Accurately Reports Urinary Stone Composition Using Attenuation Values: In Vitro Verification Using High-Resolution Micro-computed Tomography Calibrated to Fourier Transform Infrared Microspectroscopy

Zarse CA, McAteer JA, Tann M, et al (Indiana Univ, Indianapolis; Miami Univ, Oxford, Ohio: Methodist Hosp, Indianapolis, Ind)

Urology 63:828-833, 2004 4–1

Objectives.—To assess the ability of helical computed tomography (CT) to differentiate regions of known mineral composition in typical, heterogeneous urinary stones. Interest is substantial in the urologic community in using radiologic imaging to determine accurately the composition of urinary calculi. Recent advances in CT make this a viable prospect, but the heterogeneity of most stones is a complicating factor.

Methods.—The ability of micro-CT (a high-resolution laboratory instrument) to identify the mineral composition of stones was confirmed by calibrating micro-CT attenuation values to pure mineral regions of sliced stones using infrared microspectroscopy. Intact human urinary stones were then analyzed by micro-CT, and regions-of-interest of pure mineral were correlated with identical regions-of-interest from quad slice multi-detector row helical CT images. With helical CT, narrow slice widths were used to decrease volume-averaging errors, and bone windows were used so that internal stone structure was visible.

Results.—When stones were imaged using helical CT at narrow slice widths, mineral-specific regions-of-interest yielded nonoverlapping attenuation values for uric acid (566 to 632 Hounsfield units [HU]), struvite (862 to 944 HU), calcium oxalate (1416 to 1938 HU), and hydroxyapatite (2150 to 2461 HU).

Conclusions.—High resolution helical CT yields unique attenuation values for common types of stone mineral, but proper windowing is required to localize regions of homogeneity. The results of this in vitro study suggest that high-resolution helical CT may be able to identify stone composition at patient diagnosis.

► In this in vitro study, a specially designed micro-CT was used to distinguish between stone composition based on HU. The values for uric acid stones (HU 566-632) were much lower than for calcium oxalate stones (1416-1938). As the use of CT for the evaluation of urolithiasis becomes more prevalent, the ability of the scan to predict stone composition becomes important, particularly since uric acid stones may be treated medically. Despite this communication, and other in vitro studies, a simple abdominal radiograph may be able to distinguish between a uric acid stone and a calcium stone based on radiolucency. The future use of CT-assisted prediction of stone composition should try to elucidate differences between calcium oxalate dihydrate stones (SWL sensitive) and calcium oxalate monohydrate stones (SWL resistant). Unfortunately, this study shows similar HU for these stones.

S. B. Bhayani, MD

Role of Multiphasic Helical Computed Tomography in Planning Surgical Treatment for Pelvi-ureteric Junction Obstruction

El-Nahas AR, Abou-El-Ghar M, Shoma AM, et al (Monsoura Univ, Egypt)

BJU Int 94:582-587, 2004 4–2

Objective.—To evaluate the role of multiphasic helical computed tomography (CT) in planning surgical treatment for pelvi-ureteric junction obstruction (PUJO).

Patients and Methods.—Multiphasic helical CT was used in 60 consecutive patients (mean age 32 years, sd 13.72) with primary PUJO. The different images were interpreted before surgery by a urologist and radiologist. The number, type and relation of the crossing vessels to the PUJ were detected. Pyeloplasty (open or laparoscopic) was used in patients where there was a significant crossing vessel (i.e. > 2 mm in diameter and passing at the PUJ) or with ballooning of the renal pelvis. Endopyelotomy (antegrade or retrograde) was used in the other patients. Subjective and objective success rates were determined 3-6 months after treatment and then every 6 months.

Results.—Hyperdense renal stones were detected in precontrast images in 15 patients, significant crossing vessels in 33 (55%), and anterior malrotation of the renal pelvis in 23 (38%; 19 associated with significant crossing vessels, i.e. ureterovascular hydronephrosis). A large para-pelvic cyst compressing the PUJ and upper ureter was detected in one patient. Pyeloplasty was used in 45 patients, among whom the sensitivity of multiphasic helical CT in detecting crossing vessels was 97%, the specificity 92% and accuracy 96%. Uncomplicated endopyelotomy was used in 14 patients and percutaneous aspiration of the para-pelvic cyst in one.

Conclusion.—Multiphasic helical CT can accurately delineate the spatial anatomy of the renal and peri-renal area; it may be important in planning surgical treatment for PUJO, especially when endopyelotomy is considered.

▶ In this study, a CT of the ureteropelvic junction was performed in all patients prior to treatment of their PUJO. The CT was 97% sensitive in detecting crossing vessels, and in these cases, changed the therapy from endopyelotomy to pyeloplasty. As the efficacy of endopyelotomy is significantly lower with a crossing vessel (and riskier!), a CT scan of the UPJ should be considered to detect this abnormality. Ultimately, however, one must be aware that laparoscopic pyeloplasty has a higher success rate than endopyelotomy, regardless of the presence of a crossing vessel. If a laparoscopic pyeloplasty is going to be the procedure of choice, the need for a CT is questionable. If an endopyelotomy is considered, however, a CT should be performed.

S. B. Bhayani, MD

Accuracy of Computed Tomographic Angiography and Magnetic Resonance Angiography for Diagnosing Renal Artery Stenosis

Boudewijn G, for the Renal Artery Diagnostic Imaging Study in Hypertension (RADISH) Study Group (Maastricht Univ, The Netherlands; et al)

Ann Intern Med 141:674-682, 2004 4–3

Background.—Because renal artery stenosis is a potentially curable cause of hypertension and renal impairment, its accurate, prompt detection is important. The performance of CT angiography (CTA) and MR angiography (MRA) in detecting renal artery stenosis was compared with that of digital subtraction angiography.

Methods.—The prospective multicenter study enrolled 402 hypertensive patients between 1998 and 2001. All were suspected of having renal artery stenosis. Three hundred fifty-six underwent all 3 diagnostic tests and were included in the final analysis. Two panels of 3 investigators examined CTA and MRA image data.

Findings.—Clinically relevant artery stenosis was noted in 20% of the patients. Interobserver agreement was moderate. The combined sensitivities and specificities for CTA were 64% and 92%, respectively. The corresponding values for MRA were 62% and 84%.

Conclusion.—These data suggest that CTA and MRA are not sufficiently sensitive or reproducible to exclude the diagnosis of renal artery stenosis in hypertensive patients. The best method for diagnosing this disorder is DSA.

▶ Renal artery stenosis is increasingly being recognized as an important cause of renovascular hypertension and renal functional impairment. The interaction between stenotic lesions of the renal artery, the kidney's regulation of blood pressure, and the excretory function of the kidney are complex and are not easily attributable to simple cause and effect. The high prevalence of essential hypertension and renal parenchymal disease from systemic conditions such as diabetes add to the difficulty in isolating renal artery stenosis as the cause for hypertension and renal insufficiency.

Accordingly, advances in noninvasive imaging techniques, in particular CTA and MRA, have been applied to the evalution of renal artery stenosis. In theory, these imaging modalities avoid the risks associated with contrast arteriography, the "gold standard" test for renal artery stenosis. In this report, Vasbinder et al prospectively compare the diagnostic accuracy of CTA and MRA against the reference standard of digital subtraction angiography. During the 3-year study period, 356 patients underwent all 3 diagnostic tests. Two separate panels of 3 experienced radiologists reviewed the CTA and MRA studies, which were then compared to the digital subtraction angiography images.

The overall prevalence of renal artery stenosis—defined by digital subtraction angiography findings of more than 50% reduction in the luminal diameter or presence of fibrous dysplasia—was 20% in the study population. The sensitivity of CTA and MRA in identifying these lesions was approximately 63%. In contrast, the specificity of these studies was much higher, ranging from 77% to 97%. This well-done study suggests that utilization of CTA and MRA to detect renal artery stenosis may have a previously unappreciated high false negative rate and, as such, reliance on invasive techniques may be required in patients in whom there is a high clinical suspicion.

V. Krishnamurthi, MD

5 Endourology and Stone Disease

Dietary Factors and the Risk of Incident Kidney Stones in Men: New Insights After 14 Years of Follow-up

Taylor EN, Stampfer MJ, Curhan GC (Brigham and Women's Hosp, Boston; Harvard Med School, Boston)

J Am Soc Nephrol 15:3225-3232, 2004 5–1

Abstract.—Diet plays an important role in the pathogenesis of kidney stones. Because the metabolism of many dietary factors, such as calcium, may change with age, the relation between diet and kidney stones may be different in older adults. Uncertainty also remains about the association between many dietary factors, such as vitamin C, magnesium, and animal protein, and the risk of kidney stone formation. To examine the association between dietary factors and the risk of incident, symptomatic kidney stones in men and to determine whether these associations vary with age, a prospective cohort study was conducted of 45,619 men without a history of nephrolithiasis. Self-administered food frequency questionnaires were used to assess diet every 4 yr. A total of 1473 incident symptomatic kidney stones were documented during 477,700 person-years of follow-up. For men aged <60 yr, the multivariate relative risk (RR) for stone formation in the highest quintile of dietary calcium as compared with the lowest quintile was 0.69 (95% confidence interval [CI], 0.56 to 0.87; $P = 0.01$ for trend). By contrast, there was no association between dietary calcium and stone formation in men aged 60 yr or older. The multivariate RR for men who consumed 1000 mg or greater of vitamin C per day compared with those who consumed less than the recommended dietary allowance of 90 mg/d was 1.41 (95% CI, 1.11 to 1.80; $P = 0.01$ for trend). Other dietary factors showed the following multivariate RR among men in the highest quintile of intake compared with those in the lowest: magnesium, 0.71 (95% CI, 0.56 to 0.89; $P = 0.01$ for trend); potassium, 0.54 (95% CI, 0.42 to 0.68; $P < 0.001$ for trend); and fluid, 0.71 (95% CI, 0.59 to 0.85; $P < 0.001$ for trend). Animal protein was associated with risk only in men with a body mass index <25 kg/m(2) (RR, 1.38; 95% CI, 1.05 to 1.81; $P = 0.03$ for trend). Sodium, phosphorus, sucrose, phytate, vitamin B(6), vitamin D, and supplemental calcium were not independently associated with risk. In conclusion, the association between calcium intake and kidney stone formation varies with age. Magnesium intake decreases and total vitamin C intake seems to increase the risk of symptomatic nephrolithiasis. Because age and body size affect the relation between diet and kidney stones, dietary recommendations for stone prevention should be tailored to the individual patient.

▶ In this huge 14-year study of 45,619 men, dietary factors were evaluated for their effect on urolithiasis. Calcium intake decreased the risk of kidney stone formation. Vitamin C intake increased the risk of stones. Often, patients and physicians often erroneously believe that calcium stones can be eliminated by avoiding calcium rich foods. Calcium likely binds dietary oxalate, thus preventing oxalate absorption, and decreasing stone formation.

S. B. Bhayani, MD

Obesity, Weight Gain, and the Risk of Kidney Stones

Taylor EN, Stampfer MJ, Curhan GC (Harvard Med School, Boston)

JAMA 203:455-462, 2005 5–2

Introduction.—Large body size can result in increased urinary excretion of uric acid and oxalate. This can increase the risk for calcium oxalate kidney stones. What is not understood is whether obesity increases the risk of stone formation or if weight gain influences risk. A prospective investigation of 3 large cohorts was performed to ascertain whether weight gain, body mass index (BMI), and waist circumference are linked with kidney stone formation.

Methods.—The 3 large cohorts evaluated were the Health Professionals Follow-up Study (45,988 men; age range at baseline, 40-75 years), the Nurses' Health Study (93,758 older women; age range at baseline, 34-59 years), and the Nurses' Health Study II (101,877 younger women; age range at baseline, 27-44 years). The primary outcome measure was the incidence of symptomatic kidney stone.

Results.—A total of 4827 kidney stone events occurred over a combined 46 years of follow-up. After adjustments for age, dietary factors, fluid intake, and thiazide use, the relative risk (RR) for stone formation in men weighing more than 100.0 kg versus those who weighed less than 68.2 kg was 1.44 (95% confidence interval [CI], 1.11-1.86; P = .002 for trend). Among older and younger women, the RRs for these weight categories were 1.89 (95% CI, 1.52-2.36; P < .001 for trend) and 1.92 (95% CI, 1.59-2.31; P < .001 for trend), respectively. The RRs in men who gained more than 15.9 kg since age 21 years compared with men whose weight did not change was 1.39 (95% CI, 1.14-1.70; P = .001 for trend). Corresponding RRs for the same categories of weight gain since age 18 years in older and younger women were 1.70 (95% CI, 1.40-2.05; P < .001 for trend) and 1.82 (95% CI, 1.50-2.21; P < .001 for trend). BMI was linked with the risk of kidney stone formation; the RR for men with a BMI of 30 or greater compared with those with a BMI of 21 to 22.9 was 1.33 (95% CI, 1.08-1.63; P < .001 for trend). Corresponding RRs for the same categories of BMI in older and younger women were 1.90 (95% CI, 1.61-2.25; $P < .001$ for trend) and 2.09 (95% CI, 1.77-2.48; $P < .001$ for trend). Waist circumference was also positively linked with risk in men (P .002 for trend) and in older and younger women ($P < .001$ for trend for both).

Conclusion.—Both obesity and weight gain increase the risk of kidney stone formation. The magnitude of increased risk may be greater in women than in men.

▶ This study of 4827 stone episodes with follow-up of 46 years shows that obesity and weight gain are independent risk factors for kidney stone formation. Ironically, gastric bypass procedures, which are becoming increasingly popular, may also contribute to stone formation. Encourage patients to diet and exercise, not only for their general health, but also to prevent stones.

S. B. Bhayani, MD

Systematic Review of the Relative Efficacy of Non-steroidal Anti-inflammatory Drugs and Opioids in the Treatment of Acute Renal Colic

Holdgate A, Pollock T (St George Hosp, Kogarah, Australia)

BMJ 328:1401-1404, 2004 5–3

Objective.—To examine the relative benefits and disadvantages of non-steroidal anti-inflammatory drugs (NSAIDs) and opioids for the management of acute renal colic.

Data Sources.—Cochrane Renal Group's specialised register, Cochrane central register of controlled trials, Medline, Embase, and reference lists of retrieved articles.

Review Methods.—Randomised controlled trials comparing any opioid with any NSAID in acute renal colic if they reported any of the following outcomes: patient rated pain, time to pain relief, need for rescue analgesia, rate of recurrence of pain, and adverse events.

Results.—20 trials totalling 1613 participants were identified. Both NSAIDs and opioids led to clinically important reductions in patient reported pain scores. Pooled analysis of six trials showed a greater reduction in pain scores for patients treated with NSAIDs than with opioids. Patients treated with NSAIDs were significantly less likely to require rescue analgesia (relative risk 0.75, 95% confidence interval 0.61 to 0.93). Most trials showed a higher incidence of adverse events in patients treated with opioids. Compared with patients treated with opioids, those treated with NSAIDs had significantly less vomiting (0.35, 0.23 to 0.53). Pethidine was associated with a higher rate of vomiting.

Conclusions.—Patients receiving NSAIDs achieve greater reductions in pain scores and are less likely to require further analgesia in the short term than those receiving opioids. Opioids, particularly pethidine, are associated with a higher rate of vomiting.

▶ This paper analyzes 20 separate trials, comparing opiod analgesia to NSAIDs in the treatment of acute renal colic. The authors discovered that in the majority of trials, NSAID usage was associated with greater reductions in pain scores. However, not all the trials were randomized or blinded and therefore, selection bias may be present. Nevertheless, NSAID use should be considered for renal colic, as opioids can be given for breakthrough pain. However, if shock wave lithotripsy or surgery is indicated, one must be aware of the possibility of NSAID-related complications including bleeding, renal dysfunction, and peptic ulcer.

S. B. Bhayani, MD

A Multivariate Analysis of Risk Factors Associated With Subcapsular Hematoma Formation Following Electromagnetic Shock Wave Lithotripsy

Dhar NB, Thornton J, Karafa MT, et al (Cleveland Clinic Found, Ohio)

J Urol 172:2271-2274, 2004 5–4

Purpose.—Subcapsular or perinephric hematoma is one of the most frequent and potentially serious complications of extracorporeal shock wave lithotripsy (SWL). We determined the incidence of and risk factors for renal hematomas following electromagnetic shock wave lithotripsy.

Materials and Methods.—Between February 1999 and August 2003, 570 SWL treatments were performed using a Modulith SLX electromagnetic lithotriptor (Storz, St. Louis, Missouri). A total of 415 of these treatments in 317 patients were performed for stones in the renal pelvis or calices and these treatment episodes represent the study group reported. Treatment episodes were reviewed from a prospective institutional review board approved registry and analyzed for patient age, gender, body mass index, mean arterial pressure at induction, stone location, total number of shock waves and peak shock wave intensity.

Results.—Following these 415 episodes subcapsular or perinephric hematomas developed in 17 patients for an overall incidence of 4.1%. The probability of hematoma after shock wave lithotripsy increased significantly as patient age at treatment increased, such that the probability of hematoma was estimated to be 1.67 times greater for each 10-year incremental increase in patient age. None of the other variables analyzed were significantly related to the incidence of hematoma formation at the 0.05 level.

Conclusions.—The incidence of renal hematoma formation following electromagnetic SWL for renal calculus was 4.1%. The probability of hematoma increased significantly with increasing patient age but it was not associated with increasing mean arterial pressure at treatment. These findings are in contrast to previous reports of hematoma associated with electrohydraulic SWL. These differences may be a consequence of the smaller focal zone and higher peak pressure associated with Storz Modulith electromagnetic SWL and, just as importantly, a consequence of the difference in the manner in which blood pressure was defined.

► This study documents the incidence of perinephric hematoma in all patients undergoing ESWL with the Storz Modulith SLX lithotripter. All patients underwent ultrasound at 4 weeks to assess for hematoma, and the incidence was found to be 4.1%. Interestingly, hematoma formation was not correlated with mean arterial blood pressure at induction; rather the only correlating risk factor was advanced age. Treatment for caliceal stones had twice the incidence of hematoma than treatment for pelvic stones. It is important to consider that the modulith has a higher local peak energy and smaller focal zone than several other electrohydraulic units. Although the Dornier HM3 is the gold standard for treating urolithiasis, it is no longer in production, and newer machines must be assessed for both complications and stone free rates. This study did not address the stone free rate of the Storz modulith.

S. B. Bhayani, MD

Efficiency and Cost of Treating Proximal Ureteral Stones: Shock Wave Lithotripsy Versus Ureteroscopy Plus Holmium:Yttrium-Aluminum-Garnet Laser

Parker BD, Frederick RW, Reilly TP, et al (Scott, Sherwood and Brindley Found, Temple, Tex; Texas A&M Univ, Temple)

Urology 64:1102-1106, 2004 5–5

Objectives.—To compare the success rates, cost effectiveness, and efficiency of ureteroscopy (URS) and extracorporeal shock wave lithotripsy (ESWL) for proximal ureteral stones.

Methods.—In a retrospective manner, 220 patients who underwent treatment for proximal ureteral stones were included in the study. The patient records, radiographs, and billing statements of all patients treated for upper ureteral stones between January 1997 and June 2001 at Scott and White Memorial Hospital were reviewed. The patients were placed into two treatment groups according to the method of their stone's initial treatment. The stones were categorized as less than 1 cm and 1 cm or greater.

Results.—A total of 111 patients were in the ESWL group, 73 of whom had stones less than 1 cm, and 109 patients in the URS group, 81 of whom had stones less than 1 cm. In the URS group, 91% were successfully treated with one treatment intervention, and 55% of the ESWL group were successfully treated with their initial intervention (P <0.0001). Of the patients with URS failure, all but one was treated successfully with a second URS. Of the patients with ESWL failure, 52% were treated successfully by subsequent URS. The remaining patients with ESWL failure were treated with repeat ESWL, with a 62% success rate. The efficiency quotient for stones less than 1 cm for URS and ESWL was 0.79 and 0.51, respectively. For stones 1 cm or greater, URS had an efficiency quotient of 0.72 and ESWL of 0.46. The URS group required fewer days to be stone free (8 versus 25.5 days, P <0.0001).

No statistically significant difference was found in the overall complication rates ($P = 0.43$). URS had significantly lower charges for the initial procedure ($7575 dollars versus $9507 dollars, $P < 0.0001$). The total charges were also lower for URS ($9378 dollars versus $15,583, dollars $P < 0.0001$). Complications were similar in the two groups. The URS group had two ureteral strictures.

Conclusions.—The results of this study indicate that URS is more efficient and cost-effective for stones up to and larger than 1 cm with similar complication rates compared with ESWL.

▶ In this study of ESWL versus URS/laser lithotripsy of proximal ureteral stones, the ureteroscopic approach was found to be more efficacious and cheaper. Every practice should perform this study, as the results may differ based on the type of lithotripter used. For this study with a DoLi unit, URS was superior, but if an HM3 were available, I would elect for ESWL.

S. B. Bhayani, MD

Treatment of Complete Staghorn Stones: A Prospective Randomized Comparison of Open Surgery Versus Percutaneous Nephrolithotomy

Al-Kohlany KM, Shokeir AA, Mosbah A, et al (Mansoura Univ, Egypt)

J Urol 173:469-473, 2005 5–6

Purpose.—We studied the role of open surgery versus percutaneous nephrolithotomy (PCNL) in the treatment of complete staghorn stones in a prospective randomized manner.

Materials and Methods.—A total of 79 patients with 88 complete staghorn stones, defined as filling the entire collecting system or at least 80% of it, were prospectively randomized for PCNL (43) or open surgery (45). Intraoperative and postoperative morbidity, operative time, hospital stay, and stone clearance at discharge home and followup were compared for both methods. Patients with significant residuals in both groups were subjected to extracorporeal shock wave lithotripsy (Dornier Medical Systems, Inc., Marietta, Georgia) on an outpatient basis. Followup was completed for all cases with a mean duration ±SD of 4.9 ± 2.5 months (range 3 to 14). Renal function was evaluated by ^{99m}Tc-mercaptoacetyltriglycine renogram before and after treatment in both groups.

Results.—Intraoperative complications in terms of bleeding requiring blood transfusion, and pleural, vascular or ureteral injuries were recorded in 7 patients (16.3%) in the PCNL and 17 (37.8%) in the open surgery groups, a difference of significant value ($p < 0.05$). Major postoperative complications including massive hematuria requiring blood transfusion, septicemia, urinary leakage and wound infection were observed in 8 patients (18.6%) in the PCNL group and in 14 (31.1%) in the open surgery group, a difference of no significant value. PCNL was associated with shorter operative time (127 ± 30 vs 204 ± 31 minutes, $p < 0.001$), shorter hospital stay (6.4 ± 4.2 vs 10 4.2 days, $p < 0.001$) and earlier return to work (2.5 ± 0.8 vs 4.1 ± 1 weeks, p <0.001). On the other hand both treatment groups were comparable in regard to stone-free rates at discharge home (49% vs 66%) and at followup (74% vs 82%). At followup renal function improved or remained stable in 91% and 86.7% in the PCNL and open surgery groups, respectively.

Conclusions.—PCNL is a valuable treatment option for complete staghorn stones with a stone-free rate approaching that of open surgery. Moreover, it has the advantages of lower morbidity, shorter operative time, shorter hospital stay and earlier return to work.

► This study is 25 years too late. This study found that PCNL has an improved convalescence compared to open surgery for staghorn calculi. Although in several areas of the world, open surgery may be less expensive than using the disposables associated with PCNL, from a patient care perspective there is no comparison. This paper should have been published decades ago. I have not seen an open stone surgery in the last decade. Endourological approaches to kidney stone surgery are the standard of care, hopefully worldwide.

S. B. Bhayani, MD

Percutaneous Nephrostolithotomy: Predictions of Length of Stay

Matlaga BR, Hodges SJ, Shah OD, et al (Wake Forest Univ, Winston-Salem, NC)

J Urol 172:1351-1354, 2004 5–7

Purpose.—Percutaneous nephrostolithotomy (PNL) is commonly used to treat patients with complex renal calculi. A goal at our medical center is to discharge patients home less than 24 hours after PNL. We performed a study to determine factors that caused patients to be hospitalized longer than this period.

Material and Methods.—The available hospital records and office charts of 133 consecutive patients undergoing initial PNL at our institution between January 1, 1999 and December 31, 2000 were reviewed. All PNL procedures were performed by one of us using a (DGA) 1-stage technique. Mean patient age was 52 years (range 25 to 84). Of the subjects 85 were male and 48 were female.

Results.—A total of 91 patients (68%) were discharged home less than 24 hours after surgery. The overall stone-free rate was 91%. Mean length of stay in the entire group was 1.97 days. Mean length of stay in those hospitalized longer than 24 hours was 4.12 days. Mean operative time, including time to obtain access, was 188.6 minutes. Multivariate analysis demonstrated that neurogenic bladder, endocrine comorbidity and perioperative complications were factors associated with a length of stay of greater than 24 hours. Univariate analysis demonstrated that preoperative urinary tract infection and infection related calculi were also associated with a length of stay of greater than 24 hours.

Conclusions.—The majority of patients undergoing PNL can be discharged home less than 24 hours after surgery. Patients with neurogenic bladder, those with endocrine comorbidity, those who sustain significant perioperative complications and those harboring stones associated with urinary tract infection or preoperative urinary tract infection are more likely to require longer hospitalization.

► In this retrospective study, the authors assessed the predictors of the length of stay after PNL. The authors found that the only significant factors contributing to longer length of stay were neurogenic bladder, endocrine comorbidities (diabetes), and complications. All patients were sent home with a nephrostomy tube in place for several days. This study differs from others which suggest that the size of the nephrostomy tube is a factor in lengthening hospitalization. I still believe that the size of the tube is a factor in lengthening hospitalization, despite this study. My routine practice is to image patients on postoperative day 1, and if stone free, to remove the tube prior to discharge, rather than leaving it in for a week.

S. B. Bhayani, MD

6 Laparoscopy

Making Ends Meet: A Cost Comparison of Laparoscopic and Open Radical Retropubic Prostatectomy

Link RE, Su L-M, Bhayani SB, et al (Johns Hopkins Bayview Med Ctr, Baltimore, Md)

J Urol 172:269-274, 2004 6–1

Introduction.—Driven by patient requests for more minimally invasive approaches to prostatectomy, many centers worldwide are now performing a large volume of laparoscopic radical prostatectomy (LRP) procedures. The disadvantages of LRP over open radical retropubic prostatectomy (RRP) include a steep learning curve, reduced tactile feedback, little long-term data, longer operative times, and potentially greater cost. The relative cost of LRP versus RRP has received surprisingly little attention in the literature. The perioperative costs of LRP and RRP were compared at a metropolitan hospital by development of a detailed computer model.

Methods.—The predictive model incorporated institutional cost centers for operative time, operating time consumables, professional fees, hospital room and board, oral analgesics, autologous blood banking, blood transfusion, and cystography. Versions with and without pelvic lymphadenectomy (PLND) were assessed by 1- and 2-way sensitivity analyses. Operative times, length of stay, and transfusion rates were obtained from published series. Individual hospital charges were reviewed for 172 consecutive patients who underwent prostatectomy to compare and validate model predictions.

Results.—The model predicted cost premiums for LRP of 14.4% and 17.5%, respectively, without and with PLND. The actual hospital charge premium for LRP and PLND was 18.4%; this differed from the predicted cost premium by less than 1%. The most significant cost centers in order of importance were operative time, length of stay, and consumables.

To achieve cost equivalence with RRP, operative times would need to average 159 minutes (LRP and PLND) and 174 minutes (LRP), keeping other factors constant. Cost equivalence could not be achieved by shortening hospital length of stay alone, unless LRP was performed on an outpatient basis.

Conclusion.—This model predicted the perioperative costs of LRP to be greater than RRP by a factor of less than 1.2 times. If disposable instruments and trocars are eliminated, and patients undergoing LRP with PLND are discharged on postoperative day 2. The cost equivalent of RRP with PLND may be achieved with operative times of 3.4 hours.

▶ This article gives an important preliminary look at a cost comparison of LRP and RRP. It is very reassuring that cost equivalence between open and laparoscopic prostatectomy is well within reach. All surgeons need to do is learn to complete the operation more quickly (under approximately 3 hours) and to avoid use of disposable instruments. Recent reports of LRP suggest that operative times in the 2- to 3-hour range are not at all unusual. The cost will always be an advantage of laparoscopic over robotic prostatectomy.

G. L. Andriole, Jr, MD

Comparison of Early Oncologic Results of Laparoscopic Radical Prostatectomy by Extraperitoneal Versus Transperitoneal Approach

Ruiz L, Salomon L, Hoznek A, et al (Servic d'Urologie CHU Henri Mondor, Créteil cedex, France)

Eur Urol 46:50-56, 2004 6–2

Purpose.—Compare the early oncological results of laparoscopic radical prostatectomy performed by either an extraperitoneal or a transperitoneal approach.

Methods.—330 consecutive men underwent laparoscopic radical prostatectomy for localized prostate cancer, the first 165 by transperitoneal approach, and the last 165 by extraperitoneal approach. Clinical stage, serum PSA, Gleason score of biopsy were recorded, as well as operating time, surgical and medical complications, blood loss, length of hospital stay and catheterization time. The weight of the specimen, pathological stage (1997 TNM classification) and status of the surgical margins were noted. The Fisher test as well as the ξ^2-test were used for statistical analysis. Differences were considered significant when $p < 0.05$.

Results.—There were no significant differences between the two groups in terms of preoperative characteristics except for Gleason score of the biopsies which was higher in the extraperitoneal group ($p < 0.0001$). The operating time was longer with the transperitoneal approach (248.5 min vs. 220.0 min, $p < 0.0001$). There was no difference in transfusion rate (1.2% vs. 5.4%, transperitoneal vs. extraperitoneal, respectively, $p = 0.6$). There was no difference in hospital stay, medical and surgical complications. Respectively, in the transperitoneal and extraperitoneal groups, there were 108 and 88 pT2 tumors. There were no differences in terms of positive surgical margins between the two groups, 23% and 29.7% ($p = 0.21$) overall, 13.0% and 17.0% ($p = 0.42$) in pT2 tumors and 43.6% and 44.7% ($p = 0.99$) in pT3 tumors.

Conclusions.—Extraperitoneal approach offers the same early oncological results as transperitoneal approach with a shorter operative time.

► There remains a controversy about the optimal approach to laparoscopic radical prostatectomy whether it be transperitoneal or extraperitoneal. In my judgment, the data as reported in this paper and elsewhere strongly suggest that the extraperitoneal approach is superior. In my view, the extraperitoneal approach results in overall fewer complications in part because bowel injury to the small intestines may be completely avoided. There seems to be less postoperative ileus, operative times tend to be less, and many patients have quicker time to return to a normal diet. Based on these considerations, laparoscopic extraperitoneal radical prostatectomy is my preferred choice for men undergoing laparoscopic prostatectomy.

G. L. Andriole, Jr, MD

Laparoscopic Radical Prostatectomy and Body Mass Index: An Assessment of 151 Sequential Cases

Brown JA, Rodin DM, Lee B, et al (Harvard Med School, Boston)

J Urol 173:442-445, 2005 6–3

Purpose.—Little objective data are available regarding obesity and the performance of laparoscopic radical prostatectomy (LRP). We reviewed our LRP series to determine the effect of body mass index (BMI) on operative time, blood loss, anastomotic leakage, positive margins, length of stay, complications, urinary continence and erectile function.

Materials and Methods.—A single institution retrospective review was performed of 151 sequential LRPs performed by a single surgeon. Patients were separated into those who were nonobese (BMI less than 30), and those with classes I (BMI 30 to 34.9), II (BMI 35 to 39.9) and III (BMI 40 or greater) obesity according to WHO criteria.

Results.—There were 97 patients in the nonobese and 54 in the obese cohort, including 35, 14 and 5 with classes I to III obesity, respectively. A trend toward greater preoperative prostate specific antigen ($p = 0.14$), Gleason score ($p = 0.06$) and American Society of Anesthesiologists classification ($p = 0.07$) was noted in the obese (BMI 30 or greater) group. The cohorts had similar prostate size ($p = 0.11$), pathological grade ($p = 0.57$), pathological stage ($p = 0.50$), postoperative hemoglobin decrease ($p = 0.77$) and hospital stay ($p = 0.90$). The rates of positive margins ($p = 1.0$), anastomotic leakage ($p = 0.49$), prostate specific antigen recurrence ($p = 1.0$) and complication ($p = 0.14$) were also similar. Early postoperative urinary continence ($p = 1.0$) and erectile function ($p = 0.19$) appeared equivalent. Mean operative time SD was greater in obese than in nonobese patients (208 43 vs 192 34 minutes, $p = 0.02$). Mean operative time was longer in patients with classes II and III obesity (220 47 minutes, $p < 0.05$ and 249 32, $p < 0.01$, respectively). The class III group had a longer mean operative time than the class I obesity group (198 34 minutes, $p < 0.05$). Obese patients underwent a greater number of additional procedures at the time of LRP ($p = 0.01$).

Conclusions.—While obesity significantly increased LRP operative time, it did not significantly impact other intraoperative and postoperative surgical parameters. LRP should be offered to obese patients as a feasible and effective treatment option for prostate cancer.

► In this communication, the authors examine the outcomes of LRP in non-obese and obese patients. Although operative times were longer for obese patients (208 minutes vs 192 minutes), outcomes were similar with regards to oncologic efficacy, continence, potency, and complications. Most surgeons subjectively recognize that an open radical prostatectomy is more difficult in an obese patient. The authors comment that the laparoscopic approach is also more difficult subjectively. Despite similar outcomes in this study by an experienced surgeon, obesity still can be a contraindication to LRP early in the learning curve, and conversion to an open operation is very possible.[1]

S. B. Bhayani, MD

Reference

1. Bhayani SB, Pavlovich CP, Strup SE, et al: Laparoscopic radical prostatectomy: A multi-institutional study of conversion open surgery. *Urology* 63:99-102, 2004.

Survey of Urological Laparoscopic Practice Patterns in the Midwest

Wang DS, Winfield HN (Boston Univ; Univ of Iowa, Iowa City)

J Urol 172:2282-2286, 2004 6–4

Purpose.—Laparoscopic surgery is assuming a greater role in the management of many urological disorders. We performed a survey of urologists in the Midwest United States to define laparoscopic practice patterns regarding urological disease.

Materials and Methods.—Surveys were mailed to 1,450 members of the North Central Section of the American Urological Association. Questions pertained to age, practice demographics, residency training and amount of laparoscopy performed.

Results.—A response rate of 33% was obtained. A total of 49% of urologists perform no laparoscopy, 30% devote less than 5% of their practice and 21% devote 5% or more of their practice to laparoscopy. Of the responders 15% believed they were adequately trained during residency to perform laparoscopy. Among those who performed hand assisted laparoscopy (HAL), 52% used it to gain familiarity with laparoscopic techniques. There was an inverse correlation between time in practice and amount of laparoscopy performed ($p < 0.0001$). Urologists in academia perform laparoscopy at a greater proportion versus those in private practice ($p < 0.01$). Urologists who incorporated laparoscopy during fellowship performed the most laparoscopy ($p = 0.003$). Those who considered themselves adequately trained during residency were more likely to perform laparoscopy ($p < 0.0001$). Urologists who perform HAL devote more of their operating time to laparoscopy than those who do not ($p < 0.0001$). The number of laparoscopic cases performed correlated with decreased time in practice ($p < 0.0001$), academic setting ($p = 0.001$) and use of HAL ($p < 0.0001$).

Conclusions.—Urological laparoscopic surgery remains at an early stage of development in the Midwestern United States. Although HAL has widened the scope of laparoscopy among urologists, increased training for urologists and residents is necessary.

► In this study, a questionnaire was mailed to members of the North Central section of the American Urological Association to examine the surgeons' usage of laparoscopic urological surgery. Not surprisingly, younger urologists perform more laparoscopy than older urologists, and the use of hand-assistance was popular. Overall, 49.1% of urologists performed no laparoscopy. The most striking statistic was that 85% of urologists felt inadequately trained in laparoscopy during residency. One main conceptual issue in the training of urologists in laparoscopic surgery is that there is no "small learning case" such as a tubal ligation or cholecystectomy. The common urological laparoscopic procedures are all major organ removals (nephrectomy, prostatectomy, nephroureterectomy) with the chance for blood loss or injury to surrounding structures. Although the training issue will be addressed as more residents gain exposure to laparoscopy, the conundrum for practicing urologists is how to gain experience and exposure. Postgraduate courses are a start, but in an ideal case, a mentorship or miniresidency may be more effective.[1]

S. B. Bhayani, MD

Reference

1. Shalhav AL, Dabagia MD, Wagner TT, et al: Training postgraduate urologists in laparoscopic surgery: The current challenge. *J Urol* 167:2135-2157, 2002.

Prospective, Randomized Controlled Study: Transperitoneal Laparoscopic Versus Retroperitoneoscopic Radical Nephrectomy

Nambirajan T, Jeschke S, Al-Zahrani H, et al (Elisabethinen Hosp, Linz, Austria)

Urology 64:919-924, 2004 6–5

Objectives.—To evaluate the transperitoneal and retroperitoneal approaches for endoscopic radical nephrectomy in a prospective randomized manner to assess the possible differences in the outcome related to patients' morbidity and technical difficulty for the surgeon.

Methods.—A total of 40 patients with Stage cT1-T2 were randomized into two equal groups: laparoscopic radical nephrectomy (LRN) and retroperitoneoscopic radical nephrectomy (RRN). The patient demographics and tumor characteristics were comparable. Two surgeons with differing experience performed an equal number of procedures in both treatment arms. The outcome was compared, and the technical difficulty for the surgeon and assistant was assessed with the European scoring system.

Results.—All procedures were completed without a need for conversion. No statistically significant differences were found between the two approaches in terms of the number and size of the trocars used, length of incision, specimen weight, pathologic stage, operative time, need for additional procedures such as adrenalectomy and/or lymph node sampling, estimated blood loss, need for blood transfusions, analgesic requirement, length of hospital stay, or the incidence of minor or major complications. All patients in the LRN group resumed oral intake on postoperative day 1, but only 75% did so in the RRN group. The technical difficulty score for either the surgeon or the assistant did not differ significantly between the two groups. Both approaches allowed complete tumor excision. The robotic assistance system (AESOP) was more difficult with RRN compared with LRN.

Conclusions.—This first prospective randomized study comparing LRN and RRN did not find any real difference between the two approaches in relation to patient morbidity or the technical difficulty for the surgeon.

▶ This study, finally performed after more than 10 years of experience with LRN, is a prospective randomized controlled study of the retroperitoneal and transperitoneal approaches. The procedures were performed by surgeons with similar experience in both approaches. No differences were seen between the approaches for a wide variety of parameters. I strongly agree with the authors in their statement "the choice of approach depends on the individual surgeon's preference, training, and comfort level with the approach." Subjectively, I believe the transperitoneal approach allows easier orientation and more familiar landmarks, at the expense of earlier control of the hilum. I agree with the authors that the transperitoneal approach is easier for larger tumors.

S. B. Bhayani, MD

Vena Caval Transection During Retroperitoneoscopic Nephrectomy: Report of the Complication and Review of the Literature

McAllister M, Bhayani SB, Ong A, et al (Johns Hopkins Univ, Baltimore, Md; Univ of Pennsylvania, Philadelphia)

J Urol 172:183-185, 2004 6–6

Purpose.—Major vascular injuries are uncommon but serious complications of laparoscopic surgery. Early recognition and conversion to an open procedure may be required to avoid further complications. We report 2 cases in which the vena cava was transected during retroperitoneoscopic nephrectomy, and review the literature.

Materials and Methods.—All urological laparoscopic cases from 1993 to 2002 at 2 institutions were reviewed to identify major vessel transection. Two cases of inadvertent transection of the vena cava were identified. Medical records were reviewed for clinical and pathological information to identify factors leading to this complication. A MEDLINE search was performed to identify similar reports in the literature.

Results.—Two patients at 2 institutions were identified with vena caval transection during retroperitoneoscopic nephrectomy. In both cases the vena cava was misidentified as a renal vein. The injury was recognized immediately in both cases and an open repair was performed by vascular surgery. Both patients recovered with no sequelae. In both cases a rotated camera on an angled laparoscope in addition to the relative lack of retroperitoneal landmarks may have contributed to a loss of orientation within the operative field. A similar report of an aortic transection was also found in the literature.

Conclusions.—Disorientation of the operating surgeon within the surgical field secondary to rotation of the camera lens and lack of retroperitoneal landmarks may contribute to vena caval transection during retroperitoneoscopic nephrectomy. This injury has not been found in transperitoneal nephrectomy, likely because more intra-abdominal landmarks exist, aiding in maintenance of orientation. Prompt intraoperative recognition and repair of the transection results in a favorable outcome.

▶ Injury to major blood vessels is usually apparent laparoscopically, because one will see the hemorrhage. However, when the vessel is transected with the endoscopic vascular stapler, one may not recognize the injury. In this paper, both vena cava transactions were noted intraoperatively and repaired. I am also aware of transactions of the superior mesenteric artery and the aorta, some of which were recognized and others which were detected later in the postoperative course. These great vessel injuries are an unusual but recognized complication.

S. B. Bhayani, MD

En Bloc Stapling of Renal Hilum During Laparoscopic Nephrectomy and Nephroureterectomy

Rapp DE, Orvieto MA, Gerber GS, et al (Univ of Chicago; Univ of Michigan, Ann Arbor)

Urology 64:655-659, 2004 6–7

Objectives.—To evaluate the safety and advisability of en bloc mass stapling of the renal pedicle during difficult laparoscopic nephrectomy to avoid conversion to an open procedure.

Methods.—A retrospective chart review was performed of 433 consecutive patients undergoing laparoscopic simple or radical nephrectomy or laparoscopic nephroureterectomy between August 1998 and July 2003 by two surgeons. In all cases of en bloc hilar ligation, a stapler was deployed across the renal hilum without individual dissection of the renal artery and vein.

Results.—The overall incidence of en bloc ligation was 6.0% (26 of 433 patients). The reasons for en bloc ligation were a difficult hilar dissection and/or the appearance of the renal hilum in 21 cases and urgent ligation secondary to bleeding in 5 cases. No correlation was found between surgeon experience and the frequency of en bloc ligation. No immediate or short-term complications related to this method of hilar division were observed with a mean follow-up of 26 months.

Conclusions.—In this study, no cases of arteriovenous fistula development occurred after en bloc stapling of the renal pedicle. Long-term follow-up is needed, because arteriovenous fistula development may be a late complication of nephrectomy. Although we do not advocate the generalized use of en bloc division of the renal pedicle, early data suggest that en bloc stapling can be performed to avoid conversion to an open procedure with no related short-term complications.

▶ This article outlines the safety of en bloc stapling of the renal artery and renal vein during difficult hilar dissection for laparoscopic nephrectomy. In this communication, no arterio-venous fistulae were discovered at a mean follow-up of 26 months. In 21 cases, the hilar vessels could not be individually dissected and in 5 cases they were ligated urgently secondary to hemorrhage. Importantly, the authors do not advocate the routine use of this technique, but rather they only favor en bloc ligation in cases which would otherwise require open conversion. I agree that to avoid conversion, this technique is a useful "bail-out," but fistulae have been known to develop 10-20 years after ligation. It may be necessary to follow these patients for long-term consequences of the en bloc ligation, as the follow-up is not quite mature in this study.

S. B. Bhayani, MD

Intraoperative Local Anesthesia Decreases Postoperative Parenteral Opioid Requirements for Transperitoneal Laparoscopic Renal and Adrenal Surgery: A Randomized, Double-blind, Placebo Controlled Investigation

Khaira HS, Wolf JS Jr (Univ of Michigan, Ann Arbor)

J Urol 172:1422-1426, 2004 6–8

Purpose.—To determine if local anesthesia decreases discomfort following laparoscopic upper retroperitoneal surgery, we performed a randomized, double-blind, placebo controlled study in which the port sites and hand assist incision were infiltrated with bupivacaine or placebo prior to surgery.

Materials and Methods.—A total of 72 patients undergoing transperitoneal laparoscopic renal or adrenal surgery were randomly assigned to the treatment (0.5% bupivacaine) or placebo (0.9% normal saline) arm. Port and hand assist port sites were infiltrated at the outset of the procedure. Postoperative pain and opioid use were measured at consistent intervals.

Results.—A total of 37 individuals were treated with placebo (standard laparoscopy [SL] in 15 and hand assisted laparoscopy [HALS] in 22) and 35 were treated with bupivacaine (SL in 16 and HALS in 19). Mean parenteral morphine equivalents use for the placebo vs bupivacaine groups were 29.6 vs 20.0 mg at 12 hours, 50.2 vs 34.5 mg at 24 hours and 57.1 vs 36.6 mg for the total hospital stay (all $p < 0.05$). Parenteral opioid use was decreased in the bupivacaine group in the SL and HALS subgroups with a significant effect at 12 hours in the latter subgroup. On multivariate ANOVA bupivacaine use but not SL vs HALS was associated with decreased parenteral opioid use at all time points ($p < 0.05$).

Conclusions.—At the outset of transperitoneal laparoscopic urological surgery in the upper retroperitoneum, port site and other incision infiltration with long acting local anesthesia decreases postoperative parenteral opioid requirements compared with placebo controls. The effect was seen with SL and HALS and it was greater than any effect of SL vs HALS.

► This study is a prospective randomized double-blind trial involving the use of bupivicaine at port sites with transperitoneal laparoscopic renal surgery. Although hospital stays were similar between the arms, patients who received bupivicaine used less morphine at all time points. This is a relatively inexpensive intervention and should be considered.

S. B. Bhayani, MD

Laparoscopic Partial Nephrectomy: Evaluation of Long-term Oncological Outcome

Allaf ME, Bhayani SB, Rogers C, et al (Johns Hopkins Med Institutions, Baltimore, Md)

J Urol 172:871-873, 2004 6–9

Purpose.—Laparoscopic partial nephrectomy (LPN) has emerged as a viable alternative to open surgery for renal tumors less than 4 cm. We present oncological followup of patients treated with laparoscopic nephron sparing surgery at our institution.

Materials and Methods.—Between September 1996 and December 2001, 48 patients who underwent LPN for clinically localized tumors were found to have pathologically proven renal cell carcinoma. Medical and operative records were reviewed for clinical characteristics, pathological findings and followup information.

Results.—Mean patient age was 59.7 years (range 32 to 81) and mean followup was 37.7 months (range 22 to 84). Mean tumor size was 2.4 cm (range 1.0 to 4.0). Final pathological stage was pT1 in 42 patients (87.5%) and pT3a in 6 (12.5%). Histology revealed clear cell in 32 patients (66.7%), papillary in 10 (20.8%), chromophobe in 3 (6.3%), collecting duct in 1 (2.1%) and unclassified in 2 (4.2%). Intraoperative frozen section biopsies revealed negative margins in all cases. Final surgical margins were positive in 1 patient (2.1%). Followup evaluation consisting of physical examination and yearly cross-sectional imaging, which revealed no recurrences in 46 of 48 patients (95.8%). One patient with von Hippel-Lindau disease was found to have local recurrence 18 months after LPN and observation was elected. The second patient had recurrence in the same kidney away from the original tumor site approximately 4 years later.

Conclusions.—LPN is an effective treatment modality for clinically localized renal cell carcinoma. Oncological outcomes at a mean followup of 3 years are promising, although the durability of oncological outcomes must be determined.

▶ This article documents the long-term oncologic efficacy of LPN. With 48 patients and a mean follow-up of 37.7 months, 2 patients had recurrences. Both recurrences were likely unrelated to the primary tumor; one was in a patient with von Hippel Lindau disease, and one recurrence was at a site separate from the partial nephrectomy lesion. This article is critically important, as it finally establishes LPN as a reasonable alternative to open partial nephrectomy in experienced hands. Importantly, the positive margin rate was 2.1% in this series, and likely is directly related to the oncologic efficacy. When beginning one's experience with LPN, the goal should be to obtain a 5 mm to 1 cm margin. Often this requires hilar clamping and suturing of the parenchyma and collecting system. Hence, advanced laparoscopic instrumentation and techniques are needed. The beginning laparoscopist should not cut too shallow, as positive margins will probably affect long-term oncologic efficacy. For this reason, hilar dissection may be necessary, even if clamping is not anticipated, as one should be prepared to clamp if large intrarenal vessels are encountered. Furthermore, the idea of performing a hand assisted "squeeze and cut" partial nephrectomy may not be wise, as suturing may be necessary. Undoubtedly, the excellent results in this article are the result of advanced laparoscopic technique.

S. B. Bhayani, MD

Robotic-assisted Laparoscopic Partial Nephrectomy: Technique and Initial Clinical Experience With daVinci Robotic System

Gettman MT, Blute ML, Chow GK, et al (Mayo Clinic, Rochester, Minn; Univ of Innsbruck, Austria)

Urology 64:914-918, 2004 6–10

Objectives.—To develop and assess the feasibility of laparoscopic partial nephrectomy performed using the daVinci robotic system.

Methods.—Between November 2002 and August 2003, 13 patients with solid or suspicious cystic renal masses underwent robotic-assisted laparoscopic partial nephrectomy. In 8 cases, an intra-arterial catheter was inserted for renal cooling before occlusion of the renal artery. The remaining 5 patients underwent partial nephrectomy after the renal hilum had been clamped. Tumor excision and intracorporeal suturing were performed entirely with telerobotics. The perioperative data and pathologic results were retrospectively reviewed.

Results.—The mean lesion diameter was 3.5 cm (range 2.0 to 6.0). The mean operative time was 215 minutes (range 130 to 262), and the mean blood loss was 170 mL (range 50 to 300). The mean warm ischemia was 22 minutes (range 15 to 29), and the mean cold ischemia time was 33 minutes (range 18 to 43). The length of hospital stay averaged 4.3 days (range 2 to 7). The resected lesions included renal cell carcinoma in 10, oncocytoma in 2, and a complex renal cyst in 1. In 1 case, a positive margin occurred despite negative frozen sections; laparoscopic nephrectomy was performed and showed no residual tumor. One patient experienced postoperative ileus. At 2 to 11 months of follow-up, no recurrence had been observed.

Conclusions.—Robotic-assisted partial nephrectomy is feasible. Robotic partial nephrectomy can be safely performed using a transperitoneal or retroperitoneal approach. A second scrubbed assistant is mandatory to provide assistance using conventional laparoscopic instruments with this technique.

▶ Robotics is a new and exciting area of urology. The daVinci robot, which is extraordinarily expensive, has become a useful tool to perform complex reconstructive urology. Although it has been useful for prostatectomy, its usage and effectiveness over standard laparoscopic partial nephrectomy is questionable. This study shows that robotic assisted laparoscopic partial nephrectomy is feasible, but feasibility does not mean that the operation should be performed. I believe that urologists should be able to perform standard laparoscopic renal surgery without the robot. This includes nephrectomy, cryoablation, partial nephrectomy, and pyeloplasty. The robot adds extraordinary expense with no benefit in outcomes, and a fully trained laparoscopic assistant is necessary. If a laparoscopic assistant is present, why not just do the case laparoscopically? Urologists should concentrate on laparoscopic renal surgery without robotic assistance to offer the most efficient and cost effective care.

S. B. Bhayani, MD

Laparoscopic Cryoablation of Solid Renal Masses: Intermediate Term Followup

Cestari A, Guazzoni G, Dell'Acqua V, et al (San Raffaele Hosp, Milan)

J Urol 172:1267-1270, 2004 6–11

Purpose.—We report our experience with laparoscopic renal cryoablation (LRC) in select cases of small renal neoplasms. We evaluated the oncological results with the advantages of minimally invasive surgery.

Materials and Methods.—Since September 2000, at our department 37 patients with a mean age of 64 years (range 29 to 89) have undergone LRC for computerized tomography or magnetic resonance imaging (MRI) documented renal masses. Mean lesion diameter was 25.7 mm (range 10 to 60). According to tumor position in 22 cases the procedure was performed transperitoneally and in 15 it was done retroperitoneoscopically. Postoperative followup included MRI on postoperative day 1, 1, 3, 6, 12, 18 and 24 months after surgery, and annually thereafter. Moreover, 6 months following the surgical procedure biopsy of the site of the treated neoplasm was performed.

Results.—The laparoscopic procedure was successfully completed in all cases. Mean operative time was 194 minutes (range 120 to 300) and mean blood loss was 165.3 ml (range 20 to 900). Final histological evaluation revealed renal cell carcinoma in 29 cases and oncocytoma in 6, while 2 were reported as indefinite. All patients were discharged home after a mean of 3.8 days (range 3 to 7) and returned to normal social life after a mean of 7.3 days (range 5 to 9). Early and postoperative complications were evaluated. Mean diameter of the cryolesion on postoperative day 1 on MRI was 48.2 mm and it progressively decreased during followup. Of the 35 patients with at least 6 months of followup computerized tomography guided biopsy was performed in 25, who were negative for neoplasm.

Conclusions.—LRC for small renal masses appears to be a safe, reproducible, minimally invasive technique. Medium term followup in our series is encouraging, although further studies and prolonged followup are needed to access properly the role of this surgical technique.

▶ There is now substantial evidence demonstrating that the preferred treatment for most small renal masses is nephron-sparing surgery. Although laparoscopic partial nephrectomy is routinely performed by experienced laparoscopic surgeons, it remains a technically challenging procedure. Although there has been an emergence of ablative technologies for the management of small renal masses, the oncologic efficacy remains to be determined. This report along with others does demonstrate short-term efficacy of cryotherapy as determined by follow-up MRIs and needle biopsies. The long-term outcomes remain to be seen before the true efficacy of cryotherapy for renal cell carcinoma is determined. Because it is unlikely that any ablative technologies will exceed cure achieved by nephron-sparing surgery, the main theoretical advantage of cryotherapy is reduced morbidity. Findings from this report suggest that the morbidity of laparoscopic cryotherapy may not be much less than for laparoscopic partial nephrectomy. For this reason, I believe that the most valuable role for renal cryotherapy is for tumors that are amenable to percutaneous access.

D. K. Ornstein, MD

Complications of Laparoscopic Partial Nephrectomy in 200 Cases

Ramani AP, Desai MM, Steinberg AP, et al (Cleveland Clinic Found, Ohio)

J Urol 173:42-47, 2005 6–12

Purpose.—We analyzed complications of the initial 200 cases treated with laparoscopic partial nephrectomy for a suspected renal tumor.

Materials and Methods.—Since August 1999, 200 consecutive patients have undergone laparoscopic partial nephrectomy. Mean patient age was 61.6 years, mean body mass index was 29.9 and mean tumor size was 2.9 cm (range 1 to 10). There were 51 central tumors (25%) and 15 solitary kidneys (7.5%). A central tumor was defined as any tumor infiltrating up to the collecting system or renal sinus, during the excision of which entry into and repair of the collecting system was necessary. Mean estimated blood loss was 247 cc and mean operative time was 3.3 hours. Data on complications were obtained from a prospectively maintained computerized database and via telephone calls to patients and/or local referring physicians.

Results.—A total of 66 patients (33%) had 1 or more complications, which were intraoperative in 11 (5.5%), postoperative in 24 (12%) and delayed in 31 (15.5%). Overall 30 patients (15%) had a non-urological complication and 36 (18%) had a urological complication, including hemorrhage in 19 (9.5%) and urine leakage in 9 (4.5%). Hemorrhage occurred intraoperatively in 7 cases (3.5%) and postoperatively in 4 (2%), while it was delayed in 8 (4%). Of patients with urine leakage none required reoperation, 6 (3%) required a Double-J stent (Medical Engineering Corp., New York, New York) only, 2 (1%) required a Double-J stent with computerized tomography guided drainage and 1 required no treatment. Open conversion was necessary in 2 patients (1%), reoperation was done in 4 (2%) and elective laparoscopic radical nephrectomy was performed in 1 (0.5%).

Conclusions.—Laparoscopic partial nephrectomy is an advanced procedure with potential for complications. It requires considerable experience with reconstructive laparoscopy.

▶ This is the largest reported series of laparoscopic partial nephrectomy from the Cleveland Clinic. Even in the hands of an expert laparoscopist, the overall complication rate was 33%. Hemorrhage occurred in 9.5% of patients and urine leak in 4.5%. Although the urine leak rate compared favorably with open series, the incidence of hemorrhage was slightly higher. The authors have changed their practice to use a bioadhesive on the cut parenchyma, which has decreased their hemorrhage rate to 3%. Of note, 4 of 7 intraoperative hemorrhagic complications were secondary to bulldog or satinsky malfunction. Additionally, surgeons should be aware of the risk of delayed hemorrahage (4%). I agree with the authors that in 2005 laparoscopic partial nephrectomy is still an advanced laparoscopic procedure, requiring complex technical skills. However, in the hands of an experienced surgeon, the complications are comparable to the open approach.

S. B. Bhayani, MD

Tumor Seeding in Urological Laparoscopy: An International Survey

Micali S, Celia A, Bove P, et al (Univ of Modena e Reggio Emilia, Italy; Johns Hopkins Univ, Baltimore, Md)

J Urol 171:2151-2154, 2004 6–13

Purpose.—During the last 10 years laparoscopy has been applied to treat most urological pathology including malignancies. There has been concern regarding peritoneal dissemination and port site metastases. We undertook a survey to assess the incidence of this occurrence.

Materials and Methods.—A total of 50 international urology departments with experts in laparoscopic urological surgery were contacted for this study. Each site was asked to complete a 2-page survey regarding the volume of laparoscopic urological procedures and port site recurrences.

Results.—Nineteen sites elected to participate. A total of 18750 laparoscopic procedures were performed, of which 10912 were for cancer. These included 2604 radical nephrectomies, 559 nephroureterectomies, 555 partial nephrectomies, 27 segmental ureterectomies, 3665 radical prostatectomies, 1869 pelvic lymph node dissections, 479 retroperitoneal lymph node dissections, 336 adrenalectomies and 108 procedures listed as other. Tumor seeding was reported in 13 cases (0.1%), including 3 nephroureterectomies for transitional cell carcinoma, 4 nephrectomies (incidental transitional cell carcinoma), 4 adrenalectomies for metastases, 1 retroperitoneal lymph node dissection for testicular cancer and 1 pelvic lymph node dissection for cancer of the penis. Port seeding occurred in 10 cases (0.09%) and peritoneal spread in 3 cases (0.03%).

Conclusions.—The incidence of tumor seeding after laparoscopic oncological surgery is rare and does not appear greater than what has been historically reported for open surgery. Tumor seeding seems to be most commonly related to the removal of high grade tumors and deviation from oncological surgical principles.

▶ This very nice study looked at close to 20,000 laparoscopic procedures of which about half were performed for cancer. Tumor seeding secondary to the laparoscopic procedure was reported in 13 cases (0.1%). These data show that well performed laparoscopic procedures do not compromise cure. However, the authors correctly emphasize that port site or local seeding is more likely if the surgeons inadvertently violate the tumors during removal and extirpation.

G. L. Andriole, Jr, MD

Thoracic Complications During Urological Laparoscopy

Abreu SC, Sharp DS, Ramani AP, et al (Cleveland Clinic Found, Ohio)

J Urol 171:1451-1455, 2004 6–14

Purpose.—We documented thoracic related complications during urological laparoscopic surgery.

Materials and Methods.—A total of 1129 patients underwent major urological laparoscopic procedures in a 5-year period. Operative reports and postoperative radiographic reports were retrospectively reviewed to identify patients with thoracic related medical and surgical sequelae. Of the patients 619 (55%) underwent at least 1 chest x-ray in the immediate or early postoperative period. In the remaining 510 patients (45%) there was no clinical indication to perform chest x-ray.

Results.—Of 619 patients undergoing chest x-ray 438 (71%) were completely normal. Medical pulmonary complications, surgical thoracic complications and subclinical, incidentally detected gas collections in the chest were identified in 12.6%, 0.5% and 5.5% of patients, respectively. Medical complications in 12.6% of cases included pulmonary infiltrate/atelectasis in 9.7%, pleural effusion in 4.8% and pulmonary embolus in 0.3%. Surgical complications included symptomatic pneumothorax in 4 patients (0.35%), hemothorax in 1 (0.08%) and chylothorax in 1 (0.08%). Subclinical abnormal thoracic gas collections were radiographically noted in 34 of the 619 patients (5.5%) on chest x-ray, including pneumomediastinum in 19 (3.1%), pneumothorax in 10 (1.6%) and pneumopericardium in 5 (0.8%). Overall 36 of 40 (90%) thoracic surgical complications (3) and subclinical, incidentally detected gas collections (33) occurred during retroperitoneal laparoscopy. Re-intervention was necessary in 6 patients (0.5%), namely pulmonary embolus requiring vena caval filter placement in 3 (0.3%), pneumothorax requiring a chest tube in 2 (0.17%) and hemothorax requiring emergency open thoracotomy in 1 (0.08%). No patient underwent open conversion to complete the initial proposed operation.

Conclusions.—Due to its high solubility the expectant management of incidental CO_2 pneumothorax, pneumopericardium and pneumomediastinum is recommended initially in the clinically stable patient. Inadvertent diaphragmatic entry can be satisfactorily repaired laparoscopically without open conversion. Although it is rare, surgical thoracic complications are potentially life threatening, requiring prompt identification and management.

▶ The key finding in this article is that 90% of thoracic complications occurred with the retroperitoneal approach. Although most of these complications were asymptomatic, some were potentially life threatening. The authors do point out that serious thoracic complications occurred with equal incidence in transperitoneal and retroperitoneal approaches, but the serious transperitoneal complications were pneumothoraces, while the serious retroperitoneal complications included chylothorax and hemothorax. The retroperitoneal approach is certainly useful, but the laparoscopist should be aware of this potential disadvantage. The authors stress the importance of avoiding placement of a supracostal trocar.

S. B. Bhayani, MD

Pancreatic Injuries During Laparoscopic Urologic Surgery

Varkarakis IM, Allaf ME, Bhayani SB, et al (Johns Hopkins Med Institutions, Baltimore, Md)

Urology 64:1089-1093, 2004 6–15

Objectives.—To review our experience with pancreatic injury (PI) associated with urologic laparoscopy. PI associated with urologic laparoscopy is uncommon.

Methods.—From January 1999 to April 2004, 890 laparoscopic operations for upper urinary tract pathologic findings were performed, of which 574 were left-sided procedures. We reviewed the medical records for recognized intraoperative or postoperatively documented PI and recorded the patient demographic data and intraoperative and postoperative management.

Results.—Four PIs were identified, all associated with left-sided procedures. The overall rate of PI was 0.44%. Two injuries occurred during left radical nephrectomy (2.1%) and two during left adrenalectomy (8.6%). The mean tumor size was 6 ± 3.4 cm. The diagnosis was made intraoperatively in 1 patient, postoperative midepigastric pain with elevated serum amylase levels was the clinical presentation in 2 patients, and the incidental finding of pancreatic tissue in the final pathologic specimen confirmed the injury in the fourth patient. A prolonged pancreatic fistula developed only in 1 case. Three patients were treated conservatively and computed tomography-guided drainage of a pancreatic collection was required in one. The mean hospital stay was 18 days (range 4 to 57).

Conclusions.—PI is uncommon but can result in significant morbidity. Intraoperative detection and repair can minimize sequelae. Management with conservative measures and percutaneous drainage is usually successful, although a prolonged postoperative course can be expected.

▶ PIs may happen with transperitoneal laparoscopic renal surgery. Interestingly, the incidence of PI was 8.6% with left adrenalectomy and 2.1% with left nephrectomy. Conservative management was successful in the majority of cases, and drainage of a pancreatic fluid collection was successful when indicated. If a difficult dissection is encountered, a drain should be considered to treat this potential complication. Particular care should be taken in left adrenalectomy, as the pancreas lies in close proximity and may be injured by direct dissection, retraction or energy transmission.

S. B. Bhayani, MD

7 Transplantation

Mechanism of Action of Donor-Specific Transfusion in Inducing Tolerance: Role of Donor MHC Molecules, Donor Co-stimulatory Molecules, and Indirect Antigen Presentation

Kishimoto K, Yuan X, Auchincloss H Jr (Harvard Med School, Boston; Massachusetts Gen Hosp, Boston; Univ of Massachusetts, Worcester; et al)

J Am Soc Nephrol 15:2423-2428, 2004 7–1

Background.—In several transplant models, donor-specific transfusion (DST) synergizes with T cell co-stimulatory blockade to induce tolerance. However, the mechanism of DST action is not well characterized.

Methods.—The role of major histocompatibility complex (MHC) and co-stimulatory molecule expression on the immunomodulatory functions of DST was investigated with the use of specific gene knockout mice. The role of indirect recognition of antigen provided by DST was investigated using recipient mice that do not express MHC class II molecules on peripheral antigen-presenting cells but that have functional CD4+ T cells.

Findings.—In wild-type recipients of cardiac allografts, treatment with DST from wild-type donors combined with CD154 blockade induced tolerance. In this model, tolerance was induced despite the absence of MHC class I and II, CD40, or B7 molecules on transfused cells. However, when the indirect pathway was eliminated in functional CD4+ T-cell recipients, DST induction of long-term cardiac allograft survival was blocked.

Conclusion.—To date, the proximal mechanisms involving alloreactive T-cell interactions with DST have not been clear. The current experiments show that the indirect antigen recognition pathway mediates the immunomodulatory effect of DST induction of transplantation tolerance in vivo.

► During the past decade, there has been significant progress in the understanding of costimulatory signals involving T cells. The interaction between the T-cell receptor and the MHC on the antigen presenting cell (APC) is generally considered the first signal required for T-cell activation. However, this signal alone is insufficient for optimal T-cell activation.

Elegant studies have demonstrated the existence of several costimulatory molecules on T cells and their corresponding ligands on APCs, which provided a second set of signals to the T cell. These molecules tend to have distinct and overlapping roles in modulating T-cell responses and APC functions to alloantigen. The discovery of these molecules and the elucidation of their role(s) has, in turn, provided targets for therapeutic strategies, some of which have been successful in promoting transplantation tolerance in preclinical models.

The tolerogenic effect of donor-specific blood transfusions (DST) has been postulated for many years yet the mechanism by which this occurs remains unclear. A widely held belief was that donor APCs are able to promote T cell anergy through lack of costimulation signals. Additionally, and more significantly, DSTs have also had the opposite effect of sensitizing the recipient and are therefore no longer considered practical from the standpoint of clinical transplantation.

This study by Kishimoto et al aims to elucidate the mechanism of tolerance induction through DST in a murine heart transplant model. Utilizing a combined approach of DST and co-stimulatory blockade through an antibody against CD154 (a costimulatory molecule on T cells that promotes APC function), this group was able to promote indefinite survival of heart grafts across full MHC disparity as well as demonstrate tolerance to second grafts from the same donor. They further showed that the tolerizing effect of the DST was not related to direct presentation of donor antigen, as DST from MHC class I– and class II–deficient mice did not abrogate the tolerizing effect of DST and costimulatory blockade.

Similarly, DST from mice devoid of costimulatory molecules also did not abrogate the tolerizing effect. Lastly, and most significantly, recipient mice that were deficient in MHC class II APC had accelerated rejection of heart grafts, suggesting that indirect presentation of donor antigen (presentation by recipient APC) is the mechanism by which tolerance induction occurs.

The implication from these findings is that immunosuppressive strategies must avoid suppressing recipient APCs. These cells and their interaction with regulatory T cells likely plays a key role in tolerance induction.

V. Krishnamurthi, MD

Restricting Living-Donor–Cadaver-Donor Exchanges to Ensure That Standard Blood Type O Wait-List Candidates Benefit

Ross LF, Zenios S (Univ of Chicago; Stanford Univ, Calif)

Transplantation 78:641-646, 2004 7–2

Introduction.—A consortium created by Region 1 of the United Network for Sharing allows a patient waiting for a kidney transplant to take a higher priority on the list if a relative serves as a living donor to another waiting recipient. In a living paired exchange, kidneys are exchanged between 2 living-donor-recipient pairs. In a list paired exchange, kidneys are exchanged through a living-donor–cadaver-donor exchange. But a list paired exchange that allows participation of ABO-incompatible donor-recipient pairs adversely affects standard blood type O wait-list candidates, a group with the longest waiting times. Restrictions proposed in this study ensure that the standard blood type O wait-list candidates also benefit.

Methods.—The approach included 3 steps. First, a decision tree model provides a total number and the blood type frequencies of donor-recipient pairs that would participate in a list paired exchange. In the second step, these numbers are translated into organ supply-to-demand ratios for the standard cadaver wait list. In the third step, these ratios are translated into mean waiting times. Living paired exchanges occur whenever there is an ABO-compatible exchange between 2 living donor pairs. List paired exchanges would be considered only if this option fails. However, if the donor is blood-type compatible but cross-match positive, participation in the list paired exchange is permitted irrespective of donor and recipient blood types.

Results.—On the basis of 7 distinct scenarios about the number of willing donors per recipient, the national number of additional organs to be procured might range from a minimum of 414 to a maximum of 1150. Average waiting times for all the standard cadaver wait-list candidates would be reduced by the additional number of procured organs. In the various scenarios, these times might be reduced by between 5.4% and 16.0%. Standard wait-list blood type O candidates, currently those with the longest cadaver wait times, would have waiting times decreased in all 7 scenarios.

Discussion.—The restricted paired list exchange program described here could increase the number of available kidneys and decrease waiting list times. But because the model assumes that all recipients are part of a single national distribution scheme, the impact on both donor numbers and wait times would be reduced under the current regional systems.

▶ The shortage of suitable donor organs remains the single most significant hurdle in kidney transplantation today. Although the total number of kidney transplants has increased yearly since 1988, the largest proportional increase has occurred in living donor kidney transplantation. This increase can be attributed to multiple factors, including increased awareness of the improved success rates with living donor transplantation, greater emphasis on living donor transplantation by transplant programs, and diminished morbidity from improvements in surgical techniques (laparoscopic and open donor nephrectomy). One other potential source of living donor kidney transplants is in the setting of ABO incompatibility or cross-match (positive cross-match) incompatibility. Currently, the vast majority of ABO and cross-match incompatible donor-recipient pairs are prohibited from proceeding with transplantation, and, if feasible, another donor without these incompatibilities is sought. Successful kidney transplantation across ABO or cross-match incompatibility has been performed at selected centers; however, there is currently no consensus on methods to reduce preexisting antibody and on posttransplant immunosuppression. Living donor exchanges have been proposed as an alternative to transplantation across ABO and cross-match incompatibility. In this setting, 2 incompatible donor-recipient pairs would exchange donors to now-compatible recipients. As a result, 2 living-donor transplants are performed that otherwise would not have occurred. Moreover, it stands to reason that increasing the possibility of donor exchanges between multiple transplant centers will have the greatest impact on number of transplants performed. Although straightforward in theory, the realistic aspects to performing a living-donor exchange transplant are cumbersome and are mired in important practical issues, such as logistics, equality and confidentiality.

As an alternative, Ross and Zenios propose a solution in which ABO-incompatible and cross-match incompatible donor-recipient pairs would exchange with recipients on the national waiting list. Specifically, the donor in an incompatible pair would donate to the highest patient on the deceased donor waiting list and consequently, the originally intended recipient, who could not receive the organ because of incompatibility, would be given priority to receive the next deceased donor kidney. Ethical concerns have been raised for recipients of blood group O. These recipients are most likely to face ABO incompatibility and placing them at the highest positions on the waiting list will result in unfairly increasing the waiting times for already-listed O recipients. In a previous publication, Ross and Zenios showed that exclusive selection of type O blood group living donors only slightly reduces waiting times for listed blood type O recipients.[1] In this article, the same authors refine their initial proposal to include only ABO-incompatible pairs restricted to non-O recipients (A, B, and AB only) and cross-match incompatibility across all blood groups. Their analyses suggest a potential reduction of 5% to 16% of the current type O blood group recipient waiting times.

The potential impact of this approach on the supply of donor organs is significant and would greatly benefit patients on the waiting list. On a cautionary note, however, implementation of such a policy on a national level is extremely difficult because of potential disparities between living donor kidneys and deceased donor kidneys. For example, recipients added to the waiting list may have prolonged waiting times for a kidney of similar "quality." In addition, these waiting times may vary depending on local and regional numbers of deceased donors and allocation schemes. Lastly, as the waiting time increases, the possibility of changes in recipient health that preclude transplantation also increases. All of these factors may separate both in time and outcome the "exchange" aspect of a living donor renal transplant for prioritization on the waiting list.

In my impression, although somewhat cumbersome, living donor exchanges within geographic regions are most likely to facilitate ABO and cross-match incompatible transplants. In this setting, equitable "matching" schemes can be computer generated and transplants can proceed within both geographic and temporal proximity so that all donors and recipients have a view of expected outcomes.

V. Krishnamurthi, MD

Reference

1. Zenios SA, Woodle ES, Ross LF: Primum non nocere: Avoiding harm to vulnerable wait list candidates in an indirect kidney exchange. *Transplantation* 72:648-654, 2001.

Treatment of Cytomegalovirus Disease With Valganciclovir in Renal Transplant Recipients: A Single Center Experience

Babel N, Gabdrakhmanova L, Jeurgensen J-S, et al (Charité Univ, Berlin; Hoffmann-La Roche AG, Grenzach-Wyhlen, Germany)

Transplantation 78:283-285, 2004 7–3

Introduction.—IV administered ganciclovir (GCV) is highly effective when used for cytomegalovirus (CMV) prophylaxis in transplant recipients, but the IV route is inconvenient for outpatient care and costly for long-term use. Valganciclovir (VGC), a newly developed valyl ester prodrug of GCV, can be taken orally to prevent CMV. The applicability of VGC in the treatment of transplant recipients was examined in 21 patients with symptomatic CMV infection after undergoing renal transplantation.

Methods.—The mean patient age was 45.7 and the mean transplant age was 3.5 years; 67% had received a cadaver allograft and 19% received their second allograft. An extra CMV-antigen test was performed to confirm diagnosis when clinical symptoms of CMV appeared. Treatment with VGC continued until symptoms cleared and for 2 weeks after 2 CMV antigenemia assays were negative. The patients were monitored for a mean of 5.5 months for efficacy and safety of VGC.

Results.—All patients experienced a decrease in CMV antigenemia during the first 3 weeks of therapy, from mean positive levels of 5.2 to mean negative values of 0.25 positive cells per 10,000 peripheral blood mononuclear cells. The clinical symptoms associated with CMV antigenemia also resolved. Normalization of viral load required periods ranging from 3 weeks to more than 6 weeks. The efficacy of VGC was not dependent on time since transplantation or the immunosuppression used. Side effects were not serious, and there were no relapses after VGC was discontinued.

Discussion.—Valganciclovir may offer a new therapeutic option for the prevention and treatment of CMV disease in organ transplant recipients. The dosage of VGC used in this study (900 mg/d or, for patients with impaired renal function, 450 mg/d) was safe and effective. Even years after transplantation, clinical symptoms and CMV antigenemia resolved with treatment. Careful CMV monitoring during the therapy is advised.

► CMV infection remains the most important infection in transplant patients. Improvements in antiviral medications, particularly the introduction of GCV, have greatly reduced the frequency and severity of viral infections but have not completely eliminated the risk posed by CMV. VGC, the valyl ester prodrug of GCV that has nearly 10-fold greater bioavailability, has recently been shown to be equally effective as GCV for prophylaxis against CMV infection.[1] As an extension of this efficacy, however, the role of VGC in treatment of CMV infection is undetermined. IV GCV, which typically requires hospitalization and long-term central venous access, remains the mainstay of therapy for CMV infection. This article reports on the efficacy of VGC in the treatment of symptomatic CMV infection. The data show that standard doses of VGC can successfully eradicate clinical symptoms and viral "load," often within 4 weeks.

Moreover, CMV relapse did not occur when VGC was administered for 2 additional weeks after viral clearance. The implications of these findings are significant and likely to be duplicated by other groups. Effective oral therapy for the most common posttransplant infection will dramatically reduce costs, morbidity, need for hospitalization, and consequently, also increase long-term graft and patient survival after solid organ transplantation.

V. Krishnamurthi, MD

Reference

1. Akalin E, Sehgal V, Ames S, et al: Cytomegalovirus disease in high-risk transplant recipients despite ganciclovir or valganciclovir prophylaxis. *Am J Transplant* 3:731-735, 2003.

The Effects of FK778 in Combination With Tacrolimus and Steroids: A Phase II Multicenter Study in Renal Transplant Patients

Vanrenterghem Y, van Hooff JP, Klinger M, et al (Universitaire Ziekenhuizen Gasthuisberg, Leuven, Belgium; Academisch Ziekenhuis Maastricht, The Netherlands; Wroclaw Med Univ, Poland; et al)

Transplantation 78:9-14, 2004 7–4

Background.—Research using animal and in vitro models has shown that FK778 inhibits acute rejection and modifies vasculopathy. It also demonstrates antiviral activity. This study investigated the efficacy and safety of FK778 for patients receiving kidney transplants at 2 concentration-controlled ranges.

Methods.—One hundred forty-nine patients were enrolled in the randomized, double-blind study. Treatment consisted of FK778 combined with tacrolimus and corticosteroids for 12 weeks. Forty-nine patients randomly assigned to the high-level group (group H) received 2 × 600 mg/d FK778 and continued on 150 mg/day. Fifty-four patients in the low-level group (group L) received 1 X 600 mg/d followed by 75 mg/d. Forty-six patients made up the placebo group.

Subsequent doses of FK778 were adjusted to trough levels of 100 to 200 µg/mL (for group H) and 10 to 100 µg/mL (for group L). The incidence of biopsy-proved acute rejection was the primary end point.

Findings.—Targeted plasma trough levels were achieved by day 3 in 93% of group L patients and by day 9 in 50% of group H patients. Graft survival at week 16 was 89.7% in group H, 88.8% in group L, and 91.3% in the placebo group. Corresponding incidences of acute rejection were 26.5%, 25.9%, and 39.1%. Anemia was the most frequently reported adverse effect, especially in group H. However, it was reversible. Mean total cholesterol and low-density lipoprotein cholesterol concentrations were lower in the FK778 treatment groups than in the placebo group.

Conclusion.—This phase II trial in renal transplant recipients demonstrated that FK778 is pharmacologically active, well tolerated, and safe. Subsequent research is needed to optimize FK778 dosing strategies.

▶ FK778 is a developmental immunosuppressive agent that is structurally and functionally analogous to A771726, the active metabolite of leflunomide. This agent falls under the class of substances known as malononitrilamides. Malononitrilamides have been shown to prevent allograft rejection in organ transplant models through mechanisms that remain incompletely defined. FK778 binds and inhibits the enzyme dihydroorotate dehydrogenase, which is essential for pyrimidine synthesis. Lymphocyte replication, dependent exclusively on de novo pyrimidine synthesis, is profoundly suppressed by FK778. In addition to immunosuppressive effects, FK778 has also been shown to have antiproliferative effects against vascular smooth muscle as well as antiviral effects.[1,2]

This report details a multicenter, randomized, prospective, double blind (placebo-controlled) study evaluating the safety and efficacy of 2 dosing schemes of FK778 in combination with FK506 (tacrolimus) and steroids. Of the 149 low-risk adult kidney transplant recipients enrolled, approximately three fourths completed the study. Patients were randomized to high-level FK778, low-level FK778, or placebo and after a 12-week treatment period with FK778, were analyzed for rejection rates, achievement of target drug levels, and occurrence of side effects.

Although the overall rejection-free rates did not appear to be significantly different from current standard immunosuppressive protocols, the rejection rate was under 10% in patients achieving the high target trough level of FK778 within 2 weeks of transplantation. Anemia remained the most common adverse effect related to FK778 and was reversible after cessation of therapy. Interestingly, FK778-treated patients enjoyed a reduction in total cholesterol and low-density lipoprotein cholesterol levels, as compared with the placebo group.

The significance of this study is that it is the first clinical report on the safety and efficacy of a novel immunosuppressant, FK778. Notwithstanding its effects on rejection prophylaxis, the added potential long-term benefits of antiviral properties and favorable lipid profile may enable this drug to significantly reduce the number of graft losses from nonimmunologic causes.

V. Krishnamurthi, MD

References

1. Savikko J, Von Willebrand E, Hayry P: Leflunomide analogue FK778 is vasculoprotective independent of its immunosuppressive effect: Potential applications for restenosis and chronic rejection. *Transplantation* 76:455-458, 2003.
2. Zeng H, Knight DA, Shen J, et al: Cytomegalovirus (CMV) antiviral activity of malanonitrilamide, FK778. *Am J Transplantation* 3(suppl 5):393, 2003.

Blood Pressure and Renal Function After Kidney Donation From Hypertensive Living Donors

Textor SC, Taler SJ, Driscoll N, et al (Mayo Clinic, Rochester, Minn)
Transplantation 78:276-282, 2004 7–5

Introduction.—Hypertension is among the most common reasons for excluding potential living kidney donors who are otherwise suitable. With a steady lowering of the threshold for hypertension, many previously acceptable donors may no longer be considered. The basis for excluding a donor with hypertension is a concern for subsequent failure of the donor's remaining kidney. But beginning in 2001, the transplant center at Mayo Clinic has accepted moderately hypertensive white donors with normal kidney function and urine protein. The outcome for such donors was examined 1 year after kidney donation.

Methods.—Included in the study were 148 consecutive living-kidney donor candidates who completed donor nephrectomy between January 2001 and December 2002 and returned for blood pressure evaluation 6 to 12 months later. During a 2-day return visit, donors had clinic, ambulatory, and nurse blood pressure measurements recorded, and a 24-hour urine for protein and microalbumin excretion was obtained. Donors also underwent a repeat glomerular filtration rate (GFR) study (measured by iothalamate clearance).

Results.—Kidney donors were 65 men and 83 women with a mean age of 43.4 years and a mean body mass index of 27.8. Twenty-four were hypertensive and 124 were normotensive. Hypertensive and normotensive donors differed significantly in age (mean 41.4 vs 53.4 years). A family history of hypertension was present in 63.3% of donors; 18.2% were smokers. At follow-up (a mean of 282 days after donor nephrectomy), awake ambulatory blood pressure monitoring readings were unchanged in normotensive donors. Mean blood pressure in hypertensive donors fell with both drug treatment and nonpharmacologic therapy, from 145 mm Hg before nephrectomy to 132 mm Hg at follow-up, and their GFR was lower after kidney donation. Neither hypertensive nor normotensive donors had any changes in urine protein and microalbumin.

Conclusion.—In a highly selected group of white living kidney donors with modest hypertension who were evaluated during the first year after donor nephrectomy, no adverse effects were noted in terms of kidney function or urinary protein or microalbumin excretion. Clinical hypertension in these donors was able to be treated effectively. In addition, there were no differences in graft function at 1 month and 1 year in patients receiving kidneys from hypertensive versus normotensive donors.

▶ The increasing disparity between the number of deceased-donor organs and the number of patients waiting for renal transplants has led to several strategies aimed at increasing the living donor pool. Surgical advances such as laparoscopic donor nephrectomy, immunologic manipulation such as antibody reduction protocols and programmatic advances such as living donor exchanges have resulted in marked increases in the number of living kidney donors. In this article, Textor et al report on another, previously discounted, strategy to expand the living kidney donor pool. Their approach of using carefully selected white patients with documented essential hypertension enabled a 19% (24 patients) increase in their living donor renal transplant volume over a 2-year period. Most importantly, during the 12-month period after kidney donation, there was no evidence of adverse effect on blood pressure control, renal function as measured by iothalamate GFR, and urinary protein excretion implying the short-term safety of this practice. In addition, recipients of kidneys from hypertensive living donors enjoyed a renal functional outcome at 1 month and 1 year equivalent to recipients receiving kidneys from normotensive living donors. These results intimate that potential living kidney donors with hypertension may be safely used, raising the possibility of a significant increase in the living kidney donor pool and the number of patients transplanted. Although provocative, these data reflect the short-term safety and recall the need to obtain longer follow-up.

V. Krishnamurthi, MD

Predicting Coronary Heart Disease in Renal Transplant Recipients: A Prospective Study

Ducloux D, Kazory A, Chalopin J-M (Univ of Franch-Comté, Besançon, France)
Kidney Int 66:441-447, 2004 7–6

Introduction.—The disproportionately high incidence of cardiovascular events in renal transplant recipients suggests that nontraditional cardiovascular risk factors may be involved. A group of 344 consecutive renal transplant recipients, all free of vascular disease, was studied prospectively to determine their risk factors for coronary heart disease and the relevance of the Framingham Heart Study cardiovascular risk calculator in such populations.

Methods.—Patients had a transplant duration of more than 12 months and were stable at the time of enrollment. Treatment consisted of antihypertensive drugs (62.5%), angiotensin-converting enzyme (ACE) inhibitors (29.7%), beta blockers (21.4%), and statins or similar agents (37.5%); only 2% of patients took aspirin. Most patients were receiving an immunosuppressive regimen of azathioprine, prednisone, and cyclosporine or tacrolimus. Data gathered included traditional cardiovascular risk factors, nutritional status, smoking behavior, total plasma homocysteine (tHcy), and C-reactive protein (CRP).

Results.—The mean patient age was 51 years; 63% were men. The mean time lapse since transplant was 51 months. During follow-up (mean duration, 72 months), 27 coronary events occurred in 27 patients (7.8%). Five of 12 deaths were from cardiovascular causes. Cox regression analysis showed a significantly greater risk of cardiovascular events among patients in the higher quartiles of tHcy (relative risk [RR], 4.56 vs the lowest quartile) and of CRP (RR, 2.65). There was a strong relationship between the Framingham Heart Study calculated risk and cardiovascular events (RR, 9.59). With the use of the Framingham Heart Study equation, however, only 16 of 27 coronary events had been predictable during the study period. Specifically, coronary events were greatly underestimated in high-risk patients—the subgroup with a higher prevalence of the nontraditional cardiovascular risk factors.

Discussion.—In this population of renal transplant patients, none with vascular disease at enrollment, the Framingham Heart Study model predicted individual cardiovascular risk only in a high-risk subgroup. Nontraditional cardiovascular risk factors such as CRP and tHcy levels must be considered in the preventive care of renal transplant recipients.

► Cardiovascular diseases (CVD) account for the largest single cause of death after renal transplantation. Despite improvements in short-term parameters, such as rejection rates and 1-year graft and patient outcomes, the long-term success of renal transplantation remains relatively stagnant. It is highly likely that CVD and the resulting complications have a profound impact on long-term outcomes. Attempts to identify risk factors for the development of CVD in renal transplant recipients have been complicated by confounding variables, including the relatively high prevalence of hypertension, hyperlipidemia, influence of antihypertensive and antihyperlipemic therapies and, possibly, the influence of immunosuppressive medications. As such, the observed rates of CVD events (myocardial infarctions, coronary artery procedures, or death due to ischemic heart disease) transplant patients tend to be much higher than the expected rates, suggesting a greater influence by traditional risk factors and possibly also by other, less well-defined factors that are specific to renal transplant recipients.[1] In this study of 344 renal transplant recipients who had no history of CVD, CRP and serum homocysteine were found to be independent risk factors for ischemic heart disease events during the mean follow-up period of 6 years. Although traditional risk factors included in the Framingham Heart Study also conferred an increased risk, these alone frequently underestimated the likelihood of CVD events in high-risk patients. The implications of this study are that nontraditional risk factors, such as CRP and homocysteine, may account for the greater risk of CVD in transplant patients and that preventative therapies targeted toward patients with these risk factors may decrease the overall rates of CVD.

V. Krishnamurthi, MD

Reference

1. Kasiske BL, Chakkera HA, Roel J: Explained and unexplained ischemic heart disease risk after renal transplantation. *J Am Soc Nephrol* 11:1735-1743, 2000.

Campath-1H in Renal Transplantation: The University of Wisconsin Experience
Knechtle SJ, Fernandez LA, Pirsch JD, et al (Univ of Wisconsin, Madison)
Surgery 136:754-760, 2004 7–7

Background.—Immune cell depletion is known to prevent renal allograft rejection and injury. We evaluated the humanized monoclonal antibody Campath-1H (alemtuzumab; ILEX Oncology, San Antonio, Texas) in renal transplant recipients for its safety and efficacy in preventing rejection when used in combination with a calcineurin inhibitor, mycophenolate mofetil, and low-dose steroid therapy.

Methods.—One hundred twenty-six consecutive renal allograft recipients received 2 doses of Campath-1H antibody on days 0 and 1. Outcomes were compared to patients who received an anti-CD25 antibody (n = 799), Thymoglobulin (n = 160), or other antibody treatment (n = 156) in combination with a calcineurin inhibitor, mycophenolate mofetil, and higher dose steroids.

Results.—The Campath-1H group overall experienced less rejection than the other 3 groups ($P = .037$). Patients with delayed graft function experienced less rejection with Campath-1H than control groups ($P = .0096$) and improved graft survival ($P = .0119$). There was no difference in infection or malignancies between the 4 groups.

Conclusions.—Campath-1H was well tolerated in renal transplant patients and led to significant reductions in incidence of rejection. Patients with delayed graft function experienced significantly improved graft survival.

► Campath-1H, or alemtuzumab, is a humanized monoclonal antibody directed against the CD25 cell surface antigen located on T and B cells, natural killer (NK) cells, and monocytes and macrophages. Administration of a single IV dose of alemtuzumab results in a profound and long-standing lymphocyte depletion by promoting complement and antibody-dependent cytotoxic mechanisms. Currently, alemtuzumab is approved by the Food and Drug Administration for the treatment of lymphoid malignancies.

Given the effect on lymphocytes, the role of alemtuzumab in organ transplantation was initially tested in trials performed in the United Kingdom during the late 1990s. These pilot studies suggested that induction therapy with Campath-1H allowed prolonged rejection-free renal allograft survival in recipients treated with cyclosporine monotherapy, a markedly reduced immunosuppressive approach compared with current practice in the United States. Subsequently, several US transplant programs have now incorporated the use of Campath-1H in their immunosuppressive protocols for the purpose of evaluating its efficacy.

This study is one of the largest reports on the use of Campath-1H as an induction agent in renal transplant recipients treated with standard maintenance immunosuppression (calcineurin inhibitor, mycophenolate mofetil, and steroids). This group evaluated 126 renal transplant recipients treated with 2 doses of Campath-1H and standard maintenance immunosuppression and compared them with a historic cohort of nearly 1100 patients who had received the standard immunosuppressive regimens during the 6 years before this study. Their findings suggest a significant improvement in renal allograft survival and a reduction in the incidence of rejection. The freedom from rejection was most significant in patients experiencing delayed allograft function. Importantly, the beneficial effects of Campath-1H were not associated with an increased incidence of infection or malignancy.

These positive results must be balanced against several limitations of this study, specifically the retrospective nature, relatively short follow-up in the study group, and comparison with historic controls, but in the aggregate this study suggests that 2 perioperative doses of Campath-1H and calcineurin inhibitor–based immunosuppression is well tolerated and effective in preventing renal transplant rejection.

V. Krishnamurthi, MD

8 Female Urology

Incontinence and Voiding Dysfunction

Cost of Urinary Incontinence and Overactive Bladder in the United States: A Comparative Study

Hu T-W, Wagner TH, Bentkover JD, et al (Univ of California, Berkeley; Stanford Univ, Calif; Innovative Health Solutions, Brookline, Mass; et al)

Urology 63:461-465, 2004 8–1

Introduction.—Approximately 34 million community-dwelling adults in the United States have overactive bladder (OAB); fewer than 2.9 million with OAB have incontinent episodes. These individuals were compared with the approximately 17.8 million who have daily urinary incontinence (UI). The costs of UI for the year 2000 were updated and compared with costs for OAB.

Methods.—By using the cost-of-illness framework, disease epidemiologic data were combined with treatment rates, consequence probabilities, and average cost estimates to assess the total costs of UI and OAB. All costs reflect those incurred during 2000.

Results.—The total cost of UI and OAB was $19.5 billion and $12.6 billion, respectively, in 2000. In patients with UI, $14.2 billion was paid by community residents and $5.3 billion was paid by institutional residents. In patients with OAB, these costs were $9.1 and $3.5 billion, respectively.

Conclusion.—Both overall and per-person costs of UI were higher than those of OAB.

▶ This is a timely update of previous work from these authors. Notably, the costs reported in this study include direct costs, indirect costs, and intangible costs but do not include the considerable burden associated with these conditions, including the related inconvenience and psychological burden.

E. S. Rovner, MD

"Unblinding" in Randomized Controlled Drug Trials for Urinary Incontinence: Implications for Assessing Outcomes When Adverse Effects Are Evident

Dubeau CE, Khullar V, Versi E (Univ of Chicago; Imperial College, London; United Medical and Dental School of New Jersey, New Brunswick; et al)
Neurourol Urodyn 24:13-20, 2005 8–2

Aims.—To determine whether women with urinary incontinence (UI) can identify their allocation in a randomized controlled trial (RCT) of tolterodine (TOL), and whether correct identification is associated with outcomes and adverse effects (AEs).

Methods.—Exploratory analysis of a randomized, double-blind, placebo (PLC)-controlled trial of TOL 4 mg daily for 8 weeks in 743 women with urge-predominant mixed UI. Patient perception of their randomization was assessed at trial end. Main outcome measures were 7-day bladder diaries, patient perception of improvement, and UI-specific quality of life (QoL).

Results.—TOL produced a significant decrease in urge UI episodes compared to PLC (78% vs. 51%, $P = 0.0001$). Fifty-one percent of women correctly identified their randomization (58% on TOL vs. 37% on PLC, $P < 0.001$). Women who assumed they took TOL had better bladder diary outcomes than those who assumed they took PLC. Within each assumption group, patient perception outcomes were similar, regardless of actual randomization. QoL improved in all domains except general health for women on TOL. In women who assumed they took TOL, significant drug benefit was evident in three domains. Moderate-severe dry mouth was higher in those who assumed they took TOL (7.3% vs. 0%, $P < 0.0001$).

Conclusions.—Greater than fifty percent of women in this RCT of antimuscarinic treatment were "unblinded" to their randomization. Patient assumption of randomization was associated with bladder diary and perception outcomes, specific QoL domains, and dry mouth. Efficacy of urge incontinence drugs should be considered in the context of patient assumptions, expectations, and "unblinding" by easily evident side effects.

The Effect of Previous Treatment Experience and Incontinence Severity on the Placebo Response of Stress Urinary Incontinence

Yalcin I, Bump RC (Lilly Research Labs, Indianapolis, Ind)
Am J Obstet Gynecol 191:194-197, 2004 8–3

Objective.—The placebo response associated with stress urinary incontinence (SUI) is sizeable but poorly understood. The aim of this study was to examine the relationship between previous treatment experience and baseline urinary incontinence severity with placebo response.

Study Design.—Nine hundred twenty-one women ages 24 to 83 years received placebo in 4 12-week randomized trials evaluating duloxetine for SUI in 16 countries in Africa, Australia, Europe, and North and South America. Incontinence episode frequency (IEF) was calculated before and after randomization with entries from subject-completed real-time diaries. At baseline, subjects reported on their experience with previous continence surgery and with current pelvic floor muscle training (PFMT) with standardized questions. Analyses included Pearson correlations and the Wilcoxon two-sample test, and were based on intent-to-treat principles.

Results.—The placebo group averaged 17 IEF per week at baseline. Fifty-five percent of placebo-treated subjects averaged ≥14 IEF/wk, 11.8% had previous continence surgery, and 16.5% currently performed PFMT. The overall median decrease in IEF with placebo was 33%, but ranged from 11% to 57% for individual countries. The placebo response was lower in women with more severe SUI (29.6% vs 36.4%, $P = .07$), in those who had previous continence surgery (25.0% vs 33.3%, $P = .26$), and for those using PFMT (23.6% vs 33.3%, $P = .02$). There was a significant positive correlation (rho = .44; $P < .0001$) between the placebo response within a country and that country's use rate for PFMT.

Conclusion.—Treatment naivete and less severe incontinence are associated with an increased placebo response in clinical trials for stress urinary incontinence, although this difference was statistically significant only for PFMT.

► These 2 studies ask a very important question: When is a placebo treatment not a true placebo? The paper by DuBeau et al (Abstract 8–2) describes the effects of patient beliefs of whether they received placebo or active drug and the subsequent effects of that belief on their outcomes, as well as the side effects that were recorded during the trial. In this study, patients who believed they were receiving an active drug had a better response and higher rates of dry mouth compared with those who believed they were on placebo who had a poorer response and considerably less dry mouth. The obvious implication here is that when there is a well-characterized side effect in a drug trial (such as dry mouth, as in the context of antimuscarinic drug trials), then perhaps there is no true placebo arm. In the paper by Yalcin and Bump (Abstract 8–3), there were differences in placebo response rates in various groups of patients, including those with more severe stress incontinence, those who had undergone prior anti-incontinence surgery, and those who were doing pelvic floor exercises. Again, this implies that the placebo response is not a constant across all patient groups. It would be wise to characterize the placebo response, study it more completely, and elucidate how future trials can best use and optimize the placebo effect for what it is: a placebo!

E. S. Rovner, MD

Randomized, Double-blind Placebo Controlled Trial of the Once Daily Antimuscarinic Agent Solifenacin Succinate in Patients With Overactive Bladder

Cardozo L, Lisec M, Millard R, et al (King's College Hosp, London; Urologick Ambulance, Steti, Czech Republic; Prince of Wales Hosp, Randwick, Australia; et al)

J Urol 172:1919-1924, 2004 8–4

Purpose.—In this phase 3 trial we assessed the efficacy of solifenacin 5 mg and 10 mg daily in patients with symptoms related to overactive bladder. In addition, we assessed the safety and acceptability of solifenacin.

Materials and Methods.—The study was a multicenter, multinational, randomized, double-blind, placebo controlled trial. Patients were randomized to 12-week once daily treatment with solifenacin 5 mg, solifenacin 10 mg or placebo. The primary efficacy variable was changed from baseline to study end point in mean number of micturitions per 24 hours. Secondary efficacy variables included changes from baseline in mean number of urgency, nocturia and incontinence episodes per 24 hours, and mean volume voided per micturition.

Results.—Compared with changes obtained with placebo (–1.59), micturitions per 24 hours were statistically significantly decreased with solifenacin 5 mg (–2.37, p = 0.0018) and solifenacin 10 mg (–2.81, p = 0.0001). A statistically significant decrease was observed in the number of incontinence episodes with both solifenacin doses (5 mg, p = 0.002 and 10 mg, p = 0.016). This effect was also seen for episodes of urge incontinence (5 mg, p = 0.014 and 10 mg, p = 0.042). Of patients reporting incontinence at baseline, fully 50% achieved continence after treatment with solifenacin. Episodes of nocturia were statistically significantly decreased in patients treated with solifenacin 10 mg (–0.71, –38.5%) versus placebo (–0.52, –16.4%, p = 0.036). Episodes of urgency were statistically significantly reduced with solifenacin 5 mg (–2.84, –51%, p = 0.003) and solifenacin 10 mg (–2.90, –52%, p = 0.002). Mean volume voided per micturition was statistically significantly increased with both solifenacin doses (p = 0.0001). Treatment with solifenacin was well tolerated. Dry mouth, mostly mild in severity, was reported in 7.7% of patients receiving solifenacin 5 mg and 23% receiving solifenacin 10 mg (vs 2.3% with placebo).

Conclusions.—In this study treatment with solifenacin 5 mg and 10 mg once daily significantly improved all the major symptoms of overactive bladder including frequency, urgency and incontinence. Solifenacin 10 mg also decreased the frequency of nocturia. Solifenacin therapy was associated with a favorable tolerability profile and a low incidence of dry mouth, especially at the 5 mg starting dose.

► Solifenacin represents the latest salvo in the antimuscarinic battles. This once-daily antimuscarinic agent compares favorably to existing therapies, including tolterodine, oxybutynin, trospium, and darifenacin. Overall, the impressive data reported in this study include an effect on nocturia (not demonstrated with the other agents). A very high "dry" rate (although the corresponding placebo dry rate was not reported) was also reported. This compound demonstrates an excellent tolerability profile as well with dry mouth rates comparable to those reported with the tolterodine extended release formulation. Is this agent clinically and substantially better than the other agents currently available on the US market? As of yet, nobody knows.

E. S. Rovner, MD

Urodynamically Defined Stress Urinary Incontinence and Bladder Outlet Obstruction Coexist in Women

Bradley CS, Rovner ES (Univ of Iowa, Iowa City; Univ of Pennsylvania, Philadelphia)

J Urol 171:757-761, 2004 8–5

Background.—Bladder outlet obstruction in women is not well understood. Patients with urodynamic evidence of this disorder were identified in a cohort with stress urinary incontinence (SUI), and cases were analyzed to better define and determine the significance of bladder outlet obstruction in women.

Methods.—One hundred four women with SUI were identified from a videourodynamic data base. Pressure flow studies were reexamined. Bladder outlet obstruction was diagnosed in patients with a maximum flow rate of less than 12 mL/s and a detrusor pressure at maximum flow exceeding 20 cm water or a maximum detrusor pressure of more than 20 cm in women with no measurable flow. Nineteen of the eligible patients (18.3%) were given a diagnosis of bladder outlet obstruction.

Findings.—Compared with the unobstructed women, women with bladder outlet obstruction had a significantly lower maximum flow rate (13.5 and 8.7 mL/s, respectively), mean flow rate (7.9 and 5.9 mL/s, respectively), and voided volume (272 and 180 mL, respectively). In addition, women with bladder outlet obstruction had a significantly greater detrusor pressure at maximum flow, maximum detrusor pressure, and postvoid residual volume. The causes of bladder outlet obstruction were previous anti-incontinence or prolapse surgery in 6, neurologic conditions in 4, cystocele in 2, and dysfunctional voiding in 3. In the remaining 5 patients, bladder outlet obstruction was classified as idiopathic.

Conclusion.—Bladder outlet obstruction and SUI can coexist, even for patients without common causes of obstruction. These data show a similar prevalence of bladder outlet obstruction in patients with SUI as in patients with nonspecific lower urinary tract problems. Further research is warranted to determine the significance of bladder outlet obstruction in patients with SUI.

▶ Women presenting with lower urinary tract symptoms will be found to have a variety of diagnoses. These diagnoses are not mutually exclusive. In this series of patients presenting with SUI, a subset were recognized to have evidence of urodynamic outlet obstruction. Although not previously reported, it makes empiric sense that both outlet obstruction and SUI can coexist since the forces producing SUI (abdominal) are very different from that which produces urodynamic obstruction (detrusor).

E. S. Rovner, MD

Who Will Benefit From Pelvic Floor Muscle Training for Stress Urinary Incontinence?

Cammu H, Van Nylen M, Blockeel C, et al (Vrije Universiteit Brussel, Belgium)

Am J Obstet Gynecol 191:1152-1157, 2004 8–6

Objective.—The purpose of this study was to determine which patient characteristics are predictive of outcome before pelvic floor muscle training for stress urinary incontinence.

Study Design.—This was an observational study at a single-center outdoor patient clinic in Brussels, Belgium, that comprised 447 women, aged 26 to 80 years (mean, 52.7 years), who had urinary stress incontinence. All the women received individual pelvic floor muscle training under the guidance of the same physiotherapist. Twenty-two patient characteristics were considered for outcome measurements.

Results.—Forty-nine percent of the women considered their treatment to be successful; 51% of the women had experienced only some improvement, no change, or a worsening of their condition or had interrupted therapy. Three independent predictors of treatment failure were ≥ 2 leakages per day before treatment ($P < .0001$), the chronic use of psychotropic medication ($P = .002$), and a baseline positive stress test result at first cough ($P = .042$). The odds were only 15% for an individual patient to be treated successfully when these 3 predictors were present.

Conclusion.—Pelvic floor muscle training is beneficial in one half of the patients who are treated in this manner. Two or more leakages per day at baseline and the chronic use of psychotropic medication significantly predicted therapy failure.

► A vexing question in the treatment of patients with stress urinary incontinence continues to be the ability to predict who will respond to nonsurgical therapy. As surgical therapies become less and less invasive, the choice between surgery and nonsurgical therapy becomes increasingly blurred. To what types of patients should we offer nonsurgical therapy? The answer probably begins with choosing patients who will be accepting of the therapy and in whom therapy will be successful. This study did not ask quality of life questions and, furthermore, used a selected patient population but, nonetheless, begins to address the question of who will benefit from pelvic floor physiotherapy. More accurately, the study assesses the question of who may not benefit from pelvic floor physiotherapy. This may be patients with more severe incontinence at presentation, those with more chronic incontinence, and those on psychotropic medications.

E. S. Rovner, MD

The Effect of Botulinum-A Toxin on Patients With Severe Urge Urinary Incontinence

Flynn MK, Webster GD, Amundsen CL (Duke Univ, Durham, NC)

J Urol 172:2316-2320, 2004 8–7

Purpose.—We determined the effect of 150 units of botulinum-A toxin (Botox, Allergan, Irvine, California) on subjects with severe urge urinary incontinence (UUI).

Materials and Methods.—This was an open label uncontrolled clinical trial. Subjects were recruited from the female urology and urogynecology clinics at Duke University. Inclusion criteria included evidence of UUI on 3-day bladder diary, a 24-hour pad weight of 100 gm or greater, absent or minimal stress leakage, absent detrusor dysfunction, and a history of failed anticholinergic and physical therapies. Exclusion criteria included evidence of a urinary tract infection, or other correctable or neurological etiology for UUI. The detrusor of each subject was injected with 150 units of botulinum-A toxin. Evaluations were performed at 2 weeks, 6 weeks, 3 months and 6 months after injection. Outcome measures included daily incontinence episodes, Urogenital Distress Inventory and the Incontinence Impact Questionnaire, 24-hour pad weights, daily pad usage and urinalysis at all visits. Urodynamic studies were performed at the 6-week and 3-month visits.

Results.—Three subjects had uncomplicated urinary tract infections during followup. No other adverse effects occurred. Statistically and clinically significant decreases greater than 50% were seen in virtually all outcome measures at all visits up to 3 months. Most subjects showed signs of recurrent UUI by 6 months. All subjects reported remarkable subjective improvement in incontinence. No significant changes in maximal cystometric capacity, maximal detrusor pressure, peak flow or post-void residual volumes were seen.

Conclusions.—Botulinum-A toxin can significantly decrease urge urinary incontinence and improve quality of life for 3 months after injection. Additional studies are needed to determine ideal doses, dosing intervals, safety and cost-effectiveness of this therapy.

Use of Botulinum-A Toxin for the Treatment of Refractory Overactive Bladder Symptoms: An Initial Experience

Rapp DE, Lucioni A, Katz EE, et al (Univ of Chicago)
Urology 63:1071-1075, 2004 8–8

Objectives.—To define the role of botulinum toxin type A (botulinum-A) intradetrusor injections in the treatment of patients with symptoms of bladder overactivity in whom previous anticholinergic therapy has failed

Methods.—Thirty-five patients (29 women and 6 men) with frequency, urgency, and/or urge incontinence received 300 U of botulinum-A toxin injected transurethrally at 30 sites within the bladder. Patients were evaluated at 3 weeks and 6 months after treatment by completion of the short forms of the Incontinence Impact Questionnaire (IIQ-7) and the Urogenital Distress Inventory (UDI-6), as well as questions assessing global response to the treatment.

Results.—After 3 weeks, the mean IIQ-7 score decreased from 19.4 to 13.9 (P = 0.0006) and the mean UDI-6 score decreased from 16.8 to 12.8 (P = 0.0003). Overall, 21 (60%) of 35 patients reported slight to complete improvement of voiding symptoms after 3 weeks. Among the initial responders followed up for 6 months, the mean IIQ-7 score improved from 20.6 to 15.1 (P = 0.008) and the mean UDI-6 score improved from 16.9 to 13.5 (P = 0.008). Mild hematuria, pelvic pain, and dysuria were seen in 7 patients, lasting for 3 days or less after the procedure.

Conclusions.—Botulinum-A toxin injections may provide improvement in symptoms associated with bladder overactivity in a subset of patients. Improvement may be seen for at least 6 months after treatment. The procedure was well tolerated with minimal side effects. Additional study to define the role of injections in a broad group of patients with irritative voiding symptoms is warranted.

Botulinum Toxin A Has Antinociceptive Effects in Treating Interstitial Cystitis

Smith CP, Radziszewski P, Borkowski A, et al (Baylor Coll of Medicine, Houston; Warsaw School of Medicine, Poland; Univ of Pittsburgh, Pa)
Urology 64:871-875, 2004 8–9

Objectives.—To present clinical evidence with botulinum toxin A (BTX-A) suggesting an antinociceptive role in patients with interstitial cystitis (IC). Intriguing evidence in a somatic pain model has suggested that BTX-A injection may have an antinociceptive effect on both acute and chronic (inflammatory) pain.

Methods.—Thirteen female patients (6 in the United States and 7 in Poland) with IC according to the criteria of the National Institute of Diabetes, Digestive and Kidney Disease were included. Under short general anesthesia or sedation, 100 to 200 U of Dysport (Polish patients) or Botox (U.S. patients) was injected through a cystoscope into 20 to 30 sites submucosally in the trigone and floor of the bladder. Patients were evaluated with the O'Leary-Sant validated IC questionnaire or with voiding charts and a visual analog pain scale 1 month postoperatively and at subsequent 3-month intervals. The Polish patients also underwent pretreatment and post-treatment urodynamic evaluations.

Results.—Overall, 9 (69%) of 13 patients noted subjective improvement after BTX-A treatment. The Interstitial Cystitis Symptom Index and Interstitial Cystitis Problem Index mean scores improved by 71% and 69%, respectively ($P < 0.05$). Daytime frequency, nocturia, and pain by visual analog scale decreased by 44%, 45%, and 79%, respectively ($P < 0.01$). The first desire to void and maximal cystometric capacity increased by 58% and 57%, respectively ($P < 0.01$).

Conclusions.—Our results suggest that BTX-A has an antinociceptive effect on bladder afferent pathways in patients with IC, producing both symptomatic and functional (ie, urodynamic) improvements.

► It would appear that the future treatment for at least some subsets of patients with lower urinary tract dysfunction will include the use of botulinum-A toxin. Although all 3 of these papers (Abstracts 8–7 to 8–9) lack a placebo group, each shows a significant effect of the botulinum-A toxin on various groups of patients, albeit small groups in each study. Well-constructed, placebo-controlled trials (saline controlled) are desperately needed, and one of the manufacturers of the botulinum-A toxin may be in the process of sponsoring trials with this agent in both neurogenic and nonneurogenic bladder dysfunction. At present, there is no uniform consensus on the proper dosage (units) of material needed for a therapeutic effect, nor is there agreement on the optimal concentration, injection location, number of injections, or the interval required or suggested between therapeutic injection sessions.

E. S. Rovner, MD

Botulinum Toxin: A New Dimension in the Treatment of Lower Urinary Tract Dysfunction

Rajkumar GN, Conn IG (Southern Gen Hosp, Glasgow, Scotland, England)

Urology 64:2-8, 2004 8–10

Introduction.—Botulinum toxin causes flaccid paralysis in muscles by inhibiting release of acetylcholine from the nerve endings. The serotypes A and B are available for clinical use. This toxin has been pioneered as urologic therapy during the past 15 years for treatment of detrusor sphincter dyssynergia and detrusor overactivity. The rationale and efficacy of botulinum toxin treatment strategies in the lower urinary tract are reviewed.

Botulinum Toxin for Treatment of Lower Urinary Tract Dysfunction.—Inhibition of exocytosis by the botulinum toxin is a temporary process, with resolution of paralysis occurring in the affected muscle tissue occuring within a few months. Recovery occurs during 2 distinct phases: initially accessory nerve sprouting develops at the end of the affected nerve terminal with increased vesicle turnover in the terminal sprouts. In a later-stage, exocytosis seems to recover in the originally affected terminal with regression of terminal sprouts. Recovery is complete within approximately 90 days. The effect of botulinum is dose dependent and can last up to 9 months in overactive bladders. Detrusor external sphincter dyssynergia (DESD) occurs in patients with neurologic disease and classically among patients with high-level spinal cord injury. Botulinum toxin type A appears to be safe in the treatment of patients with DESD. This temporary treatment can be considerably expensive. Botulinum toxin type A appears to have good clinical efficacy in the treatment of neurogenic detrusor activity. It is a viable alternative when traditional therapies fail to provide urologic improvement or restore continence. The duration of effect appears to be longer than botulinum toxin injection in DESD; this may be attributable to the differing effects of botulinum in striated and smooth muscle. Trials should be expanded to include evaluation of patients with multiple sclerosis, interstitial cystitis, and chronic pain syndromes. Few trials have assessed the role of botulinum toxin for treatment of idiopathic detrusor overactivity; findings with small patient populations have been promising.

Conclusion.—The future uses of botulinum toxin in the treatment of lower urinary tract disorders are promising. The use of other botulinum toxin serotypes and elucidation of other mechanisms of action may provide new therapeutic indications and increased clinical efficacy.

▶ This report is an excellent overall review of the use of botulinum toxin in the treatment of lower urinary tract dysfunction. This is a concise overview that will bring the interested reader up to date on the use of this agent in the lower urinary tract. There is no doubt that we will be hearing more about this fascinating molecule in the future, and this article is an excellent introduction.

E. S. Rovner, MD

Urodynamic and Clinical Evaluation of 91 Female Patients With Urinary Incontinence Treated With Perineal Magnetic Stimulation: 1-Year Followup

Almeida FG, Bruschini H, Srougi M (Federal Univ of São Paulo-UNIFESP/EPM, Brazil)

J Urol 171:1571-1575, 2004 8–11

Purpose.—We evaluate the perineal magnetic stimulation (PMS) effect on continence and quality of life in women with urinary incontinence.

Materials and Methods.—We prospective studied 91 women with demonstrable urinary incontinence treated with 16 sessions of PMS. Pretreatment and posttreatment evaluation was done by clinical history, physical examination, voiding diary, validated quality of life survey (I-QOL) and urodynamic study (UDS). Patients with no leakage after treatment were evaluated at 3, 6 and 12 months.

Results.—Mean patient age ± SD was 60.5 ± 10.1 years. Immediately after treatment the I-QOL score increased 35% ($p < 0.001$), the number of pads daily decreased 40% ($p < 0.001$), the number of leaks daily decreased 54% ($p < 0.001$) and 34 patients (37%) became dry. Of the 91 patients 41 were evaluated before and after treatment by UDS. The average increase in vesical leak point pressure (VLPP) was 24.3% ($p = 0.001$) and initial VLPP in patients who became dry was greater than 80 cm H_2O. After treatment 77% of patients with initial low pressure detrusor overactivity on UDS became free of this condition. One year after discontinuing PMS 94% of patients who became dry immediately after treatment had recurrence.

Conclusions.—Immediately after 16 sessions of PMS women with urinary incontinence have significant improvement in the I-QOL score with decreased daily pad use and leakage episodes but 63% had failure. Therapy is more effective in patients with a VLPP of greater than 80 cm H_2O. The beneficial effect is temporary with high and early recurrence after discontinuing treatment.

▶ The importance in this study lies not with the relatively poor short-term results of magnetic therapy, but, rather, the dismal long-term effects of this therapy. The poor long-term effects associated with this therapy are not unexpected. However, it should be noted that it remains unclear whether long-term therapy or long-term intermittent therapy, or even reapplication of this same therapy, might be effective in the long term in maintaining continence. An alternative to magnetic therapy would be intensive pelvic floor physiotherapy, and there is very little data on the long-term effectiveness of this therapy either.

E. S. Rovner, MD

Treatment of Primary Bladder Neck Obstruction in Women With Transurethral Resection of the Bladder Neck

Blaivas JG, Flisser AJ, Tash JA (Cornell Univ, New York; Lenox Hill Hosp, New York; Mount Sinai Med Ctr, New York)

J Urol 171:1172-1175, 2004 8–12

Background.—Primary bladder neck obstruction (PBNO) is uncommon in women, diagnosed in 1% to 16% of women with bladder outlet obstruction. It is far more common in men, for whom more experiences with therapy have been reported. The presentation, clinical characteristics, treatment, and follow-up of a group of women with PBNO were described.

Methods.—Thirty-seven women undergoing transurethral resection for bladder outlet obstruction diagnosed by videourodynamic study (VUDS) between 1993 and 2002 were identified from a patient data base. After exclusion of patients with neurogenic, traumatic, anatomical, or iatrogenic causes of obstruction, 7 patients remained for analysis. All had a diagnosis of PBNO and underwent transurethral bladder neck resection.

Findings.—The 7 patients ranged in age from 39 to 81 years. Six women initially had symptoms of obstruction, including weak or intermittent stream and urinary hesitancy. In these 6 patients, physical examination was unremarkable, with normal perianal sensation, anal sphincter tone, and lower extremity reflexes. One woman had abdominal swelling on presentation, which was found to be a markedly distended bladder filled with more than 1000 cc urine. On VUDS, all patients were seen to have overt urethral obstruction. Obstruction was seen clearly at the vesical neck in 6 patients. In the remaining patient, the obstruction site was not clear.

Treatment consisted of α-blockers in 3 patients and intermittent self-catheterization in all 7. Subsequently, transurethral bladder neck resection at the vesical neck and proximal urethra was done. At a median follow-up of 3 years, 6 patients reported that they were cured of lower urinary tract symptoms, and 1 reported improvement. The mean flows before and after surgery were 5 and 30 mL/s, respectively. Average voided volumes were 194 and 416 mL/s, and average postvoid residual urine volumes were 680 and 173 mL, respectively.

Conclusion.—In women, PBNO is very rare but easily treated when diagnosed by VUDS. The proportion of patients in this series presenting with urinary retention in middle age suggests that PBNO may be more common in less apparent forms than has been recognized previously.

▶ This article describes a small series of women with PBNO. At the authors' tertiary care clinic, this diagnosis was noted in a very small number of patients, and the authors estimate that approximately only 5% of women who are found to have obstruction have the obstruction located at the level of the bladder neck. Nevertheless, these authors note successful treatment of this condition with transurethral resection, with only 1 of 7 women having symptomatic stress incontinence. Notably, only 3 of the 7 patients in this study had pharmacologic therapy, although all were on clean intermittent catheterization prior to definitive surgical resection.

Overall, this is an important but rare cause of bladder outlet obstruction in females and can only be diagnosed using VUD. Other common etiologies of bladder outlet obstruction in females include vaginal prolapse, prior anti-incontinence surgery, detrusor-external sphincter dyssynergia, and urethral diverticulum.

E. S. Rovner, MD

Efficacy and Morbidity of Autologous Fascia Lata Sling Cystourethropexy

Latini JM, Lux MM, Kreder KJ (Univ of Iowa, Iowa City)

J Urol 171:1180-1184, 2004 8–13

Background.—Sling cystourethropexy for intrinsic sphincter deficiency is now accepted as an effective strategy for all types of stress urinary incontinence. An experience using autologous fascia lata for sling cystourethropexy was reported.

Methods.—The retrospective study included data on 100 women who had had autologous fascia lata sling cystourethropexy performed by 1 surgeon between 1993 and 2002. Patients were followed up for a mean of 4.4 years. In addition, a follow-up survey was conducted using Black and Urogenic Distress Inventory–6 questionnaires in combination with questions on pad use, satisfaction, and leg morbidity.

Findings.—Eighty-five percent of the women said they were dry or improved. Ninety-three percent were pain free at the harvest site at day 7. No harvest site infections nor lower extremity thrombotic complications occurred. Eighty-three percent of patients reported that the procedure had positively affected their life. Only 4% felt it had a negative effect. Seventy-seven percent were satisfied with the procedure, 82% said they would recommend the treatment to a friend with incontinence, and 83% said they would have the procedure again.

Conclusion.—Autologous fascia lata sling cystourethropexy results in high patient satisfaction in women with stress urinary incontinence. The efficacy is comparable to that of other sling cystourethropexy materials, and harvest site morbidity is low. This approach should be considered a primary surgical approach for this patient population.

Abdominal Sacral Colpopexy Using Autologous Fascia Lata

Latini JM, Brown JA, Kreder KJ (Univ of Iowa, Iowa City)

J Urol 171:1176-1179, 2004 8–14

Background.—Many techniques and materials have been used to treat vaginal vault prolapse. The authors reported their experience with autologous fascia lata in abdominal sacral colpopexy.

Methods.—Ten women undergoing abdominal sacral colpopexy with autologous fascia lata for vaginal vault prolapse between 1999 and 2001 were identified for the retrospective analysis. All had at least 18 months of follow-up, with a range of 19 to 42 years. Patients ranged in age from 55 to 82 years.

Findings.—Preoperatively, pelvic organ prolapse quantification stages were II in 3 patients, III in 5, and IV in 2. Postoperatively, the scores were stage II or lower in all 10 patients. Operating time was a mean of 182 minutes, and blood loss was a mean of 107.5 cc. None of the patients had morbidity from fascia lata harvest. All 8 women returning a survey said they would have the procedure again and recommend it to a friend.

Conclusion.—The efficacy of autologous fascia lata is comparable to that reported for other materials in the literature. The use of autologous fascia lata does not result in significant morbidity. In this series, patient satisfaction was high.

▶ These 2 articles (Abstracts 8–13 and 8–14) demonstrate acceptably low morbidity and excellent success with the use of autologous fascia lata as a material for vaginal reconstruction. There are few reports of the use of autologous fascia lata in the literature, although one would expect it to be no different in terms of its efficacy than the more commonly used autologous material of rectus fascia. The use of fascia lata does require a specialized instrument for harvest of the fascia (a Crawford fascial stripper or Masson fascial stripper).

Although the authors speculate in the articles that the morbidity associated with the use of fascia lata is equivalent to, or perhaps even less than, that associated with rectus fascia, a prospective study comparing the 2 materials would be necessary to make a definitive conclusion. It is clear that fascia lata is a suitable material for vaginal reconstruction and incontinence surgeries and represents a reasonable alternative to synthetic materials and rectus fascia as well as allograft and xenograft materials.

E. S. Rovner, MD

Delayed Treatment of Bladder Outlet Obstruction After Sling Surgery: Association With Irreversible Bladder Dysfunction

Leng WW, Davies BJ, Tarin T, et al (Univ of Pittsburgh, Pa)

J Urol 172:1379-1381, 2004 8–15

Purpose.—Our urethrolysis cohort demonstrated an unusual delay time to surgical treatment of bladder outlet obstruction. We determined whether urethrolysis outcomes, ie persistent bladder symptoms, were associated with time between sling and urethrolysis surgeries.

Materials and Methods.—Retrospective analysis of all patients who underwent urethrolysis for post-sling voiding dysfunction between June 1997 and June 2002 was performed. We excluded from study 6 patients with a known history of overactive bladder symptoms, neurogenic bladder dysfunction and use of anticholinergic pharmacotherapy before stress incontinence surgery. The remaining 15 patients were stratified into 2 outcomes groups based upon the absence or presence of post-urethrolysis bladder storage symptoms. Patients (7) in group 1 have no current bladder symptoms. Patients (8) in group 2 still require anticholinergic drug therapy for significant bladder symptoms of frequency and urgency. Data collected for the 2 groups included mean age, existence of urinary retention before urethrolysis, mean time to urethrolysis in months, urethrolysis outcome based upon subjective bladder symptoms and followup duration. For comparison of mean age between groups the standard t test was used. Fisher's exact test was used to compare frequency of urinary retention before urethrolysis between groups. Lastly the Mann-Whitney U test was conducted to compare time to urethrolysis between groups. All statistical analyses were conducted using the SPSS software package (SPSS, Inc., Chicago, Illinois).

Results.—There was no statistically significant difference between the groups with respect to age or frequency of urinary retention before urethrolysis. Time to urethrolysis for the whole cohort ranged from 2 to 66 months. Mean followup after urethrolysis was 17.3 ± 22.9 months. Comparison of mean time between incontinence and urethrolysis surgeries between group 1 (9.0 ± 10.1 months) and group 2 (3125 ± 21.9 months) demonstrated a statistically significant difference (p = 0.01).

Conclusions.—This urethrolysis population demonstrated an unusual delay time to surgical treatment of bladder outlet obstruction. We categorized the cohort according to absence or presence of persistent bladder storage symptoms, and found a strong association between persistent bladder symptoms and greater delay to urethrolysis.

▶ In this very small study of patients with bladder outlet obstruction secondary to prior surgery, these authors have noted that the patients who do not respond to urethrolysis have a relatively longer delay between the initial anti-incontinence surgery and the subsequent urethrolysis. The implication is that some degree of bladder dysfunction occurs secondary to the obstruction caused by the original incontinence surgery. Furthermore, the authors suggest that more aggressive earlier intervention in obstructed patients might reduce the incidence of long-term bladder dysfunction and, therefore, improve the results of urethrolysis. This can probably only be proven in a prospective trial, but the theory is intriguing and, furthermore, suggests that practitioners should be more aware of the possibility of bladder outlet obstruction after anti-incontinence surgery and the importance of addressing this condition promptly when recognized.

E. S. Rovner, MD

Tension Free Vaginal Tape/Transobturator Tape

A Prospective Randomized Trial Comparing Tension-Free Vaginal Tape and Transobturator Suburethral Tape for Surgical Treatment of Stress Urinary Incontinence

deTayrac R, Deffieux X, Droupy S, et al (Kremlin-Bicêtre Hosp, France)
Am J Obstet Gynecol 190:602-608, 2004 8–16

Introduction.—A large number of surgical procedures are available for the treatment of female stress urinary incontinence (SUI); few have been objectively evaluated in prospective trials. Tension-free vaginal tape (TVT) was compared with transobturator suburethral tape (TOT) in the surgical treatment of SUI in women.

Methods.—Sixty-one women with SUI were randomly assigned to treatment with either TVI or TOT. Preoperative assessment included a quality of life questionnaire and a urodynamic examination. One-year outcome evaluation included a pressure-flow urodynamic study for comparison of bladder outlet obstruction in both treatment groups.

Results.—Patient characteristics, preoperative quality of life, and urodynamic assessment were similar for the TVT and TOT groups. The mean surgical time was significantly shorter in the TOT group (15 minutes vs 27 minutes; $P < .001$). The incidence of bladder injury was 0% in the TOT group compared with 9.7% in the TVT group (0 and 3 patients, respectively; $P >$ .05). The incidence of postoperative urinary retention was 25.8% and

13.3% in the TVT and TOT groups, respectively (8 and 4 patients, respectively; $P > .05$). The rates of cure (83.9% vs 90%), improvement (9.7% vs 3.3%), and failure (6.5% vs 6.7%) were similar in the TVT and TOT groups, respectively. The 1-year outcome data were available in 29 women in the TVT group and in 27 in the TOT group. No vaginal erosion or bladder outlet obstruction was observed in either group.

Conclusion.—It appears that TOT is equally efficient as TVT in the surgical treatment of SUI in women, with no between-group differences in bladder outlet obstruction at 1-year follow-up.

▶ This well-done and well-structured study demonstrates essentially no difference in efficacy between TVT and TOT at 1 year. Interestingly, urodynamics done postoperatively also demonstrated no difference between the incidence of obstruction in the 2 groups. There was 1 complication in each group that required a secondary procedure: 1 patient in the TOT group required a transection of the sling for urinary retention, and 1 patient in the TVT group had a urethral erosion requiring partial resection of the sling material. It is hoped that both of these series of patients will be followed in the coming years to determine their long-term relative efficacy and associated safety.

E. S. Rovner, MD

A Randomized Comparison of Tension-Free Vaginal Tape and Endopelvic Fascia Plication in Women With Genital Prolapse and Occult Stress Urinary Incontinence

Meschia M, Pifarotti P, Spennacchio M, et al (Univ of Milan, Italy)

Am J Obstet Gynecol 190:609-613, 2004 8–17

Introduction.—Women with severe genital prolapse may also have stress urinary incontinence (SUI). Usually, they are stress continent primarily because of urethral kinking or compression. A prophylactic anti-incontinence procedure is recommended during prolapse repair to prevent postoperative SUI. No consensus has formed regarding the optimal prophylactic procedure for enhancing postoperative continence rates and reducing morbidity. Two anti-incontinence procedures (tension-free vaginal tape [TVT] and bladder neck endopelvic fascia plication) were compared in women with severe genital prolapse and potential SUI.

Methods.—In addition to vaginal reconstructive surgery, 50 patients with stage II or higher anterior defect and a positive stress test result with prolapse reduction underwent either a TVT or plication of the endopelvic fascia procedure. Patients underwent preoperative history, physical examination, stress test, and urodynamic evaluation.

Results.—Median follow-up was 26 and 24 months in the TVT and fascia plication groups, respectively. The subjective (96% vs 64%; $P = 01$) and objective (92% vs 56%; $P < .01$) continence rates were higher after the TVT compared with the fascia plication procedure. Both groups had similar rates of spontaneous voiding, urinary retention, and de novo urge incontinence.

The anatomic outcome was unsatisfactory for 15 women (30%): 7 in the fascia plication group and 8 in the TVT group.

Conclusion.—Women with severe pelvic organ prolapse and occult SUI can be offered TVT at the time of prolapse repair.

► This is a well-designed and very powerful study demonstrating the lack of durability of the anterior repair or Kelly plication for the treatment of occult SUI compared with the TVT procedure. It is notable that all stress incontinence failures were noted in the first year, implying that if the fascial plication is successful over the first year it may have some properties of durability. Clearly, longer term follow-up is necessary to test this hypothesis. Based on this well done study and analysis, it would be difficult to recommend a simple plication for the treatment of occult SUI today.

E. S. Rovner, MD

Pelvicol™ Pubovaginal Sling Versus Tension-Free Vaginal Tape for Treatment of Urodynamic Stress Incontinence: A Prospective Randomized Three-Year Follow-up Study

Abdel-Fattah M, Barrington JW, Arunkalaivanan AS (Torbay Hosp, Torquay, Devon, England)

Eur Urol 46:629-635, 2004 8–18

Objectives.—The aim of this study was to compare the long-term success rates, complication rates and patient satisfaction rates for Pelvicol™ pubovaginal sling (Bard) versus TVT™ (Gynecare) in surgical treatment of urodynamic stress incontinence (USI) in women.

Design.—Prospective randomized cohort trial.

Setting.—District General Hospital, South West of England.

Methods.—One hundred and forty-two women with urodynamic stress incontinence were randomized to either surgical procedure (Pelvicol™ = 74, TVT™ = 68) with median follow-up of 36 months. A postal questionnaire was sent to all women and the response rate was excellent at approximately 90% in both groups.

Results.—Cure of incontinence, as identified by a quality of life improvement >90%, and/or patient-determined continent status as dry, were comparable in both groups. When the cure rates were adjusted assuming the non-respondents as failures the figures were almost identical ($p > 0.05$). Preoperative continence pad usage was similar for both groups. Overall, a postoperative significant decrease in pad score was noted in both groups ($p = 0.01$) but there was no significant difference between the groups ($p > 0.05$). Statistical analysis failed to detect significant differences between both groups as regards complication rates such as frequency, nocturia, de-novo urgency or dyspareunia.

Conclusion.—Pelvicol™ sling is a safe procedure in the surgical management of USI with similar success rate and patient satisfaction rate to TVT™ up to three years of follow-up.

▶ This is one of the few randomized prospective trials for the surgical treatment of stress urinary incontinence in women. A median follow-up of 36 months suggests that all of the early failures have been identified. It is important to note that this study demonstrates equivalence between polypropylene and biologic material at 3 years. If longer term follow-up and other studies corroborate these findings, then patient choice and surgical familiarity and comfort with any given sling material may be the ultimate determinants in the choice of anti-incontinence surgery material.

E. S. Rovner, MD

Tension-Free Vaginal Tape Procedure for Urinary Incontinence With Low Valsalva Leak Point Pressure

Paick J-S, Ku JH, Shin JW, et al (Seoul Natl Univ, Korea)

J Urol 172:1370-1373, 2004 8–19

Purpose.—We evaluated the outcome of the tension-free vaginal tape (TVT) procedure for stress urinary incontinence with low Valsalva leak point pressure (VLPP) and identified factors predicting the outcome.

Materials and Methods.—A total of 221 women 29 to 80 years old (mean age 55.2) were included in the study. The TVT procedure was performed mostly using local anesthesia. Mean followup was 10.5 months (range 6 to 52). Patients were divided into 61 with low (less than 60 cm H_2O) and 160 with higher (60 cm H_2O or greater) VLPP. Cure of incontinence was defined as an absent subjective complaint of leakage and absent objective leakage on stress testing.

Results.—The overall cure rate was significantly lower in patients with low vs higher VLPP (82.0% vs 93.1%, $p = 0.013$). In women with low VLPP multivariate analysis indicated that urge symptoms and low maximal urethral closure pressure were independent factors for treatment failure (OR 15.12, 95% CI 1.90 to 120.61, $p = 0.010$ and OR 0.92, 95% CI 0.86 to 099, $p = 0.018$, respectively).

Conclusions.—The cure rate after the TVT procedure is lower in women with VLPP less than 60 cm H_2O compared to those with higher VLPP. Our findings suggest that women with urge symptoms and low maximal urethral closure pressure should be considered to be at high risk for failure after the TVT procedure.

Does Valsalva Leak Point Pressure Predict Outcome After the Distal Urethral Polypropylene Sling? Role of Urodynamics in the Sling Era

Rodríguez LV, de Almeida F, Dorey F, et al (Univ of California, Los Angeles; Federal Univ of Sao Paulo, Brazil)

J Urol 172:210-214, 2004 8–20

Purpose.—Recently sling procedures have been shown to be effective in the treatment of all types of incontinence. In this study we evaluated the role of preoperative Valsalva leak point pressure (VLPP) in predicting the outcome of sling surgery.

Materials and Methods.—We prospectively evaluated 174 consecutive patients who underwent a distal polypropylene sling procedure for the treatment of stress urinary incontinence (SUI). Using SEAPI scores patients were divided by VLPP into group 1—60 patients who did not leak on urodynamics, group 2—27 patients with VLPP greater than 80 cm H_2O, group 3—71 patients with VLPP 30 to 80 cm H_2O and group 4—16 patients with VLPP less than 30 cm H_2O. Surgical outcomes were determined by symptom, bother and quality of life questionnaires filled out by patients. The physicians were blinded to patient response.

Results.—Mean followup was 14.7 months (range 12 to 30) and mean patient age was 62 years (range 32 to 88). The groups were well matched before surgery with respect to age, number of previous surgeries, and severity of SUI symptoms and urge incontinence. The percentage of patients who were cured or improved was similar among groups. After surgery there was no statistical difference among patient mean self-reported symptoms of or bother from SUI or urge incontinence.

Conclusions.—The distal urethral polypropylene sling provides similar symptom improvement in all patients regardless of preoperative VLPP. VLPP is helpful in the diagnosis of SUI but appears to be of minimal benefit in predicting the outcome of the distal urethral polypropylene sling procedure.

► Minimally invasive polypropylene slings are here to stay. These 2 large series (Abstracts 8–19 and 8–20) show excellent results independent of Valsalva leak point pressure. Although the study by Paick et al (Abstract 8–19) suggests a lower overall cure rate in patients with a lower Valsalva leak point pressure (< 60 cm H_2O), they still had an excellent cure rate in this group of 82%. These findings bring up an interesting point: Should we be doing Valsalva leak point pressures, or urodynamics, at all in patients considering anti-incontinence surgery? I believe, however, that until there is a better test for diagnosing and evaluating detrusor dysfunction, urodynamics should continue to be done before irreversible surgical treatment of urinary incontinence.

E. S. Rovner, MD

How Important Is TVT Location?

Dietz HP, Mouritsen L, Ellis G, et al (Univ of Otago, Dunedin, New Zealand)

Acta Obstet Gynecol Scand 83:904-908, 2004 8–21

Background.—The tension-free vaginal tape (TVT) is claimed to be a midurethral procedure, but data on sling placement are scarce to date. The aim of this study was to investigate tape position and mobility and correlate this with postoperative symptoms of bladder dysfunction.

Methods.—One hundred and forty-one women 5 weeks to 2.1 years (mean 0.66 years) after TVT placement took part in a prospective clinical observational study. Appointments consisted of standardized symptom questionnaire, clinical stress test flowmetry and translabial ultrasound. The main outcome measures were patient symptoms, subjective satisfaction and cure/improvement. Paired *t*-test and ANOVA statistics were employed for continuous, normally distributed parameters.

Results.—Tape position varied from 30 mm above to 12.7 mm below the symphysis at rest and between 15 mm above to 18.7 mm below the symphysis on Valsalva. The horizontal distance of the tape from the symphysis pubis was weakly associated with recurrent stress incontinence ($p = 0.048$). More cranial tapes were weakly associated with urge incontinence ($p = 0.03$), frequency ($p = 0.048$) and symptoms of voiding dysfunction ($p = 0.029$). There was no association between tape placement and patient satisfaction or subjective cure/improvement.

Conclusions.—Position and mobility of the TVT vary markedly. This may be explained by varying degrees of dissection, localization of incisions and the preoperative degree of anterior vaginal wall prolapse. However, variations in placement seem to have relatively little effect on symptoms.

When the Sling Is too Proximal: A Specific Mechanism of Persistent Stress Incontinence After Pubovaginal Sling Placement

Poon C, Zimmern P (Univ of Texas, Dallas)

Urology 64:287-291, 2004 8–22

Objectives.—To review a series of patients with persistent stress urinary incontinence (SUI) after pubovaginal sling (PVS) placement because of an excessively proximal position of the graft on the bladder neck.

Methods.—Four women, who had previously undergone PVS placement for SUI, presented for evaluation of persistent SUI. All underwent investigations, including history, symptom questionnaire, quality-of-life assessment, physical examination, voiding cystourethrography, and multichannel urodynamic studies. Subsequently, takedown of the primary PVS and placement of an autologous fascial PVS were performed on all patients. A detailed case review of one of the patients is presented.

Results.—All patients had persistent severe SUI confirmed by a positive supine stress test and Valsalva leak point pressure determination. Malposition of the graft was diagnosed preoperatively on the basis of severe distortion of the bladder base and a wide-open bladder neck at rest on the lateral standing voiding cystourethrography images. The diagnosis was confirmed on operative exploration. All patients were continent after takedown of the prior PVS and placement of an autologous fascial sling.

Conclusions.—Persistent SUI after PVS placement may occur secondary to positioning of the graft excessively proximally on the bladder neck. True lateral voiding cystourethrography views are essential for the precise diagnosis. In our experience, optimal management involves takedown of the primary PVS and placement of an autologous fascial PVS.

► Where exactly are we putting polypropylene slings, or fascial slings for that matter, when we are doing transvaginal anti-incontinence surgery? Based on these 2 studies (Abstracts 8–21 and 8–22), it may not be exactly where we think they ought to be. Despite the wide variation in the placement of slings in the report by Dietz et al (Abstract 8–21), there did not appear to be any difference in the overall efficacy of the procedure and outcomes with respect to symptoms. Perhaps the success of anti-incontinence surgery with slings is less a function of exactly where we put the sling on the urethra than operating on the correct patient, adhering to good surgical technique to minimize morbidity, and, finally and perhaps least importantly, placing the sling somewhere along the urethra within a reasonable "zone of safety" (ie, avoiding placement at the level of the trigone, as in the report by Poon and Zimmern, Abstract 8–22).

E. S. Rovner, MD

Tape Related Complications of the Tension-Free Vaginal Tape Procedures

Tsivian A, Kessler O, Mogutin B, et al (Edith Wolfson Med Ctr, Holon, Israel; Tel Aviv Univ, Israel)

J Urol 171:762-764, 2004 8–23

Background.—The tension-free vaginal tape (TVT) procedure for treating stress urinary incontinence in women is rapidly gaining in popularity worldwide. However, few reports about its complications have been published. The diagnosis and treatment of tape-related complications after the TVT procedure were described.

Methods.—Fourteen patients who had had the TVT procedure and had related complications were seen during the past 4 years. Twelve patients underwent additional surgery for TVT-related complications, and 1 is scheduled for such surgery. The remaining patient continues under observation. Patients' records were reviewed.

Findings.—Eight patients had an obstructed urethra after TVT surgery. Five had tape erosion into the vagina, 1 of whom had erosion concomitant with urethral obstruction. Another patient had tape erosion into the bladder. The most common initial symptoms were persistent urethral pain, recurrent infection of the urinary tract, urgency, urge incontinence, and vaginal discharge. Twelve patients needed partial tape removal or tape incision. This was performed transvaginally in 11 women. The remaining patient required cystotomy with excision of the intravesical part of an eroded tape.

None of the women underwent formal urethrolysis. During a mean 4.8-month follow-up after corrective surgery in 12 patients, 10 remained continent and all were symptom free.

Conclusion.—Tape-related complications after a TVT procedure occur in at least 6% of women. Urologists must be alert to the signs and symptoms of such complications to ensure timely and appropriate treatment.

▶ Although many authors have reported complications related to the TVT procedure, most of these have been isolated case reports or tertiary care centers with referred cases. This report describes a total of 14 complications related to the TVT procedure of which the authors relate that 12 came from their own series of approximately 200 women undergoing the TVT procedure. This gives a unique insight into these complications.

The authors allude to a possible learning curve as the cause of some of these complications but do not explore any other possible etiologic or predictive factors. Importantly, the authors note that the vast majority of these complications were evident almost immediately after surgery, although the authors chose to delay evaluation and correction in the majority of these patients.

E. S. Rovner, MD

Surgical Treatment of Female Stress Urinary Incontinence With a Trans-Obturator-Tape (T.O.T.) Uratape: Short Term Results of a Prospective Multicentric Study

Costa P, Grise P, Droupy S, et al (Academic Hosp CAREMEAU, Nîmes, France; Hosp Nicole, Rouen, France; Hosp Bicêtre, Le Kremlin-Bicêtre, France; et al)

Eur Urol 46:102-107, 2004 8–24

Objective.—The aim of the study was to assess the efficacy and safety of a new minimally invasive surgical procedure using the Trans-Obturator-Tape Uratape to treat female stress urinary incontinence.

Patients and Methods.—183 women with stress urinary incontinence (SUI) associated with urethral hypermobility, underwent the T.O.T. procedure (October 2001 to March 2003). 26 patients were previously operated for incontinence. 26 patients were operated at the same time for their genital prolapse. Mean age was 56 years (29–87). 50/183 patients were having mixed incontinence. A non-elastic, polypropylene tape (UraTape, Mentor-Porgès) with a silicon coated central part was placed under the mid-urethra. The surgical placement technique utilises a trans-obturator percutaneous approach. All patients underwent post-operative clinical examination, cough-stress test (full bladder), uroflowmetry, and post-voiding residual assessment.

Results.—Mean follow-up was 7 months (1–21). At 1 year follow-up 80.5% of the patients were completely cured and 7.5% were improved. The overall peri-operative complication rate was 2.2% with no vascular, nerve or bowel injury. 6 patients (3.3%) had post-operative urinary retention.

Conclusion.—The present multicentric study confirms the results obtained by the instigator of the technique, E. Delorme, and allows us to consider T.O.T. as an effective and safe technique for the treatment of female stress urinary incontinence, alone or in combination with prolapse repair.

Bladder Injury During Transobturator Sling

Minaglia S, Özel B, Klutke C, et al (Univ of Southern California, Los Angeles; Washington Univ, St Louis)

Urology 64:376-377, 2004 8–25

Introduction.—One of the proposed advantages of the new, minimally invasive transobturator sling for surgical treatment of female genuine stress urinary incontinence is that it avoids the risk of bladder injuries that commonly occur during retropubic needle passage. This approach is designed to reproduce the natural suspension of the urethral fascia. The 2 anatomic trials and 1 case report to date have revealed that bladder injuries may still occur with this new transobturator approach. Described are 3 cases in which bladder injury occurred with the transobturator sling approach.

Case Report 1.—A 66-year-old woman was seen for bothersome stress urinary incontinence after vaginal hysterectomy and posterior colporrhaphy for symptomatic vaginal prolapse 4 years previously. She had a hypermobile urethra, stable cystometrography findings, and normal voiding. Passage of the Emmett needle during surgery was difficult because of the patient's habitus. The nonwoven polypropylene mesh was inserted. Cystoscopy showed a right anterior lateral bladder perforation. The mesh was removed after the bladder was drained. A second insertion was performed and verified to be without complication by cystoscope; posterior colporrhaphy was performed. She was discharged the following day and a Foley catheter was maintained for 7 days postoperatively. At 6-week follow-up, she had no problems.

Case Report 2.—A 50-year-old woman was seen for bothersome stress urinary incontinence after vaginal hysterectomy and anterior and posterior colporrhaphy for treatment of symptomatic vaginal prolapse 2 years previously. She had a hypermobile urethra, stable cystometrography, and normal voiding. After uneventful insertion of the Emmett needle, cystoscopy showed a right anterior lateral bladder perforation. The bladder was drained and the mesh was removed. A second insertion was performed and verified to be without complication by cystoscopy. She was discharged home the same day. Transurethral bladder drainage by Foley catheter was maintained for 7 days. Postoperative 6-week follow-up was normal.

Case Report 3.—A 66-year-old woman seen for bothersome stress urinary incontinence several years after hysterectomy and 3 months after abdominal sacrocolpopexy 3 months previously. During surgery, passage of the Emmett needle was accompanied by leakage of urine from the vaginal incision. Cystoscopy showed a perforation at the bladder neck. The mesh was removed and a second insertion was performed; it was verified to be without complication by cystoscopy. Transurethral bladder drainage by Foley catheter was performed for 5 days. Recovery was uneventful.

Conclusion.—Routine intraoperative cystoscopy is recommended for the identification of bladder injuries during the transobturator sling procedure.

► Early reports on the use of transobturator slings for treatment of stress urinary incontinence have been excellent. The report by Costa et al (Abstract 8–24) represents a short-term experience with a very large series of patients. Nevertheless, the short-term results are quite good. It is not clear whether this procedure will replace mid-urethral polypropylene slings placed through the retropubic space. Nevertheless, as evidenced by the article by Minaglia et al (Abstract 8–25), the risk of bladder injury still exists even with a transobturator approach. Other complications with the transobturator tape, including tape extrusion and urinary retention, seem to be similar to that reported with other polypropylene mid-urethral slings.

E. S. Rovner, MD

Sling/Pelvic Prolapse

Pelvic Organ Descent in Young Nulligravid Women

Dietz HP, Eldridge A, Grace M, et al (Royal Prince Alfred Hosp, Sydney; Queensland Inst of Med Research, Brisbane, Australia; Royal Women's Hosp, Brisbane, Australia)

Am J Obstet Gynecol 191:95-99, 2004 8–26

Objective.—There is little information available on what constitutes "normal" pelvic organ mobility. This study presents normal values for urethral, bladder, cervical, and rectal descent on Valsalva.

Study Design.—One hundred eighteen nulligravid white women aged 18 to 24 years were recruited for a prospective observational study. Translabial ultrasound was undertaken supine and after voiding, with the most effective of at least 3 Valsalva maneuvers used for evaluation.

Results.—Urethral rotation on Valsalva varied from 0 to +90 degrees (mean 32 degrees), bladder neck descent from 1.2 to 40.2 mm (mean 17.4 mm). The cervix descended to between 59 and 0 mm above the symphysis pubis (mean 30.8 mm); the rectal ampulla descended to between 54 mm above and 22 mm below the symphyseal margin (mean 7.8 mm). In a test-retest series, intraclass correlations were between 0.64 and 0.89, implying good-to-excellent repeatability of the ultrasound assessment.

Conclusion.—A wide range of values was obtained for all parameters. A significant congenital contribution to the phenotype of female pelvic organ prolapse appears likely.

▶ Although some of the patients in this study were symptomatic, all were nulliparous. The range of "normal" is quite wide according to this report and brings into question some strongly held beliefs regarding what is, therefore, abnormal. That is, until we can firmly decide what is "normal," we will continue to have problems defining what is "abnormal."

E. S. Rovner, MD

Osseous Complications After Transvaginal Bone Anchor Fixation in Female Pelvic Reconstructive Surgery: Report From Single Largest Prospective Series and Literature Review

Frederick RW, Carey JM, Leach GE (Tower Urology Inst for Continence, Los Angeles)

Urology 64:669-674, 2004 8–27

Objectives.—To report, from our prospective database and review of published studies (including primary reported patient series and case reports for osseous complications after transvaginal bone anchor fixation in female pelvic reconstructive surgery), our results and those from previously reported patient series to determine the incidence of osteitis pubis and osteomyelitis.

Methods.—A total of 440 patients from our database of cadaveric transvaginal sling (n = 127) and cadaveric prolapse repair with sling (n = 313) procedures had at least 3 months of examination follow-up and were included in this report. We found 15 primary reported patient series involving transvaginal bone anchor fixation in published studies, for a total of 788 patients. The combined patient population of 1228 was assessed for the incidence of osteitis pubis and osteomyelitis.

Results.—Of our 440 patients included in this study, 2 developed osteitis pubis (0.45%), and none had osteomyelitis (0%). In the published studies we reviewed, no case of osteitis pubis and 1 case of osteomyelitis (1 of 788, 0.13%) were reported. One additional case of osteomyelitis with transvaginal bone anchor fixation was reported. The combined incidence of osteitis pubis was 2 (0.16%) of 1228, and the combined incidence of osteomyelitis was 1 (0.08%) of 1228.

Conclusions.—In procedures using transvaginal bone anchor fixation in female pelvic reconstructive surgery, the combined incidence, from our experience and that reported in published studies, of osteitis pubis and osteomyelitis was 2 (0.16%) and 1 (0.08%) of 1228, respectively. The infectious osseous complication rate associated with transvaginal pubic bone anchor fixation appears to be less than that previously reported for suprapubic bone anchor placement. In our experience, when using careful surgical technique and proper prophylactic precautions, infectious osseous complications have not been encountered.

Complications From Transvaginal Pubovaginal Slings Using Bone Anchor Fixation

Fialkow MF, Lentz GM, Miller EA, et al (Univ of Washington, Seattle)

Urology 64:1127-1132, 2004 8–28

Objectives.—To evaluate the history and management of complications from transvaginally placed pubovaginal slings using bone anchor fixation.

Methods.—During a 3-year period, 10 patients were referred to us for complications related to transvaginally placed pubovaginal slings using bone anchor fixation.

Results.—The patient age ranged from 42 to 73 years. All women had a vaginally introduced bone anchor sling for stress urinary incontinence. The presenting symptoms after surgery included fever, pain, and difficulty ambulating in 1; pain and/or vaginal dyspareunia with discharge in 5; pain or dyspareunia alone in 2; and vaginal discharge alone in 2 patients. Two patients ultimately developed bone lesions on radiologic studies consistent with osteomyelitis. Six patients developed sinus drainage tracts associated with granulation tissue from at least one bone anchor that was unresponsive to outpatient management. One of the patients with pain alone had a permanent suture extending into the bladder neck. Nine patients underwent surgery, of whom five had resolution of their presenting complaint. Four of these patients were continent at last follow-up.

Conclusions.—Transvaginally placed pubovaginal slings using bone anchors can be associated with serious complications that may be intractable to common therapies. This knowledge may enable practitioners who use this technique to better counsel their patients regarding these significant complications.

► These 2 articles (Abstracts 8–27 and 8–28) describe 2 vastly different results with transvaginal bone anchor fixation for anti-incontinence surgery. In neither series is the actual denominator of patients operated on actually known, and therefore the actual rates of pubic osteomyelitis is unknown. In the series by Frederick et al (Abstract 8–27), the authors had no episodes of osteomyelitis in their own patient series. This may represent the results of a master surgeon using flawless technique. Can we expect these type of results with the "occasional" practitioner of anti-incontinence surgery using bone anchors? If this is not the case, this represents the crux of the argument against the use of bone anchoring systems in general.

E. S. Rovner, MD

Efficacy and Safety of a Novel System (NASHA/Dx Copolymer Using the Implacer Device) for Treatment of Stress Urinary Incontinence

van Kerrebroeck P, ter Meulen F, Larsson G, et al (Univ Hosp Maastricht, The Netherlands; Västerås Central Hosp, Sweden; Huddinge Univ, Stockholm)

Urology 64:276-281, 2004 8–29

Objectives.—To investigate the efficacy and safety of non-animal-stabilized hyaluronic acid/dextranomer (NASHA/Dx) copolymer for transurethral injection using a new guiding instrument (the Implacer) for stress urinary incontinence.

Methods.—In an open, prospective, multicenter study, 42 invasive therapy-naive female patients with stress urinary incontinence were given 4 × 1.0 mL or 4 × 0.7 mL of NASHA/Dx copolymer using the Implacer. The efficacy parameters, measured at baseline and 1, 3, 6, and 12 months after treatment, included cough-induced leak point pressure, urine leakage by provocation test, number of incontinence episodes in 24 hours, and patient perception of bladder condition, rated on a 6-point scale.

Results.—The collected cough-induced leak point pressure data were not judged to be valid and reliable. Statistically significant reductions in median urine leakage were observed (P <0.0001), from 36 g (range 0.0-300) after 20 "jumping jacks" or vigorous coughs at baseline to 55 g (range 0.0–98) at 3 months and sustained at 12 months (7.0 g, range 0.0–98). Of the 42 patients, 32 (76%) demonstrated a degree of improvement in urine leakage at 3 and 12 months. The median number of incontinence episodes in 24 hours decreased significantly from 1.9 (range 0.0–24) at baseline to 0.4 (range 0.0–24) at 12 months (P <0.0001). At both 3 and 12 months, 29 patients (69%) had improved by at least one category on the 6-point patient perception scale. Treatment was well tolerated, and no complications were reported with use of the Implacer.

Conclusions.—The results of this study indicate that a novel system (NASHA/Dx copolymer insertion using the Implacer) is an effective and well-tolerated treatment for invasive therapy-naive patients with stress urinary incontinence, with improvement sustained for at least 12 months. These encouraging results warrant additional study.

▶ This noncontrolled noncomparative study of this new periurethral injectable agent seems to provide reasonable results at 12 months. This is a novel delivery system that does not require a cystoscope for delivery. A blinded comparative trial with collagen is currently underway in the United States.

E. S. Rovner, MD

A Randomized, Double-blind, Placebo-controlled Comparison of the Effect of Nitrofurantoin Monohydrate Macrocrystals on the Development of Urinary Tract Infections After Surgery for Pelvic Organ Prolapse and/or Stress Urinary Incontinence With Suprapubic Catheterization

Rogers RG, Kammerer-Doak D, Olsen A, et al (Univ of New Mexico, Albuquerque; Univ of Iowa, Iowa City; Obstetric and Gynecological Associates, Houston; et al)

Am J Obstet Gynecol 191:182-187, 2004 8–30

Objective.—The purpose of this study was to determine if antibiotic prophylaxis with nitrofurantoin monohydrate macrocrystals (study drug) after pelvic organ prolapse and/or urinary incontinence surgery with suprapubic catheterization (SPC) decreases urinary tract infection (UTI) compared with placebo in a randomized, double-blind, multicenter trial.

Study Design.—Six centers participated in this study. After a negative preoperative urine culture, history, surgical and postoperative course, urine culture and symptoms at SPC removal, and at 6 to 8 weeks postoperative, any other UTI and adherence were recorded. To demonstrate a 50% decrease in the bacteruria rate from 20%, with 80% power and α of 0.05, 438 patients were required. Data were evaluated with Student t test and Fisher exact test.

Results.—Of 449 patients enrolled, 211 randomized to study drug, and 224 randomized to placebo. No pre- or perioperative differences existed between groups (all $P > .05$). Antibiotic prophylaxis decreased positive urine cultures compared with placebo (46% vs 61%, $P = .002$), symptomatic UTI at SPC removal (7.2% vs 19.8%, $P = .001$), and any other symptomatic UTI 6 to 8 weeks postoperatively (18.9% vs 32.6%, $P = .002$). Antibiotic prophylaxis did not decrease symptomatic UTI at the 6- to 8-week postoperative visit (1.8% vs 5.4%, $P = .10$)

Conclusion.—Antibiotic prophylaxis with nitrofurantoin monohydrate macrocrystals decreases UTI compared with placebo after pelvic organ prolapse and/or urinary incontinence surgery with suprapubic catheterization.

▶ This study clarifies an issue in clinical medicine that heretofore was in dire need of evidence-based recommendations. This trial suggests that patients with indwelling catheters after anti-incontinence or pelvic organ prolapse surgery do benefit from low-dose urinary prophylaxis until removal of the catheter. Morbidity related to the medication was minimal; there was essentially no development of "resistant organisms" with the use of the prophylactic agent compared with that noted with placebo. Finally, there was a definite clinical effect. Whether these results are transferable to other conditions requiring urinary catheter drainage, especially those requiring long-term urinary catheter drainage, is unclear.

E. S. Rovner, MD

Sexual Function

Sexual Function After Surgery for Stress Urinary Incontinence and/or Pelvic Organ Prolapse: A Multicenter Prospective Study

Rogers RG, Kammerer-Doak D, Darrow A, et al (Univ of New Mexico, Albuquerque; Univ of Iowa, Iowa City; Cleveland Clinic Found, Ohio)

Am J Obstet Gynecol 191:206-210, 2004 8–31

Objective.—The purpose of this study was to assess sexual function in women after surgery for stress urinary incontinence and/or pelvic organ prolapse (UI/POP) at 3 and 6 months with the Pelvic Organ Prolapse Urinary Incontinence Sexual Questionnaire (PISQ).

Study Design.—Of 269 eligible women participating in a trial of prophylactic antibiotic use with suprapubic catheters, 102 (37.9%) agreed to participate in a sexual function study. Women underwent a variety of anti-incontinence and reconstructive surgeries. Sexual function and urinary incontinence were assessed preoperatively and at 3 and 6 months postoperatively with the PISQ and Incontinence Impact Questionnaires (IIQ-7). Paired t tests compared changes over time. Logistic regression compared worsening PISQ vs other variables. Generalized McNemar's test compared individual questions pre- and postoperatively. Significance was set at $P < .05$.

Results.—Mean age was 47.1 (23 to 85) years, and 64% of women were premenopausal. Seventy-five (74%) women completed questionnaires at 3 or 6 months. Sexual function scores declined after surgery despite improvement in IIQ-7 scores (PISQ = 86 vs 78, $P < .001$; IIQ-7 = 52 vs 13, $P < .001$). Behavioral Emotive domain scores worsened at 3 to 6 months compared with preoperative scores, while the Physical domain improved (all $P < .001$). Worsening PISQ scores were independent of age, type of surgery, hysterectomy, complications, or hormonal status (logistic regression, all $P < .05$).

Conclusion.—Sexual function scores in women after surgery for UI/POP do not improve despite improvement of incontinence at 3 to 6 months after surgery.

Sexual Function in Women Before and After Suburethral Sling Operation for Stress Urinary Incontinence: A Retrospective Questionnaire Study

Glavind K, Tetsche MS (Aalborg Sygehus, Denmark)

Acta Obstet Gynecol Scand 83:965-968, 2004 8–32

Background.—The aim of this questionnaire study dealing with women with stress urinary incontinence was to find out what influence incontinence and operation for incontinence in the form of tension-free vaginal tape (TVT) or intravaginal slingplasty operation (IVS) had on the patient's sexuality and if there were any adverse effects on sexuality after the operation.

Methods.—Eighty-four patients were operated on from April 1998 to September 2002. A questionnaire was sent to all patients with questions concerning their sexuality before and after the operation.

Results.—Sixty-seven patients (81%) answered the questionnaire. Before the operation 53 patients (79%) were sexually active and 26 patients (49%) experienced incontinence during intercourse. Only one patient (0.01%) stated the incontinence as the reason for not being sexually active. No patients developed de novo incontinence during intercourse after the operation. Half of the patients who were cured of their incontinence during intercourse experienced a better sexual life. Five patients (7%) cited reduced libido after the operation and two patients (3%) felt the operation to be the cause.

Conclusion.—Among sexually active women with stress urinary incontinence referred for suburethral sling operation 49% experienced incontinence during intercourse and half of the cured patients in this group experienced a better sexual life after the operation. Incontinence affects sexual life to a great extent. Two patients (4%) experienced less libido after the operation and found the operation to be the cause of this. The risk of deterioration of sexual life after the operation is very small. Further investigation into this subject is needed.

► These 2 studies came to the opposite conclusions. How can this be? Perhaps it has something to do with sexual attitudes on either side of the Atlantic Ocean, or perhaps it is related to the fact that sexual function in the female is multifactorial and, to a large degree, difficult to measure accurately. Furthermore, both studies have methodologic flaws in that the patients in both had a variety of different operations for a variety of different indications and, because these were questionnaire-based studies, there was not an optimal participation and response rate. Sexual function in the female is a very complex and multifactorial process. It is likely that urinary incontinence affects patients' sexual functioning in an extremely variable fashion. Furthermore, the amount and type of urinary incontinence, as well as the wide range of sexual habits, may have also accounted for the disparate findings in these 2 studies. Nevertheless, it is clear that urinary incontinence can have an effect on sexual function in women and, furthermore, the surgical treatment of this condition may not invariably affect sexual functioning in a positive way. Preoperative counseling in this regard may be helpful in tempering patient expectations in these cases.

E. S. Rovner, MD

9 Urinary Tract Infection

Antibody Responses and Protection From Pyelonephritis Following Vaccination With Purified Escherichia Coli PapDG Protein

Roberts HA, Kaack MB, Baskin G, et al (Tulane Univ, New Orleans, La; Washington Univ, St Louis)

J Urol 171:1682-1685, 2004 9–1

Purpose.—A critical early step in the establishment of Escherichia coli pyelonephritis is bacterial attachment via the tip protein of P fimbriae. This adhesin, PapG, binds to glycolipid receptors present on vaginal and kidney epithelial surfaces. In this study, we investigated the efficacy of vaccination with purified PapDG protein complex in preventing pyelonephritis caused by *E. coli.*

Materials and Methods.—Mature cynomolgus monkeys were intraperitoneally vaccinated with 100 μg purified PapDG protein. Following 3 identical boosters serum antibody titers to PapDG were measured by enzyme-linked immunosorbent assay. Vaccinated and unvaccinated animals were urethrally inoculated with 1 × 10 cfu of *E. coli* strain DS17, which was isolated from a child with acute pyelonephritis. The infection course was monitored by catheterized urine cultures, and by histological examination of the kidneys, bladder and kidney tissue culture 28 days after infection.

Results.—Intraperitoneal administration of purified PapDG vaccine resulted in the development of specific antibody responses in cynomolgus monkeys. In contrast to control monkeys, vaccinated monkeys did not show histological evidence of pyelonephritis after subsequent urethral challenge with pyelonephritogenic *E. coli* expressing P fimbriae.

Conclusions.—Purified PapDG is a tractable vaccine candidate that in our small study demonstrated the ability to elicit adequate serum antibody levels to prevent *E. coli*-mediated pyelonephritis.

► The authors vaccinated primates to block bacterial adhesion to urothelial P-fimbriae receptors. This adhesion is required for the development of pyelonephritis in this primate model. Vaccinated monkeys did not develop histologic evidence of pyelonephritis. The vaccination did not decrease the incidence of bacteruria. This is a promising new modality and may have significant clinical utility, as antimicrobial resistance becomes an increasingly significant concern.

D. E. Coplen, MD

10 Sexually Transmitted Disease

Prevalence of Chlamydial and Gonococcal Infections Among Young Adults in the United States

Miller WC, Ford CA, Morris M, et al (Univ of North Carolina, Chapel Hill; Univ of Washington, Seattle)

JAMA 291:2229-2236, 2004 10–1

Context.—Chlamydial and gonococcal infections are important causes of pelvic inflammatory disease, ectopic pregnancy, and infertility. Although screening for *Chlamydia trachomatis* is widely recommended among young adult women, little information is available regarding the prevalence of chlamydial and gonococcal infections in the general young adult population.

Objective.—To determine the prevalence of chlamydial and gonococcal infections in a nationally representative sample of young adults living in the United States.

Design, Setting, and Participants.—Cross-sectional analyses of a prospective cohort study of a nationally representative sample of 14,322 young adults aged 18 to 26 years. In-home interviews were conducted across the United States for Wave III of The National Longitudinal Study of Adolescent Health (Add Health) from April 2, 2001, to May 9, 2002. This study sample represented 66.3% of the original 18,924 participants in Wave I of Add Health. First-void urine specimens using ligase chain reaction assay were available for 12,548 (87.6%) of the Wave III participants.

Main Outcome Measures.—Prevalences of chlamydial and gonococcal infections in the general young adult population, and by age, self-reported race/ethnicity, and geographic region of current residence.

Results.—Overall prevalence of chlamydial infection was 4.19% (95% confidence interval [CI], 3.48%-4.90%). Women (4.74%; 95% CI, 3.93%-5.71%) were more likely to be infected than men (3.67%; 95% CI, 2.93%-4.58%; prevalence ratio, 1.29; 95% CI, 1.03-1.63). The prevalence of chlamydial infection was highest among black women (13.95%; 95% CI, 11.25%-17.18%) and black men (11.12%; 95% CI, 8.51%-14.42%); lowest prevalences were among Asian men (1.14%; 95% CI, 0.40%-3.21%), white men (1.38%; 95% CI, 0.93%-203%), and white women (2.52%; 95% CI, 1.90%-3.34%). Prevalence of chlamydial infection was highest in the south (5.39%; 95% CI, 4.24%-6.83%) and lowest in the northeast (2.39%; 95% CI, 1.56%-3.65%). Overall prevalence of gonorrhea was 0.43% (95% CI, 0.29%-0.63%). Among black men and women, the prevalence was 2.13% (95% CI, 1.46%-3.10%) and among white young adults, 0.10% (95% CI, 0.03%-0.27%). Prevalence of coinfection with both chlamydial and gonococcal infections was 0.030% (95% CI, 0.18%-0.49%).

Conclusions.—The prevalence of chlamydial infection is high among young adults in the United States. Substantial racial/ethnic disparities are present in the prevalence of both chlamydial and gonococcal infections.

▶ This study evaluates the prevalence of these sexually transmitted diseases in young adults in the United States. These data were prospectively obtained in a population followed from adolescence into adulthood. The incidence of untreated chlamydial infection (4%) is high in both men and women, suggesting that both populations should be screened to decrease the potential morbidity of pelvic inflammatory disease, infertility, and chronic pelvic pain. The incidence of gonorrhea is lower (0.43%), but there is a very large racial disparity in the incidence of both STDs. The increased incidence in blacks correlates with the increased incidence of ectopic pregnancy in this population. Current screening protocols exclude males, but this population is the larger reservoir for infection of the general population.

D. E. Coplen, MD

11 Benign Prostatic Hyperplasia

Epidemiology

Longitudinal Changes in Lower Urinary Tract Symptoms Among a Cohort of Black American Men: The Flint Men's Health Study

Sarma AV, McLaughlin JC, Jacobsen SJ, et al (Univ of Michigan Health System, Ann Arbor; Mayo Clinic, Rochester, Minn; GlaxoSmithKline Research and Development, Greenford, England)

Urology 64:959-965, 2004 11–1

Objectives.—To examine the progression of lower urinary tract symptoms in a longitudinal population-based cohort of black men. Population-based studies of prostatism and longitudinal data regarding changes in lower urinary tract symptom severity have largely focused on white men, with little attention directed toward black men.

Methods.—In 1996, a probability sample of 369 black men, aged 40 to 79 years, residing in Genesee County, Michigan, and without a prior history of prostate cancer/surgery participated in a prostate cancer screening protocol that included completing the American Urological Association Symptom Index (AUASI). Four years after baseline, 175 of the 369 men agreed to participate in the follow-up protocol. Of the 175 men, 149 had not reported undergoing treatment for benign prostatic hyperplasia and had complete symptom data. These men were included in this study. Differences between baseline and follow-up AUASI scores were examined.

Results.—The mean and standard deviation AUASI scores at baseline and follow-up were 7.1 (6.4) and 7.0 (6.8), respectively. Although overall no statistically significant change was found in the mean AUASI during the 4 years of follow-up (−0.11; SD 6.2; $P = 0.7$), the average change in the symptom score and the variability in the change increased with patient age at baseline from a mean of −0.42 (SD 5.0) among men in their 40s to 2.1 (SD 6.6) among men in their 70s. Of the 91 men (61.1%) who reported mild to no symptoms (AUASI score 7 or less) at baseline, 24 (26.4%) reported moderate to severe symptoms (AUASI score 8 or more) at follow-up. This progression of symptom severity was observed across all ages.

Conclusions.—In this population-based study of longitudinal changes in urinary symptoms in black men, we found a substantial percentage of men demonstrated a measurable progression in urinary symptom severity over time. Additional studies are needed to examine critically any racial differences in lower urinary tract symptom progression.

▶ Despite the ever-growing body of literature regarding cross-sectional and longitudinal incidence and prevalence rates of lower urinary tract symptoms in men, there is a paucity of data from ethnic minorities in the United States. The Flint Men's Health Study attempts to address this issue under the leadership of Drs Wei and Sarma from the University of Michigan. In 1996, a sample of 369 black men aged 40 to 79 years participated in prostate cancer screening and were followed up 4 years later. One hundred and seventy-five of the 369 men agreed to participate in the follow-up protocol, of which the majority had not undergone treatment for benign prostatic hyperplasia since that time. The authors demonstrated that a significant percentage of men demonstrated a measurable progression of urinary symptoms and severity over time. The average change in the symptom score and the variability of the change increased with patient age to baseline from a mean of −0.42 among men in their 40s to a mean of 2.1 among men in their 70s. A total of 26.4% of the men who reported mild or no symptoms at baseline reported moderate to severe symptoms at follow-up.

It is important to continually follow up cohorts of this nature to understand the subtle differences between ethnic groups in terms of likelihood of stabilization or progression of lower urinary tract symptoms.

C. G. Roehrborn, MD

Longitudinal Study of Men With Mild Symptoms of Bladder Outlet Obstruction Treated With Watchful Waiting for Four Years

Djavan B, Fong YK, Harik M, et al (Univ of Vienna; LKH Bregenz, Austria; Royal Free Hosp, London; et al)

Urology 64:1144-1148, 2004 11–2

Objectives.—To determine the risk of clinical progressions in men with mild lower urinary tract symptoms of bladder outlet obstruction and identify the predictors for progression in this group of men.

Methods.—A total of 397 men who presented to the urology clinics with mild symptoms of bladder outlet obstruction (International Prostate Symptom Score less than 8) were analyzed in this longitudinal study conducted during a 4-year period. They began with the watchful waiting protocol and were followed up every 3 months for 48 months. Age, International Prostate Symptom Score (IPSS), divided into obstructive symptom score and irritative symptom score, serum prostate-specific antigen level, total prostate volume, transitional zone volume, urinary flow rates, and postvoid residual urine volume were documented.

Results.—The cumulative incidence of clinical progression, defined as worsening of the IPSS with migration to the moderate symptom group (IPSS 8 to 18) or severe symptom group (IPSS 19 to 35) and an increase in IPSS of more than 2 points, was 6%, 13%, 15%, 24%, 28%, and 31% at 6, 12, 18, 24, 36, and 48 months, respectively. Nineteen patients (4.9%) developed acute urinary retention within the 48-month follow-up period. Of these 19 patients, only 2 (0.6%) required transurethral resection of the prostate. The variables of importance for disease progression in the artificial neural network analysis were, in order of statistical significance, prostate-specific antigen level, obstructive symptom score, and transitional zone volume.

Conclusions.—The risk for men with mild symptoms of bladder outlet obstruction to progress clinically and develop complications such as acute retention of urine is moderate. Prostate-specific antigen, obstructive symptom score, and transitional zone volume were identified as important risk factors.

► The group from Vienna followed a cohort of 397 men presenting with mild lower urinary tract symptoms for a 4-year period. These men were offered a watchful waiting or surveillance protocol and followed up every 3 months for 48 months. They observed a cumulative incidence of clinical progression defined as worsening of the IPSS with migration to the moderate or severe symptom group, and an increase in IPSS score of more than 2 points in 6%, 13%, 15%, 24%, 28%, and 31% of men at 6, 12, 18, 24, 36, and 48 months, respectively. A total of 4.9% of the men developed acute urinary retention within 4 years, however, only 2 required transurethral resection. The authors drew the conclusion that the risks for men to progress to moderate or severe symptoms is quite high over time; however, the risk of episodes of urinary retention remains low. The authors furthermore observed that serum prostate-specific antigen and the transition zone of the prostate were important parameters to predict symptomatic worsening. For example, baseline prostate-specific antigen was 2.2 in those men who experienced progression versus 0.83 for those who did not experience progression, and the transition zone volume was highly significantly greater at 16.4 versus 8.9% cm^2 (P = .001). Observation of such nature enhances our knowledge about parameters that can be used when counseling men regarding watchful waiting versus active intervention and complements the knowledge we have gained from placebo-controlled groups in large medical trials such as PLESS and MTOPS.

C. G. Roehrborn, MD

Is Questionnaire Enough to Assess Number of Nocturic Episodes?: Prospective Comparative Study Between Data From Questionnaire and Frequency-Volume Charts

Ku JH, Hong SK, Kim HH, et al (Seoul Natl Univ, Republic of Korea)

Urology 64:966-969, 2004 11–3

Objectives.—To determine whether the voiding symptom questionnaire provides information regarding nocturia as accurate as that provided by frequency-volume (FV) charts, we evaluated patients with lower urinary tract symptoms.

Methods.—We prospectively analyzed 164 patients (62 men and 102 women, mean age 53.6 years, range 20 to 83) referred for the evaluation of lower urinary tract symptoms. At the initial visit, all patients answered the International Prostate Symptom Score (IPSS) questionnaire to quantify nocturia and subsequently were requested to complete a 3-day FV chart.

Results.—The differences in age between the men and women were not statistically significant. The total IPSS and IPSS bother scores were similar between the sexes. For all patients, the actual number of nightly voids in the FV charts and the IPSS nocturia score were modestly intercorrelated (r = 0.609, P <0.001). However, large individual differences were found in the nighttime diuresis rate (67.7%) between the IPSSs and FV charts. No statistically significant differences were found between men and women, but agreement was achieved in only 39.2% of patients younger than 60 years old and 22.4% of those 60 years old or older for the number of voids per night recorded by the FV charts and reported by the IPSS (P = 0.024). Overestimation of the number of nocturic episodes in the IPSS was more common than underestimation, especially in patients 60 years old or older (P = 0.014).

Conclusions.—The findings of the present study revealed poor agreement between the subjectively estimated nocturnal frequency and chart-determined nocturnal frequency. Our results suggest that FV charts should be included as an integral part of evaluating nocturia in both sexes.

▶ While the use of the IPSS or the AUA Symptom Score is extremely prevalent among urologists and even primary care providers, concerns have been raised regarding the validity of the answers and their relationship to the actual presence of these symptoms. Nowhere is this more true than regarding the number of nocturnal urination episodes or nocturia. The IPSS score simply asks how often a patient has gotten up to urinate from the time he went to bed until the next morning. Several attempts have been made in the past to relate the answers given by patients to the data obtained from FV charts or other more quantitative assessment tools. A group of investigators from Korea prospectively studied 164 patients with lower urinary tract symptoms and gave them FV charts over 3 days as well as the IPSS. They documented that agreement was achieved in only roughly 40% of patients younger than 60 years, and only 22% of those 60 years old for the number of voiding episodes per night between the FV chart and the IPSS score. The study raises considerable doubt regarding the validity of the answers given on the IPSS score, particularly regarding the number of nocturnal voiding episodes. This might appear to be a minor issue; however, the IPSS score is utilized for baseline assessment and also to document progression of the disease, worsening of symptoms, and response to treatment. Since nocturia is one of the leading irritative symptoms in men with benign prostatic hyperplasia, one would desire to have as valid as possible information regarding the actual number of nocturnal voiding episodes.

Therefore it seems that for physicians concerned about these particular symptoms or the validity of the symptom assessment in general, the use of the FV chart might be a better way to obtain a more correct assessment.

C. G. Roehrborn, MD

Diagnostics

The 24-h Frequency-Volume Chart in Adults Reporting No Voiding Complaints: Defining Reference Values and Analysing Variables

van Haarst EP, Heldeweg EA, Newling DW, et al (Sint Lucas Andreas Hosp, Amsterdam; Onze Lieve Vrouwe Gasthuis, Amsterdam; Vrije Universiteit, Amsterdam)

BJU Int 93:1257-1261, 2004 11–4

Objective.—To determine the variables (e.g. voiding frequency, voided volumes, urine production) and their mutual relationships and differences between age groups and genders, using a frequency-volume chart (FVC) in an adult population (representing all age groups) who denied having any voiding complaints.

Subjects and Methods.—In all, 1152 men and women aged >20 years completed a 24-h FVC; registration started with the first voided volume in the morning and concluded with the first voided volume the next morning. The time of voiding and volume were both recorded, and bedtime hours noted. Each participant claimed to have no voiding complaints. The statistical analysis was aimed at discerning the relationships between the FVC variables, gender and age.

Results.—There was a linear increase in mean 24-h voiding frequency and nocturia in men, from 6.0 and 0.5 in the third decade to 8.5 and 1.6 in those aged >70 years (Table 1). Contrary to men, in women the mean 24-h frequency declined slightly in the older decades; it increased from 6.9 in the third to 8.2 in the sixth, declining to 7.8 in those aged >70 years. Nocturia in women increased linearly, although slower than in men, from 0.7 in the third decade to 1.4 in those aged >70 years. The mean volume/void decreased significantly in both genders, from 313 to 209 mL in men, and from 274 to 240 mL in women. The mean 24-h volume was 1718 and 1762 mL in men and women, respectively. For both genders there was a strong linear association between 24-h urine production and voided volumes.

Conclusion.—The volume/void and maximum voided volume decreased significantly with age in both sexes, but more prominently in men. As a result, in men the frequency increased with age, probably reflecting subclinical

TABLE 1.—Characteristics of Frequencies and Volumes per Age Decade and Gender

Age Decade	Sex	N	Mean (SD) Frequency			Mean (SD) Volume/Void, mL				
			24-h	Day	Night	24-h*	Day*	Night*	Nocturnal	Maximum
20-29	M	85	6.01 (2.00)	5.53 (1.88)	0.48 (0.63)	1690 (747)	297 (92)	390 (161)	469 (258)	491 (152)
	F	102	6.92 (2.54)	6.20 (2.31)	0.73 (0.82)	1677 (860)	258 (101)	361 (176)	473 (231)	479 (186)
30-39	M	114	6.46 (2.31)	5.80 (1.97)	0.66 (0.77)	1707 (720)	298 (142)	380 (178)	472 (239)	510 (201)
	F	127	7.14 (2.11)	6.38 (1.83)	0.76 (0.84)	1739 (767)	257 (110)	335 (172)	473 (286)	475 (172)
40-49	M	128	6.63 (2.33)	5.95 (2.10)	0.67 (0.81)	1765 (839)	280 (112)	387 (170)	514 (268)	503 (184)
	F	119	7.65 (2.29)	6.75 (2.06)	0.84 (0.86)	1711 (711)	243 (90)	349 (158)	510 (260)	475 (169)
50-59	M	83	7.81 (2.99)	6.83 (2.65)	0.98 (0.91)	1794 (758)	258 (112)	339 (142)	539 (327)	465 (196)
	F	98	8.20 (2.66)	6.97 (2.31)	1.23 (0.96)	1853 (805)	241 (108)	356 (191)	582 (314)	470 (183)
60-69	M	67	8.03 (2.67)	6.70 (2.01)	1.33 (1.17)	1738 (745)	227 (95)	323 (134)	602 (309)	414 (156)
	F	81	8.12 (2.29)	6.86 (2.12)	1.26 (1.00)	1852 (780)	226 (92)	355 (169)	620 (359)	445 (181)
≥70	M	83	8.55 (2.44)	6.90 (1.95)	1.65 (1.37)	1602 (604)	189 (69)	276 (107)	579 (315)	349 (131)
	F	65	7.78 (2.26)	6.43 (1.85)	1.35 (1.04)	1655 (566)	216 (89)	324 (145)	612 (270)	439 (170)

*Volume/void over the indicated period.

(Courtesy of Van Haarst EP, Heldeweg EA, Newling DW, et al: The 24-h frequency-volume chart in adults reporting no voiding complaints: Defining reference values and analysing variables. *BJU Intl* 93:1257-1261, 2004. Reprinted by permission of Blackwell Publishing.)

changes associated with the development of prostatic enlargement. In contrast to men the frequency in women increased initially and decreased in the older groups. A higher 24-h urine production was associated with a higher mean volume/void.

► These investigators gave 1152 men and women older than 20 years a 24-hour urine frequency-volume chart and used the data obtained to establish normative parameters and reference values. Table 1 shows the characteristics of frequency in volumes per decade of age and gender from men and women in their 20s to those older than 70 years. It is quite apparent that the mean frequency increases, particularly at night, from 0.48 to 1.65 in men and from 0.73 to 1.35 in women, while the mean voided volume over a 24-hour period does not seem to change perceptibly. Of interest, the nocturnal voided urine seems to increase in both men and women; hence, the increased episodes of nocturia. These normative tables might be useful for physicians engaged in the counseling of patients with lower urinary tract symptoms and suspected benign prostatic hyperplasia as well as women with voiding dysfunction.

C. G. Roehrborn, MD

Noninvasive Assessment of Bladder Contractility in Men

McIntosh SL, Drinnan MJ, Griffiths CJ, et al (Univ of Newcastle upon Tyne, England)

J Urol 172:1394-1398, 2004 11–5

Purpose.—Preoperative assessment of detrusor function by pressure flow study (PFS) improves outcome from prostatectomy but is invasive and uncomfortable for the patient. We report on a large scale validation of a novel noninvasive assessment of detrusor contractility.

Materials and Methods.—A flexible cuff placed around the penis was inflated automatically during voiding until flow interruption. Cuff pressure at interruption ($p_{cuff.int}$) reflects isovolumetric bladder pressure ($p_{ves.isv}$), a measure of detrusor contractility. For comparison 151 symptomatic men performed the cuff test with simultaneous PFS monitoring. Test/retest agreement was assessed in 91 subjects who performed a cuff test without PFS on 2 occasions.

Results.—For the 117 (77%) subjects with an acceptable cuff pressure flow trace, Bland Altman analysis showed that $p_{cuff.int}$ overestimated $p_{ves.isv}$ by a mean (s.d.) of 16.4 (27.5) cm H_2O, predominantly due to the cuff being positioned below the bladder. For test/retest analysis 52 (57%) of the men who were able to attend twice provided acceptable cuff data on both occasions with a mean (s.d.) difference in $p_{cuff.int}$ of −3.3 (32.0) cm H_2O, improving to 0.0 (20.3) cm H_2O in a subgroup of 39 subjects who voided more than 150 ml. On questionnaire assessment 121 (80%) subjects preferred the cuff test to PFS.

Conclusions.—The cuff test gives a valid and reproducible estimate of isovolumetric bladder pressure in a manner acceptable to patients, although test failure and variability of agreement require improvement. The test may be of value in the assessment of urinary symptoms and may aid in patient selection for prostatectomy.

An Automated Penile Compression Release Maneuver as a Noninvasive Test for Diagnosis of Bladder Outlet Obstruction

Harding CK, Robson W, Drinnan MJ, et al (Univ of Newcastle, Newcastle upon Tyne, England)

J Urol 172:2312-2315, 2004 11–6

Purpose.—We tested the hypothesis that the previously described penile urethral compression release (PCR) maneuver provides a valid diagnosis of bladder outlet obstruction (BOO) using automated rather than manual penile compression by controlled inflation of a penile cuff. We also investigated urodynamic events underlying generation of the PCR index.

Materials and Methods.—A total of 150 subjects attending for pressure flow studies were studied using conventional and noninvasive cystometry. Patients were classified into urodynamic diagnostic groups using standard invasive studies. The PCR index was calculated for each individual from noninvasive penile cuff data and the results were summarized for each group. ROC analysis of the PCR index was performed to define an optimum threshold for BOO diagnosis. Simultaneous invasive and noninvasive data were used to define the relationship between the PCR index, bladder contractility and the maximum flow rate.

Results.—The mean PCR index ± SD was significantly higher in the BOO group compared to the normal cystometry group (215% ± 84% vs 93% ± 39, p <0.01). ROC analysis showed that a PCR index of greater than 160% diagnosed BOO with 78% sensitivity, 84% specificity and a positive predictive value of 69%. There was a strong positive correlation between the PCR index and isovolumetric detrusor pressure, which is a measure of bladder contractility (r = 0.44, p <0.01).

Conclusions.—The results of this study suggest that the PCR index combines valid estimates of bladder contractility and the maximum flow rate, and it represents a clinically useful, noninvasive urodynamic parameter for the diagnosis of BOO.

► It is widely accepted that invasive urodynamic studies are the only way to reliably determine whether a man with lower urinary tract symptoms and clinical benign prostatic hyperplasia is obstructed at the level of the bladder neck or prostate. Urodynamic experts claim that the outcomes of surgery are superior in those men with obstruction compared to those who do not have obstruction. This argument justifies the performance of invasive urodynamic testing before prostatectomy or other surgical procedures according to international guidelines. However, the invasive nature of the PFS has been a major hindrance to its widespread acceptance in practice in addition to the considerable variability among investigators, technicians, and even within 1 patient from day to day.

The group from Newcastle upon Tyne has recently published 2 articles (Abstracts 11–5 and 11–6) in *The Journal of Urology* describing a new noninvasive assessment of bladder contractility in men. This consists of a flexible cuff placed around the penis, which is inflated automatically during voiding until flow interruption. The cuff pressure interruption reflects the isovolumetric bladder pressure, which is a measure of detrusor contractility. In both studies, a cohort of about 150 patients is described who underwent invasive urodynamic testing as well as testing with the noninvasive PCR method. It turns out that the mean PCR index was significantly higher in the obstructed versus the nonobstructed group, with an area under the curve of greater than 160% to diagnose BOO with the sensitivity of 78% and a specificity of 84%.

This reviewer wonders whether urodynamic experts in general would accept a sensitivity of 78% with a specificity of 84% and the inherent false-negative rate of 16%. This would imply that when testing men as to whether they are obstructed, in 22% of truly obstructed men the tests would be negative, that is, these patients might not be referred for a prostatectomy based on the outcome of the tests, while indeed they are obstructed and they would likely benefit from such intervention. Second, this reviewer wonders whether the tests would be easily transferable from a single site to other investigative sites and, ultimately, to acceptance and widespread practice. Nonetheless, any effort to obtain the results of invasive urodynamic studies by noninvasive means would certainly be a welcome addition to our diagnostic armamentarium.

C. G. Roehrborn, MD

Correlation Between Detrusor Collagen Content and Urinary Symptoms in Patients With Prostatic Obstruction

Mirone V, Imbimbo C, Sessa G, et al (Univ "Federico II," Naples, Italy; G Moscati Hosp, Avellino, Italy)

J Urol 172:1386-1389, 2004 11–7

Purpose.—We used computerized imaging analysis to compare the collagen content of detrusor specimens between patients affected with symptomatic obstructive benign prostatic hyperplasia (BPH) and asymptomatic controls.

Materials and Methods.—In our study we enrolled 36 patients with symptomatic urodynamically obstructed BPH undergoing transurethral resection of the prostate. We also enrolled 28 men (mean age 61.3, range 55 to 70) undergoing transurethral resection of the bladder for primitive, singular Ta bladder cancer, with no significant urinary symptoms, as the control group. During the transurethral surgical procedure in controls and in patients with BPH, a biopsy was performed deep through the muscular layer from either of the lateral bladder walls. Computerized morphometric analysis of the stained sections was performed with an image analysis system, and a percentage of collagen fibers was extracted through morphological filtering and expressed as a mean percentage of the total bioptic area.

Results.—Collagen content in bladder detrusor specimens was significantly higher in patients with BPH compared to controls (48% and 17% of bioptic area, respectively, $p < 0.001$). Mean detrusor collagen content was clearly higher in patients with severe symptoms than in patients with moderate symptoms (50.45 ± 8.22% and 43.09% ± 7.05%, respectively).

Conclusions.—Our study supports the important role of detrusor collagen neo-deposition in determining lower urinary tract symptoms in obstructive BPH. Detrusor collagen content correlates with urodynamic obstruction, the presence and severity of symptoms and, given that collagen neoformation is irreversible could probably have a role in the postoperative persistence of lower urinary tract symptoms in patients undergoing surgery for BPH.

▶ It has been understood for many years that the lower urinary tract symptoms in the aging men are not necessarily exclusively caused by the growth and enlargement of the prostate with subsequent obstruction at the level of the bladder neck. Rather, significant changes take place in the aging bladder, among them deposition of collagen leading to a less-efficient behavior of the detrusor muscle. These investigators enrolled 36 patients with urodynamically proven obstruction, all of whom underwent a transurethral resection of the prostate. A biopsy was performed through the muscular layer from either one or both of the lateral bladder walls. The authors show that the total collagen content in bladder detrusor specimens was significantly higher in patients with BPH compared with a control group of patients who underwent a transurethral resection of a bladder tumor without evidence of lower urinary tract symptoms or BPH. This relatively simple, yet convincing, study supports the important role of collagen deposition in the detrusor muscle in the development of lower urinary tract symptoms in men with obstructive BPH. The collagen content of the detrusor indeed correlates with the urodynamic obstruction and the presence and severity of the symptoms, and may very well have a role in the postoperative persistence of symptoms in those men who do not respond to surgical therapy.

A logical question from this study would be whether biopsies of the bladder wall are warranted in men before subjecting them to transurethral resection of the prostate if indeed it is suspected that the detrusor may already have shown significant alteration. In such cases, transurethral resection of the prostate often is unsuccessful in relieving most of the irritative, and occasionally the obstructive, symptoms. The unfortunate flip side of this observation is, however, that no alternative therapies exist for these unfortunate men and thus many of them will choose to undergo transurethral resection of the prostate even if the odds of having significant improvement are less than optimal.

C. G. Roehrborn, MD

Association of Prostatic Inflammation With Down-Regulation of Macrophage Inhibitory Cytokine-1 Gene in Symptomatic Benign Prostatic Hyperplasia

Taoka R, Tsukuda F, Ishikawa M, et al (Kagawa Univ, Kita-gun, Japan)

J Urol 171:2330-2335, 2004 11–8

Purpose.—Our previous DNA microarray analyses revealed that the macrophage inhibitory cytokine-1 (MIC-1) gene was significantly down-regulated in symptomatic benign prostatic hyperplasia (BPH) samples. We compared the histopathological features of inflammatory changes in prostate adenoma tissues from individuals with symptomatic and asymptomatic (histological only) BPH using MIC-1 mRNA levels.

Materials and Methods.—Prostate adenoma tissues were obtained from 25 patients who underwent transurethral prostatectomy to relieve lower urinary tract symptoms due to BPH and 6 patients with bladder cancer who underwent cystoprostatectomy due to bladder cancer. Inflammatory changes in the prostate were examined histopathologically and immunohistochemically, and classified according to the consensus classification system of the Chronic Prostatitis Collaborative Research Network and International Prostatitis Collaborative Network advocated in 2001 with some modification. MIC-1 mRNA was assessed quantitatively by real-time reverse transcriptase-polymerase chain reaction.

Results.—MIC-1 gene down-regulation was observed in 16 of 25 symptomatic BPH samples (64.0%), whereas MIC-1 mRNA was high in 6 of 6 prostate adenoma samples from patients with bladder cancer ($p = 0.0006$). MIC-1 gene down-regulation correlated with the grade of glandular/periglandular inflammatory changes with statistical significance ($p = 0.0387$). MIC-1 gene down-regulation was found in only 1 of 7 BPH samples with a glandular predominant pattern, whereas it was found in 15 of 24 BPH samples with a mixed type or stromal predominant pattern ($p = 0.0373$).

Conclusions.—Gland destruction by inflammatory infiltrates, followed by replacement of the stromal component in symptomatic BPH may be induced by the down-regulation of the MIC-1 gene.

▶ The exact pathophysiology of BPH is very complex and still poorly understood. It has always been stated that BPH consists of a proliferation of stromal and epithelial components, with the ratio of stromal to epithelial cells varying from gland to gland and between populations. A common observation in BPH tissue specimens are chronic inflammatory infiltrates. The authors investigate the role and pathophysiology of these inflammatory infiltrates by studying adenomatous tissue from 25 patients undergoing transurethral prostatectomy for BPH, and from patients who underwent cystoprostatectomy for bladder cancer, the latter prostates serving as controls. They focused their attention on the MIC-1 gene and identified it as downregulated in BPH in a previous communication.[1] In this article, they observed that in 16 of 25 symptomatic BPH samples, the MIC-1 gene was downregulated, while its mRNA was high in all prostatic adenoma samples from patients with bladder cancer. The downregulation was correlated with the grade of glandular/periglandular inflammatory changes and was found in only 1 of 7 samples determined with the glandular pattern but in 15 of 24 samples with a stromal predominant pattern.

This article is of considerable interest and is a continuation of the work performed by the senior author with Dr Getzenberg at the University of Pittsburgh and published in *Prostate* in 2004. Recent data from MTOPS suggests that inflammatory infiltrates do indeed play a major role not only in the pathophysiology, but also in the natural history of BPH. The future will show whether these observations warrant diagnostic assessments inclusive of tissue sampling in men suffering from lower urinary tract symptoms, as the finding of inflammatory infiltrates may have therapeutic implications.

C. G. Roehrborn, MD

References

1. Kakehi Y, Segawa T, Wu XX, et al: Down-regulation of macrophage inhibitory cytokine-1/prostate derived factor in benign prostatic hyperplasia. *Prostate* 59:351, 2004.

Quantitative Morphometric Analysis of Individual Resected Prostatic Tissue Specimens, Using Immunohistochemical Staining and Colour-Image Analysis

Phipps S, Habib FK, McNeill A (Univ Dept of Oncology; Western Gen Hosp, Edinburgh, Scotland)

BJU Int 94:919-921, 2004 11–9

Objective.—To develop a method for obtaining morphometric measurements representative of individual chips from transurethral resection of the prostate (TURP).

Materials and Methods.—In all, 232 sections were cut in pairs from 25 TURP chips, collected from four patients undergoing TURP for benign prostatic hyperplasia. Individual tissue chips were processed, embedded in paraffin wax and pairs of neighbouring sections cut from the specimens at intervals of 300 μm throughout the thickness of the specimen. Of each pair, the epithelial tissue (ET) of one and the smooth muscle (SM) of the other section were stained immunohistochemically with anti-prostate-specific antigen and anti-SM myosin, respectively. Proportions of ET and SM within the sections were measured with colour-image analysis and calculated within the TURP chips using all pairs of sections cut from the specimen, and the first pair of sections only. The differences between the sets of results were analysed using descriptive statistics.

Results.—From each TURP chip, 3–7 pairs of sections were cut; for both ET and SM within each chip the differences between the results calculated using data from all pairs of sections and the first pair alone were small, as were the distributions of these differences within each prostate.

Conclusions.—Morphometric measurements from one section from a processed TURP chip, as opposed to serial sections, can be used to reliably assess the morphology of tissue within that specimen. This permits a considerable saving of resources when undertaking morphometric image analysis of resected prostatic tissue specimens.

► A fundamental question in tissue-based research in benign prostatic hyperplasia (BPH) has always been what amount of tissue is needed to obtain reliable information regarding the tissue composition of the entire gland. Multiple authors have analyzed stromal to epithelial ratios based on one or multiple core biopsies. Given the heterogeneity of prostate tissue, it has always seemed unlikely that a single core or even several cores would truly be representative of the tissue composition of the entire prostate. These authors examined 232 sections in pairs from 25 TURP chips, which they collected from 4 patients undergoing TURP for BPH. They demonstrated that morphometric measurement from 1 section from a prostate TURP chip could be used to reliably assess the morphology of tissue within that specimen.

This reviewer is somewhat critical of the sweeping conclusions from the observations made inasmuch as the tissue was collected from only 4 patients, and we do not know whether these 4 patients represented the entire spectrum of possible observations and, thus, are representative for a larger cohort of BPH patients. Nonetheless, any and all efforts to determine what type of tissue and what amount of ET is needed for analysis to be representative for the entirety of the gland is useful in a multitude of translational research efforts in BPH. Tissue bank collections such as baseline biopsies from the MTOPS study are useful only if and when it can be demonstrated that the samples obtained are indeed representative for the entire gland.

C. G. Roehrborn, MD

Molecular Profiling of Benign Prostatic Hyperplasia Using a Large Scale Real-Time Reverse Transcriptase-Polymerase Chain Reaction Approach

Fromont G, Chene L, Latil A, et al (Université Paris 7; Université Paris 5; Hôpital Tenon, Paris)

J Urol 172:1382-1385, 2004 11–10

Purpose.—Benign prostatic hyperplasia (BPH) is characterized by a hyperplastic growth of epithelial and stromal cells in the prostate. Despite the high prevalence of the disease little is known regarding the molecular etiology of BPH. Therefore, a comparison of gene expression patterns between normal prostate, BPH and prostate cancer could provide insights into the pathogenic mechanisms of the disease and identify candidate genes that could be targeted for therapeutic use.

Materials and Methods.—Prostate tissue specimen were obtained from 30 patients undergoing adenomectomy for BPH. Adenoma weight was less than 60 gm in 15 patients and more than 60 gm in the remainder. Normal prostate tissue was obtained from 15 patients undergoing radical prostatectomy for cancer from areas selected for absent tumor and BPH. Two pools of organ confined prostate cancer were also analyzed. We quantified in the 5 pools of tissues the expression of 327 genes using real-time quantitative reverse transcriptase-polymerase chain reaction.

Results.—A total of 23 genes showed increased expression in BPH with a fold change of at least 2.5 between normal prostate and the 2 BPH groups, of which most were normal or down-regulated in prostate cancer. Seven genes showed decreased expression in BPH with a fold change of at least 3.5 between normal prostate and BPH. Most of them were also normal or down-regulated in prostate cancer.

Conclusions.—We identified a set of genes up-regulated in BPH compared to normal prostate tissue and often prostate cancer, including genes previously implicated in BPH and others not previously linked to this disease to our knowledge. Further investigations are now warranted to determine the clinical relevance and therapeutic potential of these genes.

▶ Molecular profiling has become a fashionable word in basic and molecular research in a variety of disease processes. It should surprise no one that molecular profiling of BPH is of as much interest as it is in other disease processes. In this study, prostate tissue specimens from 30 patients who underwent an adenomectomy for BPH were compared with normal tissues from 15 patients undergoing radical prostatectomy for cancer. The authors carefully selected those areas that did not show a tumor or BPH. The expression of a total of 327 genes was analyzed by using real-time quantitative reverse transcriptase polymerase chain reaction (RT-PCR). A total of 23 genes showed increased expression in BPH, and 7 genes decreased in expression in BPH according to the criteria set forth by the investigators before initiating the study. Among the genes that are overexpressed are insulin-like growth factors, fibroblast growth factors, and other genes that in the past have been reported as being involved in the pathophysiology of BPH. Similarly, some of the underexpressed genes had previously been reported. Of note, most of the upregulated genes identified in BPH showed higher expression in prostates larger than 60 g compared with those less than 60 g. This supports the hypothesis that overexpressed genes could be directly associated with increased prostate volume, that is, the actual event leading to the term BPH. A majority of the genes overexpressed in BPH compared with normal tissue were also normal or underexpressed in cancer, which points to the fundamental difference between benign and malignant overgrowth.

While this reviewer believes that perhaps the use of cystoprostatectomy specimens and prostates that do not contain any element of cancer would have been a better control, the findings are certainly of interest and, perhaps, allow the development of future therapeutic targets in the disease process itself. Some of the genes may lend themselves to develop targeted medical interventions, which would increase our therapeutic armamentarium for patients with lower urinary tract symptoms and BPH.

C. G. Roehrborn, MD

Serenoa Repens Treatment Modifies BAX/BCL-2 Index Expression and Caspase-3 Activity in Prostatic Tissue From Patients With Benign Prostatic Hyperplasia

Vela-Navarrete R, Escribano-Burgos M, Farré AL, et al (Autonomous Univ of Madrid; Univ Madrid)

J Urol 173:507-510, 2005 11–11

Purpose.—Permixon is a lipidosterolic extract of Serenoa repens (SR) widely used to treat men with benign prostatic hyperplasia (BPH). We tested the effect of this drug on molecular mechanisms associated with apoptosis, such as the Bax-to-Bcl-2 expression ratio and caspase-3 activity, in prostatic tissue from men with symptomatic BPH treated for 3 months before surgery.

Materials and Methods.—An open, multicenter pilot study of 2 parallel groups of patients with BPH was done. They were randomized to be followed for 3 weeks without any treatment before surgery (control group) or to receive 160 mg SR orally twice daily for a 3-month period preceding the same surgery. Surgery was ultimately performed in 17 controls and 12 patients by transurethral prostate resection or retropubic adenomectomy. Bax and Bcl-2 expression, and caspase-3 activity were determined by Western blot in 15 controls and 10 patients, and reported in blinded fashion.

Results.—The Bax-to-Bcl-2 ratio, which is used as an apoptotic index, was significantly increased in the prostatic tissue of treated patients The level of the intact 116 kDa poly (adenosine diphosphate-ribose) polymerase form, an enzyme involved in the cell death apoptotic pathway, was also found to be decreased in prostatic tissue from SR treated patients, suggesting increased caspase 3 activity in the prostate.

Conclusions.—Permixon increased molecular markers involved in the apoptotic process, ie the Bax-to-Bcl-2 expression ratio and caspase-3 activity. This could have clinical relevance due to the improvement in symptoms produced by treatment with this drug.

▶ The debate of whether phytotherapeutic agents are of any benefit in patients with lower urinary tract symptoms and BPH has been ongoing for years. Our understanding of the exact mechanisms by which these phytotherapeutic agents might work is very limited. *Serenoa repens* is one of the most widely used phytotherapeutic agents for the treatment of lower urinary tract symptoms and BPH, and Permixon is one of the most widely used brand names representing a lipidosterolic extract of *Serenoa repens*. In this study, the effect of this agent on molecular mechanisms associated with apoptosis was examined by using the Bax-to-Bcl-2 expression ratio and, as a second measure, the activity of caspase-3 in prostate tissue from men with symptomatic BPH treated for 3 months before undergoing surgery. This report involved an open, multicenter study of 2 parallel groups of patients treated with either 160 mg *Serenoa repens* extract twice daily for a 3-month period or having no treatment before surgery. The authors demonstrated that molecular markers involved in the process of apoptosis were significantly increased, that is, the Bax-to-Bcl-2 expression ratio and the caspase-3 activity.

In the past, *Serenoa repens* has been speculated to act as a 5_{α}-reductase inhibitor, α-receptor blocker, and an anti-inflammatory agent or through a variety of poorly defined mechanisms. This study adds another possible mechanism of action to this list, namely an effect on apoptosis.

Apoptotic activity has been shown in the past for the quinazoline derivative doxazosin and other α-receptor blockers in laboratory experiments as well as in human beings. Nonetheless, long-term studies demonstrated that the prostate growth rates are similar when comparing doxazosin with placebo-treated patients over a period of 4 to 5 years in the MTOPS study. It leads one to wonder whether the apoptotic effect seen on a molecular level indeed may have a significant impact on symptoms, flow rate, or progression of the disease.

C. G. Roehrborn, MD

Medical Treatment

Alfuzosin Once Daily Facilitates Return to Voiding in Patients in Acute Urinary Retention

McNeill SA, for the Alfaur Study Group (Western Gen Hosp, Edinburgh, Scotland; et al)

J Urol 171:2316-2320, 2004 11–12

Purpose.—We confirmed the beneficial effect of the α1-blocker alfuzosin for the acute management of acute urinary retention (AUR) related to benign prostate hyperplasia (BPH), and further identified factors influencing the success of a trial without catheter (TWOC).

Materials and Methods.—A total of 360 patients presenting with a first episode of spontaneous AUR related to BPH underwent emergency catheterization and were then randomly and blindly assigned to receive 10 mg alfuzosin once daily or placebo at a ratio of 2:1 for 3 days. The primary efficacy criterion of this large study was the rate of successful TWOC within 24 hours after catheter removal. The influence of factors such as age, urine retention volume, fluid consumption, constipation and urinary tract infection on TWOC outcome was also assessed.

Results.—Successful TWOC was recorded in 61.9% of the 236 patients treated with alfuzosin vs 47.9% of the 121 receiving placebo ($p = 0.012$). Elderly patients (65 years or older) and patients with a drained volume of 1000 ml or greater had significantly greater chances of TWOC failure (success vs failure OR 0.309, 95% CI 1.182 to 0.514 and OR 0.361, 95% CI 0.225 to 0.571, respectively). Nevertheless, even in the presence of these 2 factors 10 mg alfuzosin once daily almost doubled the likelihood of successful TWOC (OR 1.98, 95% CI 1,226 to 3,217). Alfuzosin (10 mg) once daily was well tolerated.

Conclusions.—Alfuzosin (10 mg) once daily significantly improved the rate of successful TWOC in patients with AUR related to BPH, even in elderly patients and those with a large drained volume who were at increased risk for TWOC failure. This should contribute to decrease the morbidity and mortality associated with emergency surgery and avoid the discomfort and potential morbidity associated with an in situ catheter.

► Several smaller studies have demonstrated in the past that the use of α-receptor blocking agents in the setting of AUR increases the success rate of TWOC. This is particularly true in those episodes of urinary retention that are precipitated by unrelated surgery, intake of cold medications, and so forth. This rather large study of 360 patients presenting with a first episode of spontaneous AUR related to BPH demonstrates that the use of alfuzosin 10 mg once daily results in an improved success rate of TWOC in 61.9% compared with 47.9% in those receiving placebo. Of note, patients with a drain volume of greater than 1000 mL or patients older than 65 years had a significantly lesser chance of succeeding in TWOC.

This is the largest study thus far to examine the role of α-blockers in the setting of AUR and strongly suggests that clinicians engaged in the care of such patients should give a 2- to 3-day course of an α-blocker before attempting TWOC.

C. G. Roehrborn, MD

Intermittent Tamsulosin Therapy in Men With Lower Urinary Tract Symptoms

Yanardag H, Goktas S, Kibar Y, et al (Gulhane Military Med Acad, Ankara, Turkey)

J Urol 173:155-157, 2005 11–13

Purpose.—We investigated in what is to our knowledge the first prospective study the safety and efficacy of intermittent tamsulosin therapy in patients with lower urinary tract symptoms.

Materials and Methods.—This study was performed between January 2001 and February 2003 in 140 patients. In phase 1 of this study patients received 1, 0.4 mg tamsulosin capsule daily for 3 months and were reevaluated after 3 months. At this assessment uroflowmetry, International Prostate Symptom Score and ultrasonographic estimation of residual urine were determined. In phase 2 responders to tamsulosin therapy were then randomized into 1 of 3 groups, namely group 1—continued 4 mg tamsulosin once daily every day, group 2—0.4 mg tamsulosin once daily every other day and group 3—discontinued tamsulosin. Efficacy assessments were done again at 4, 12 and 24 weeks.

Results.—There were no statistically differences among the patients in groups 1 and 2 at 6 months for International Prostate Symptom Score, maximum or average urine flow, or residual urine. Differences between patients in groups 1 and 3 were statistically significant at 6 months. Differences between patients in groups 2 and 3 were also statistically significant at 6 months for these parameters.

Conclusions.—Tamsulosin at a dose of 0.4 mg once daily and 0.4 mg once daily every other day for lower urinary tract symptoms provide comparable improvements in urinary flow and symptoms. Each treatment was well tolerated.

▶ Given the waxing and waning of lower urinary tract symptoms, and the costs associated with the medical therapy for lower urinary tract symptoms and benign prostatic hyperplasia, it is only understandable that particularly in countries with limited resources, the concept of intermittent use of such medication resonates with the prescribing doctor. A group of investigators from Turkey studied this concept in a prospective manner by giving 140 patients 0.4 mg tamsulosin daily for 3 months, then randomized them into 3 groups: a group with continued tamsulosin daily, a group with tamsulosin every other day, and a third group in which tamsulosin was discontinued. Efficacy assessment was continued for another 24 weeks. The authors found no statistically significant difference among the patients in groups 1 and 2 at 6 months; however, there were significant differences at 6 months between groups 1 and 3 and groups 2 and 3, indicating that those who discontinued tamsulosin altogether had worse outcomes. The authors suggest that tamsulosin every other day provided comparable improvements and lower urinary tract symptoms compared with taking it every day.

This reviewer urges caution. First, the pharmacokinetic data relating to every other day use of tamsulosin 0.4 mg are not studied and, second, if the alternating intake of tamsulosin is not controlled by a placebo tablet, it might not be fair to compare the 3 regimens altogether. For example, the patients taking at least 1 tablet every other day have a much stronger placebo response than those patients in whom no tablet, either active or placebo, is given. To perform this study properly, patients would have to be given a placebo on alternating days or a placebo every day, not just be discontinued. Nonetheless, it is understandable that in countries where health care resources are limited efforts such as these are made, but it seems comparatively easy to perform studies in such a setting in a proper manner.

C. G. Roehrborn, MD

5-Alpha Reductase Inhibition Provides Superior Benefits to Alpha Blockade by Preventing AUR and BPH-Related Surgery

Boyle P, Roehrborn C, Harkaway R, et al (European Inst of Oncology, Milan, Italy; Univ of Texas, Dallas; Albert Einstein School Med Ctr, Philadelphia; et al)
Eur Urol 45:620-627, 2004 11–14

Objectives.—This analysis examines the relative effectiveness of current medical therapies for BPH in preventing AUR, AUR-related catheterisation and surgery in real-life clinical practice.

Methods.—This is a retrospective analysis of observational data from the General Practice Research Database (UK) (GPRD). The cohort contains 4500 patients experiencing BPH or lower urinary tract symptoms strongly suggestive of BPH, aged over 50 years, who were prescribed a 5ARI (finasteride) or an alpha-blocker (alfuzosin, doxazosin, indoramin, prazosin, tamsulosin, terazosin) as their first BPH treatment between 1996 and 1999 inclusive. Cox regression and competing risks analyses, adjusted for age and year of first treatment, followed patients from the start of their first BPH treatment to AUR, catheterisation or surgery, or censoring.

Results.—Patients prescribed an alpha-blocker were significantly more likely to experience AUR (hazard ratio 2.32, 95%CI 1.37, 3.94) or surgery (hazard ratio 1.78, 95%CI 1.30, 2.44) than patients prescribed a 5ARI. These differences were sustained with sensitivity analyses.

Conclusion.—Real-life clinical practice shows that significantly fewer BPH patients prescribed a 5ARI experienced serious complications associated with the progression of BPH compared with those prescribed an alpha-blocker.

► Studies such as PLESS and MTOPS have demonstrated that 5-α reductase inhibitors are capable of reducing the incidence rates of AUR and BPH-related surgery. In this retrospective analysis of observational data from the General Practice Research Database from the United Kingdom, a cohort of 4500 patients with BPH and lower urinary tract symptoms aged 50 years and older was analyzed. These patients were either prescribed finasteride as a 5ARI or an α-blocker (alfuzosin, doxazosin, prazosin, tamsulosin, or indoramin). It turns out the patients prescribed an α-blocker were significantly more likely to experience AUR, with a hazard ratio of 2.32, or surgery, with a hazard ratio of 1.78, compared with patients prescribed a 5ARI.

It is heartening to see that real-life clinical practice corroborates the findings from controlled clinical trials in that fewer BPH patients treated with a 5ARI experienced serious complications such as AUR and surgery compared with those taking an α-blocker. This study does not address the question regarding risk factors of AUR and progression or whether the cost-effectiveness might be even better in certain subgroups of patients.

C. G. Roehrborn, MD

Efficacy and Safety of Long-term Treatment With the Dual 5α-Reductase Inhibitor Dutasteride in Men With Symptomatic Benign Prostatic Hyperplasia

Debruyne F, Barkin J, van Erps P, et al (Univ Hosp Nijmegen, The Netherlands; Univ of Toronto; Middelheim Hosp, Antwerp, Belgium; et al)

Eur Urol 46:488-495, 2004 11–15

Objectives.—Dutasteride, a dual inhibitor of Type 1 and Type 2 5α-reductase, has been shown to improve disease measures in patients with symptomatic benign prostatic hyperplasia (BPH) in three randomised, placebo-controlled, large-scale, 2-year Phase III clinical studies. This paper reports the pooled results of a 2-year open-label extension of the three randomised studies assessing the long-term efficacy and safety of dutasteride.

Methods.—Patients randomised to dutasteride or placebo in the double-blind portion of the Phase III studies were eligible for a 2-year open-label extension, where all patients received dutasteride 0.5 mg daily (dutasteride/dutasteride [D/D] group and placebo/dutasteride [P/D group]).

Results.—Significant improvements in AUA-SI score and Q_{max} were observed from Month 24 to 48 in both study groups. At Month 48, patients in the D/D group had significantly greater improvements in AUA-SI score and Q_{max}, and significantly greater reductions in prostate volume, than those in the P/D group. Acute urinary retention and BPH-related surgery occurred in a small percentage of patients during the open-label phase. No new safety issues were noted with long-term therapy. Onset of new drug-related adverse events were reported most frequently at the start of therapy and declined over time in patients receiving dutasteride.

Conclusions.—Long-term treatment with dutasteride results in continuing improvements in urinary symptoms and flow rate, and further reductions in TPV, in men with symptomatic BPH. The reduction in risk of AUR and BPH-related surgery, seen in the double-blind phase, was durable over 4-year treatment. Dutasteride was also well tolerated in long-term use.

► Use of the 5α-reductase class of medications for treatment of symptomatic BPH has become well established. The introduction of dutasteride potentially allowed for even greater efficacy because of dual receptor inhibition. This study demonstrates a remarkable continued improvement in flow rates and symptom scores in men participating in the open-label extension trial. While there are biases introduced in such open-label studies, these findings do suggest that men who continued to take dutasteride obtained sustainable and greater symptomatic benefit. In fact, the curves plotting the average AUA-SI over time suggests that symptom relief in the latter 42 months of treatment was equal to the first 6 months of treatment with an average drop of 3 AUA-SI points. This calls into question the typical practice of discontinuing 5α-reductase inhibitors after only 3 to 6 months if patients do not show a response. In reality, it may take much longer and, given the relatively benign adverse effects profile of this medication class, the primary considerations clinically would be cost to the patient and cost to society.

J. T. Wei, MD, MSc

► The two 5-α reductase inhibitors, finasteride and dutasteride, are relatively comparable in terms of their clinical efficacy as well as safety. Finasteride has been tested in 2 long-term studies, namely the 4-year PLESS trial and the 5-year MTOPS trial. The phase III development program for dutasteride consisted of 3 randomized, placebo-controlled 2-year studies followed by an open-label 2-year extension study. This paper describes the findings from baseline to month 48, ie, patients who were either treated with dutasteride for 4 years or who had dutasteride therapy following an initial treatment with placebo. Perhaps, the most striking finding is that the D/D group experienced an improvement of 4.4 points at the end of the randomized placebo-controlled phase of the trial and an improvement of 6.5 points at the end of the open label trial, ie, this group of patients had an ongoing and sustained improvement in symptoms (as well as in urinary flow rate) when continuing on the open label dutasteride that exceeded the improvement seen in the placebo-dutasteride switch patients.

One can speculate what may lead to this increased improvement in symptoms and flow rate after the end of the randomized placebo-controlled phase of the trial. It is possible that this represents a responder bias, which is, however, unlikely as the group of patients at the end of the 2-year study period who elected to either continue or not continue in the open label extension study had very similar characteristics. It is also possible that the patients chosen for the dutasteride phase III trial program, namely men with particularly large prostates and higher PSA values, had a larger reservoir of potential improvement compared to patients in other clinical trials. Without a head-to-head comparison and without having comparable patients treated with finasteride and dutasteride, one will not be able to ultimately answer the question however intriguing these data might be.

C. G. Roehrborn, MD

Comparison of Doxazosin With or Without Tolterodine in Men With Symptomatic Bladder Outlet Obstruction and an Overactive Bladder

Lee JY, Kim HW, Lee SJ, et al (Catholic Univ of Korea, Seoul; Univ of Pittsburgh, Pa)

BJU Int 94:817-820, 2004 11–16

Objective.—To assess the efficacy of combined treatment with doxazosin and tolterodine, as although α-blockers are commonly used and generally effective in men with symptomatic bladder outlet obstruction (BOO), a subset of men with BOO and overactive bladder (OAB) symptoms often complain of persistent symptoms.

Patients and Methods.—In a prospective study of 144 consecutive men with BOO at one tertiary urology centre, all had a baseline pressure-flow urodynamic study and were then subdivided into those with BOO or BOO + OAB, based on absence or presence of involuntary detrusor contractions. The Abrams-Griffiths nomogram was used to determine obstructive BOO. After the initial evaluation, all patients were treated with doxazosin 4 mg/day for 3 months. In patients with no symptomatic improvement, tolterodine 2 mg twice daily was added for an additional 3 months.

Results.—Of the 144 patients, 76 (53%) were diagnosed as having BOO and 68 (47%) BOO + OAB. The patients with BOO + OAB were older ($P <$ 0.05) and had a higher International Prostate Symptom Score. After 3 months of treatment with doxazosin, 60 (79%) with BOO and 24 (35%) BOO + OAB reported a symptomatic improvement. In those patients with no improvement, six of 16 with BOO and 32 of 44 (73%) with BOO + OAB improved after adding tolterodine. Acute urinary retention developed in only two of 60 men (3.3%) treated with the combined therapy.

Conclusion.—About half of men with symptomatic BOO had an OAB; while about three-quarters of men with symptomatic BOO and no OAB improved with doxazosin, only a third with BOO + OAB were helped with doxazosin alone Combining tolterodine with doxazosin was effective in three-quarters of men with BOO + OAB. Overall, most men with BOO with or with no OAB were helped with doxazosin alone or with the addition of tolterodine.

▶ It was only recently that the new paradigm of medical therapy for lower urinary tract symptoms and benign prostatic hyperplasia was accepted as a combination of 5-α reductase inhibitors with α-receptor blocking agents based on the strength of the MTOPS study. Now, a new type of combination therapy is becoming more and more popular, namely the combination of an α-receptor blocker with anticholinergic agents to treat men with symptomatic benign prostatic hyperplasia, lower urinary tract symptoms, and particularly those with OAB or very prevalent irritative symptoms. In this prospective study, 144 men with BOO were divided into those with BOO or BOO + OAB based on the absence or presence of involuntary detrusor contractions noted on invasive urodynamic studies. The patients were given doxazosin 4 mg daily for 3 months, and in those patients with no symptomatic improvement, tolterodine 2 mg twice daily was added for an additional 3 months. As it turned out, 53% of the patients had BOO and 47 had associated OAB. In general, those patients were older and had a higher symptom score. Seventy-nine percent of the BOO patients and 35% of the BOO + OAB patients reported improvement. Of those without improvement, but BOO + OAB, 73% improved after adding tolterodine. Fortunately, acute urinary retention developed in only 2 of the 60 men treated with combined therapy.

This and other studies of a similar nature suggest that it may very well be safe when properly monitored to add an anticholinergic agent in a patient already treated with an α-receptor blocker for benign prostatic hyperplasia in case the therapeutic benefit is not what was hoped for. This is particularly true for patients who suffer concomitantly from OAB symptoms or a high prevalence of irritative symptoms. It is anticipated that additional studies will be done to verify this hypothesis and, most likely, in the future when talking about combination medical therapy for benign prostatic hyperplasia, we may not only refer to 5-α reductase inhibitors together with α-receptor blocking agents to treat symptoms and prevent progression, but also a combination of anticholinergic or antimuscolenic agents together with α-receptor blockers to treat BOO in men who also suffer from OAB.

C. G. Roehrborn, MD

Surgical Treatment

Transurethral Ethanol Injection Therapy for Prostatic Hyperplasia: 3-Year Results

Goya N, Ishikawa N, Ito F, et al (Tokyo Women's Med Univ)
J Urol 172:1017-1020, 2004 11–17

Purpose.—We assessed the medium-term (3-year) efficacy of transurethral ethanol injection therapy of the prostate (EIP) for benign prostatic hyperplasia.

Materials and Methods.—A total of 34 patients were followed for a median of 4.3 years after EIP. Mean age was 68.1 years and mean baseline prostate volume was 49.3 ml. With the patient under combined sacral and urethral anesthesia, dehydrated ethanol was injected into the prostate with endoscopic guidance. A urethral catheter was inserted postoperatively.

Results.—Mean total ethanol dose was 6.4 ml and a catheter was required for a mean of 7.6 days postoperatively. Mean International Prostate Symptom Score was 21.8 points before EIP (in 34 patients), and decreased to 13.1 points after 3 years (in 17, $p < 0.01$). Mean quality of life index decreased from 5.0 points before EIP to 2.8 points after 3 years ($p < 0.001$). Mean peak urine flow rate was 8.3 ml per second before EIP and increased to 12.7 ml per second after 3 years ($p < 0.01$). Mean residual urine volume decreased from 93 ml before EIP to 28 ml after 3 years ($p < 0.01$). Mean prostate volume decreased from 49.3 ml before EIP to 45.7 ml after 1 year ($p < 0.001$), but increased to 51.4 ml after 3 years. No major complications were experienced. By 3 years after surgery 59.0% of patients had not required further treatment.

Conclusions.—Transurethral EIP caused minimal complications while maintaining improvement of the prostate symptom score and an increased peak urine flow after 3 years.

▶ Among the minimally invasive interventions becoming somewhat popular in the late 1990s was the injection of ethanol into the prostate, which resulted in a demonstrable coagulative necrosis in animal experiments as well as in human beings. This study from Japan examines the outcome on 34 patients who were followed for up to 4.3 years after ethanol injection. The patients required postoperative catheterization for about 1 week and experienced a decrease in their symptom score from 22 points to 13 points after 3 years. The prostate volume decreased from about 50 mL to 45 mL after 1 year, but then grew back to 51 mL after 3 years. The authors suggest that the complication rate was minimal and that the symptom score improvement was maintained up to 3 years.

American Medical Systems in the United States had embarked on a dose-finding study using ethanol injection into the prostate. At present, however, these developments are on hold. There have been reports of a few significant complications that were observed in controlled clinical trial settings in the United Kingdom. In one such patient, the coagulation involved the bladder, leading to a significant morbidity. It remains to be seen whether the injection of absolute alcohol, either in its aqueous form or in a gel form, is a viable minimally invasive treatment option for men with benign prostatic hyperplasia.

C. G. Roehrborn, MD

Evaluation of the Transurethral Ethanol Ablation of the Prostate (TEAP) for Symptomatic Benign Prostatic Hyperplasia (BPH): A European Multi-Center Evaluation

Grise P, Plante M, Palmer J, et al (Höpital Charles Nicolle, Rouen, France; Univ of Vermont, Burlington; Medway Maritime Hosp, Gillingham, Kent, England; et al)

Eur Urol 46:496-502, 2004 11–18

Introduction.—Benign prostatic hyperplasia (BPH) causes a number of lower urinary tract symptoms (LUTS) that affect quality of life. Minimally invasive therapies such as laser ablation were developed to reduce the complication rates associated with invasive therapies such as transurethral resection of the prostate (TURP). A longitudinal, multicenter European study examined the safety and efficacy of a transurethral ethanol injection system used to ablate prostatic tissue in men with BPH.

Methods.—The prospective study used the ProstaJect device to treat LUTS. Eligible patients were older than 50 years, had experienced symptoms for at least 6 months, and had a normal prostate-specific antigen level. Treatment dosages were based on prostate volume, prostatic urethral length, and median lobe involvement. Patients were evaluated 4 to 7 days after the procedure and at follow-up periods of 1, 3, 6, and 12 months.

Results.—The transurethral ethanol ablation of the prostate (TEAP) procedure was performed in 115 men; 46 received general anesthesia and 69 had conscious and/or local sedation. Patients had an average age of 66.9 years, a mean prostate volume of 45.9 g, and an average LUTS duration of 44.0 months. The procedure required an average of 25 minutes, and the average total amount of ethanol injected per procedure was 14.0 mL. By 4 days after treatment, 98% of patients voided spontaneously. The significant reduction in LUTS noted 1 month after TEAP was maintained at 12-month follow-up, and the International Prostate Symptom and Quality of Life scores decreased by more than 50%. Prostate volume was reduced by an average of 16%. Adverse events included discomfort or irritative voiding symptoms and hematuria, occurring in 26% and 16% of patients, respectively. Fewer than 3% experienced retrograde ejaculation and erectile dysfunction. Seven percent of patients underwent TURP, mainly for continued obstructive symptoms, and 2 patients required open surgery after bladder necrosis developed.

Conclusion.—Results of the first large-scale study evaluating the safety and efficacy of TEAP to treat BPH confirm the advantages of the procedure, which is minimally invasive, easy to learn, cost-effective, and performed quickly in office. No dose-response relationship and no pretreatment predictors of response were identified.

► Historically, TURP was the most commonly performed operation among the elderly, second only to cataract surgery. It was associated with significant blood loss, blood transfusions, urinary incontinence, and even impotence. As a result, tremendous efforts have been put forth to develop new surgical therapies that have fewer side effects. Over the past 15 years, we have witnessed the introduction of many minimally invasive therapies for BPH, including balloon dilations, urethral stents, TUNA, TUMT, and lasers in all configurations. Although not all of these have stood the test of time, many continue to be used with some demonstrable efficacy. The injection of ethanol into the prostatic urethra is one of the more recent concepts to be moved forward into clinical practice. The premise is that dehydrated ethanol will cause tissue necrosis in the prostate and thereby relieving obstruction; however, it has also been proposed that relief of symptoms may be due to disruption of nerve endings. Mechanism notwithstanding, this large multi-institutional study has prospectively shown that ethanol will result in significant reduction of lower urinary tract symptoms and improve urinary flow rates. However, 2 of 115 patients or nearly 2% experienced significant adverse effects, including bladder necrosis and subsequent reconstructive surgery. Although infrequent, these adverse effects require significant resources to manage and have devastating effects on the patients. Clearly, as we consider what therapies we will offer to our BPH patients, the possibility of such devastating side effects must be weighed against the potential benefits of treatment. As we refine the use of ethanol and other approaches, it is imperative that we conduct well-designed, adequately powered, clinical trials to demonstrate efficacy and also observational studies to define adverse effects.

J. T. Wei, MD, MSc

Three-Year Follow-up of Feedback Microwave Thermotherapy Versus TURP for Clinical BPH: A Prospective Randomized Multicenter Study

Wagrell L, Schelin S, Nordling J, et al (Uppsala Univ Hosp, Sweden; Kalmar County Hosp, Sweden; Herlev Hosp, Denmark; et al)

Urology 64:698-702, 2004 11–19

Objectives.—To compare, in a prospective randomized multicenter study, the efficacy and safety of transurethral microwave thermotherapy with ProstaLund Feedback Treatment (PLFT), using the CoreTherm device, with transurethral resection of the prostate (TURP) 36 months after treatment.

Methods.—The study was conducted at 10 centers in the United States and Scandinavia. A total of 154 patients with benign prostatic hyperplasia were randomized to PLFT or TURP in a 2:1 ratio. The treatment outcome was evaluated on the basis of the International Prostate Symptom Score (IPSS), the quality-of-life question (QOL) of the IPSS, peak urinary flow rate (Qmax), urodynamics, and adverse events. The microwave power and treatment time were adjusted according to each patient's response to the supplied energy (ie, the intraprostatic temperature guided the PLFT).

Results.—Statistically significant improvements in both the TURP and the PLFT groups were observed for IPSS, QOL, and Qmax at 36 months. The average value for the PLFT group was 8.2, 1.2, and 11.9 mL/s for IPSS, QOL, and Qmax, respectively. The corresponding values for the TURP group were IPSS 5.0, QOL 1.0, and Qmax 13.5 mL/s. The difference in IPSS outcome was statistically significant; however, no statistically significant differences were found in QOL or Qmax between the two treatment groups. The degree of improvement was in the same range as that observed after 12 and 24 months for both groups. During the 12 to 36-month period, the most frequent adverse events in the TURP group were impotence (15%), micturition urgency (13%), and urethral disorder (8%); in the PLFT group, impotence (8%), prostate-specific antigen increase (5%), and hematuria (4%) were the most common.

Conclusions.—The clinical outcome 3 years after microwave thermotherapy with PLFT was comparable to the results seen after TURP. The safety of PLFT compared favorably to that of TURP in this study.

▶ The ProstaLund microwave feedback treatment using the CoreTherm device is unique among the microwave thermotherapy treatment devices for benign prostatic hyperplasia in that it is equipped with a needle mounted on the catheter and pushed into the prostate that provides direct real-time feedback during the treatment and thereby allows a treatment duration and intensity adjustment to the local condition. The device has been developed in Sweden and is marketed in the United States under the brand name CoreTherm. A multicenter trial was conducted in Scandinavia and in the United States randomizing patients to either PLFT or TURP in a 2:1 ratio. This study reports 3-year follow-up and demonstrates significant improvement in both TURP and PLFT groups for a symptom score, quality-of-life score, and peak urinary flow rate. At the end of 3 years in the PLFT group, the IPSS score had decreased from 21 to 8.2 points, and in the TURP group from 20.4 to 5.0 points. Peak urinary flow rate had improved in the PLFT group from 7.6 to 11.9 mL/s, and in the TURP group from 7.9 to 13.5 mL/s. The authors claim that the clinical outcome was comparable to the results seen after TURP, while the safety compared favorably to TURP. Clearly, a sustained symptom improvement from 21 to 8.2 points is a very significant improvement, and perhaps greater than reported with many of the other minimally invasive treatments. It nearly matches the improvement seen with the TURP. Of note, 68 patients were available at 3 years for a follow-up of an original cohort of 99 patients, which seems to be a very representative cohort. Concerning the flow rate improvements, which are less pronounced, this reviewer wonders why the TURP cohort had such a seemingly small increase in peak urinary flow rate. Most TURP series result in peak urinary flow rates after therapy close to or above 20 mL/s, while the improvement noted here amounts to 13.5 mL/s at the 3-year mark. Nonetheless, the significant improvements in QOL and symptom score demonstrate what appears to be a very significant and sustained improvement utilizing the CoreTherm device. Of note, the CoreTherm device does not provide cooling, and thus patients treated by this device in general wear a catheter during the postoperative period and may experience hematuria, urgency, and occasionally tissue sloughing. Regrettably in this particular article, no data are provided regarding the number of patients requiring catheterization and/or the duration of such catheterization.

C. G. Roehrborn, MD

Long-term Pooled Analysis of Multicenter Studies of Cooled Thermotherapy for Benign Prostatic Hyperplasia: Results at Three Months Through Four Years

Trock BJ, Brotzman M, Utz WJ, et al (Johns Hopkins School of Medicine, Baltimore, Md; Univ of Minnesota; Abbott-Northwestern Hosp, Minneapolis, Minn; et al)

Urology 63:716-721, 2004 11–20

Objectives.—To determine the long-term efficacy of cooled thermotherapy in the treatment of lower urinary tract symptoms of clinical benign prostatic hyperplasia.

Methods.—A total of 541 men underwent cooled thermotherapy treatment in six multicenter studies in the United States, England, and Canada. Both fixed and random effects models were used to pool the data across the six studies. The treatment response was measured as the difference between the urinary tract symptoms at baseline versus those at 3, 12, 24, 36, and 48 months after therapy. The treatment response included changes in the American Urological Association Symptom Score (AUA symptom score), peak urinary flow rate in milliliters per second (Qmax), and quality of life (QOL).

Results.—The baseline measures were comparable across the studies. At 3 months, the AUA symptom score had improved by a mean of 11.6 (55%), Qmax by a mean of 4.0 (51%), and QOL by a mean of 2.3 (53%). These changes persisted with only slight attenuation through 48 months (corresponding mean changes of 43%, 35%, and 50%). These changes were highly statistically significant (P <0.0001 to 0.01). An improvement of at least 25% was achieved for the AUA symptom score and QOL by more than 85% of men and by more than 65% of men for Qmax.

Conclusions.—This pooled analysis of six multicenter studies of cooled thermotherapy, involving 541 men, found highly significant improvements in AUA symptom score, Qmax, and QOL. The results were highly consistent across the studies. The improvements reflected changes from baseline values of 45% to 50% for AUA symptom score and QOL and 35% to 40% for Qmax at a follow-up duration up to 48 months after therapy. The level of improvement for all three measures remained high at 48 months, indicating that the response is durable.

► The TARGIS cooled thermotherapy system is a transurethral microwave device, which includes a urethral cooling device to presumably protect the urethral mucosa from sloughing. This report on 541 men includes patients treated in 6 multicenter studies in the United States and Canada. While the baseline parameters were comparable, the patients were treated under different treatment conditions in multiple centers during different periods. The AUA score decreased overall from 21 points to about 9 points at 3 months, and in the 171 patients remaining at 4 years, remained at 11.5 points, a highly significant improvement from baseline. Peak urinary flow rate improved from 7.9 to 11.96 mL/s at 3 months and remained at 10.94 mL/s at 4 years, albeit in only 67 patients available for follow-up. The authors conclude that highly significant improvement in symptom score, Qmax, and QOL was achieved in up to 4 years' duration, and that the results were highly consistent across the various studies and centers. Because of the nature of the studies, however, only numerical minorities of patients were in fact available for follow-up at 4 years. Nonetheless, the 3-year data are very comparable to the 4-year data, and at that time point, at least 229 patients were available for symptom assessment. It therefore appears that the data are stable and that the improvements indeed are sustained.

C. G. Roehrborn, MD

Transurethral Needle Ablation Versus Transurethral Resection of the Prostate for the Treatment of Symptomatic Benign Prostatic Hyperplasia: 5-Year Results of a Prospective, Randomized, Multicenter Clinical Trial

Hill B, Belville W, Bruskewitz R, et al (Univ of Maryland, Baltimore; Univ of Michigan, Ann Arbor; Univ of Wisconsin, Madison; et al)

J Urol 171:2336-2340, 2004 11–21

Purpose.—We report the 5-year efficacy and safety of transurethral needle ablation of the prostate (TUNA) compared to transurethral resection of the prostate (TURP) for the treatment of lower urinary tract symptoms (LUTS) secondary to benign prostatic hyperplasia (BPH).

Materials and Methods.—A total of 121 men 50 years or older with LUTS secondary to BPH a minimum of 3 months in duration were enrolled in this prospective, randomized clinical trial at 7 medical centers across the United States. Of the participants 65 (54%) were randomly selected to receive TUNA and 56 (46%) were selected to receive TURP. International Prostate Symptom Score, quality of life, peak urinary flow rate, post-void residual urinary volume, and prostate size and configuration were evaluated before the procedure and then annually for 5 years after the procedure. Adverse events were also recorded throughout the study.

Results.—Improvement from baseline for TUNA and TURP retained statistical significance at each interval for International Prostate Symptom Score, quality of life and peak flow rate. Post-void residual volume was statistically significant at all time points for TURP and at year 5 for TUNA. The TURP group reported 41% retrograde ejaculation, while the TUNA group reported none. The incident of erectile dysfunction, incontinence and stricture formation was also greater in TURP than in TUNA cases with significantly fewer adverse events for TUNA than for TURP.

Conclusions.—The results of this study demonstrate stable treatment outcomes after 5 years of followup and suggest that TUNA is an attractive treatment option for men with LUTS due to BPH.

► The other minimally invasive treatment that became very popular in the 1990s is the TUNA procedure. In the United States, a randomized trial was conducted in 5 centers comparing TUNA and TURP. In this study, 5-year efficacy and safety data are reported on the original 121 patients randomized to TUNA or TURP. The AUA Symptom Score improvement in the TUNA group was from 24 points at baseline to 11.7 points at year 1 and 10.7 points at year 5, while the improvement was from 24.1 points to 7.8 points at year 1 and 10.8 points at year 5 in the TURP group. Peak flow rate improved from 8.8 to 11.4 mL/s at year 5 in the TUNA group and from 8.8 to 18.6 mL/s in the TURP group. The results of this study demonstrate stable treatment outcomes in terms of symptom improvement after 5 years of therapy, although the peak urinary flow rate improvements are clearly inferior to that achieved with TURP.

It is important to observe that for both the microwave thermotherapy and the TUNA treatment, symptom improvements are maintained in those patients available for follow-up at 3 to 5 years after the original procedure. From a health care cost point of view, however, it is important to understand what may have happened to those patients who were not available for follow-up at 3 to 5 years. A significant number of those patients may have been placed on medical therapy, while others may have undergone additional treatment. It is notoriously difficult to determine the number of patients who undergo additional treatment, including surgery for BPH, in those studies. Without these data, however, a true cost-effectiveness analysis cannot be performed, as it is indeed the re-treatment rate that drives the cost of such therapies.

C. G. Roehrborn, MD

Photoselective Vaporization of the Prostate for the Treatment of Benign Prostatic Hyperplasia: 12-Month Results From the First United States Multicenter Prospective Trial

Te AE, Malloy TR, Stein BS, et al (Cornell Weill Med Coll, New York; Univ of Pennsylvania, Philadelphia; Brown Univ, Providence, RI; et al)

J Urol 172:1404-1408, 2004 11–22

Purpose.—We report the 1-year efficacy and safety of photoselective vaporization of the prostate (PVP) for symptomatic and obstructive benign prostatic hyperplasia (BPH).

Materials and Methods.—A prospective clinical trial was performed in 139 men clinically diagnosed with symptomatic bladder outlet obstruction secondary to BPH who were enrolled and treated with a high power, 80 W, quasicontinuous wave potassium-titanyl-phosphate laser at 6 American medical centers across the country. Efficacy parameters were mean and percent changes from baseline in the American Urological Association Symptom Index (AUA-SI) score, quality of life score (QOL), peak urinary flow rate (Qmax), post-void residual urine volume (PVR) and transrectal ultrasound prostate volume measurement. Patients were evaluated 1, 3, 6 and 12 months following treatment. At each followup evaluation side effects were elicited.

Results.—Significant improvements in AUA-SI score, QOL score, Qmax and PVR were noted as early as 1 month after PVP treatment. At 12 months the mean AUA-SI score decreased from 23.9 to 4.3 ($p < 0.0001$) and the QOL score decreased from 4.3 to 1.1 ($p < 0.0001$), while mean Qmax increased from 7.8 to 22.6 ml per second ($p < 0.0001$). PVR decreased from 114.3 to 24.8 ml ($p < 0.0001$), while the transrectal ultrasound volume reduction went from 54.6 ml at baseline to 34.4 ml. There was no significant blood loss or fluid absorption during or immediately after PVP. Complications consisted of transient hematuria, dysuria and urinary retention in 12 (8.6%), 13 (9.3%) and 7 (5%) patients, respectively.

Conclusions.—PVP is a unique, safe and effective outpatient modality that provides immediate symptomatic and urodynamic relief of bladder outlet obstruction secondary to BPH. Long-term followup is needed to validate further the maintenance of clinical efficacy beyond 1 year.

▶ One of the newer modifications of the standard transurethral resection of the prostate is the use of the potassium-titanyl-phosphate (KTP) laser to vaporize prostate tissue. This treatment is also referred to as the "bloodless" TURP, or Green-Light laser prostatectomy. Indeed, it is an attractive treatment that in some way mimics the right-angle neodymium YAG laser, which was abandoned because of the high proportion of patients reporting postoperative irritative voiding symptoms. In this trial, 139 men with BPH were enrolled in a prospective clinical trial in several centers in the United States and treated with the GreenLight laser. These patients experienced significant improvement in symptom score, quality of life score, peak flow rate, and postvoid residual urine volume. As promised, there is truly no significant blood loss or fluid absorption noted with the KTP or GreenLight laser. The serum sodium decrease observed was 1.3 mEq/L, and the surgical time was 38.7 minutes, with a range from 9 to 140 minutes. It should be noted that the vaporization of tissue is not terribly efficient with the KTP laser and, thus, to effectively treat larger glands may require prolonged periods of time. The cost for operation room utilization in some cases may offset the savings associated with the lack of blood loss and the shorter hospitalization. Along these lines, the postoperative catheterization time ranged from no catheter to 72 hours and, on average, was 14 hours. Forty-four patients (32%) did not require any catheterization at all.

This reviewer has used the KTP laser over the last 6 months and is impressed with its ability to improve symptoms and flow rate, while not being associated with any significant or noticeable blood loss. The learning curve is rather short, but very large prostates may require the use of 2 or even more laser fibers, which limits the cost effectiveness of the device to some degree.

C. G. Roehrborn, MD

Holmium Laser Resection of the Prostate Versus Transurethral Resection of the Prostate: Results of a Randomized Trial With 4-Year Minimum Long-term Followup

Westenberg A, Gilling P, Kennett K, et al (Tauranga Hosp, New Zealand; Christchurch School of Medicine, New Zealand)

J Urol 172:616-619, 2004 11–23

Purpose.—It has previously been shown that holmium laser resection of the prostate (HoLRP) is superior to transurethral resection of the prostate (TURP) with regard to perioperative morbidity and is equivalent to TURP in the short term. We present the long-term results of a randomized, prospective trial comparing HoLRP to TURP since information regarding the durability of holmium prostatectomy is lacking in the literature to date.

Materials and Methods.—A total of 120 patients with urodynamic obstruction were randomized (April 1996 to August 1997) into 2 comparable groups and assigned to HoLRP or TURP. All patients were assessed preoperatively and followed prospectively at 3 weeks, 3, 6, 12, 24 and 48 months postoperatively with an American Urological Association symptom score, quality of life score, peak urinary flow rate, and questionnaires concerning sexual function and continence. Preoperative pressure flow studies, ultrasound prostatic volume assessment and post-void residual volume measurement were repeated at the 6-month visit. All adverse events were noted.

Results.—Of 120 patients 73 completed the 48-month assessment. HoLRP and TURP resulted in significant improvements in all parameters. There was no difference between the 2 techniques in terms of urodynamic parameters, potency, continence and symptom scores at the 48-month assessment. HoLRP took significantly longer to perform but perioperative morbidity, catheter time, nursing contact time and hospital stay were significantly less for HoLRP compared to TURP.

Conclusions.—HoLRP and TURP give equivalent and satisfactory long-term results, with no differences noted in major morbidity. This confirms the durability of these 2 treatments. Peri-operative morbidity is less with HoLRP.

Transurethral Holmium Laser Enucleation of the Prostate Versus Transurethral Electrocautery Resection of the Prostate: A Randomized Prospective Trial in 200 Patients

Kuntz RM, Ahyai S, Lehrich K, et al (Auguste Viktoria Hosp, Berlin; Cairo Univ)

J Urol 172:1012-1016, 2004 11–24

Purpose.—Transurethral electrocautery resection (TURP) is generally regarded as the gold standard surgical treatment for bladder outflow obstruction due to benign prostatic hyperplasia despite its rather high morbidity. The high powered holmium:YAG laser can be used endoscopically to enucleate obstructing prostatic tissue in a relatively bloodless manner. The technique of transurethral holmium laser enucleation of the prostate (HoLEP) was compared to standard TURP for the surgical management of prostate adenomas in a randomized, prospective clinical trial.

Materials and Methods.—A total of 200 urodynamically obstructed patients with a prostate of less than 100 gm on transrectal ultrasound were randomized to HoLEP or TURP. All patients were assessed preoperatively, and 1, 6 and 12 months postoperatively. Patient baseline characteristics, perioperative data and postoperative outcome were compared. All complications were noted.

Results.—HoLEP was significantly superior to TURP in terms of catheter time, hospital stay and hemoglobin loss but operative time was longer. HoLEP and TURP resulted in a significant improvement in American Urological Association symptom scores, peak urinary flow rates and post-void residual urine volumes with symptoms scores and residual volume significantly better in the holmium group. Effects on continence and potency were similar in the 2 groups but adverse events were less frequent in the holmium group.

Conclusions.—HoLEP and TURP are highly effective procedures for removing obstructing prostatic adenomas. HoLEP resulted in significantly better micturition parameters and less perioperative morbidity.

▶ By now, HoLRP and HoLEP have become standard treatment protocols in many centers around the world. In the first of these contributions, the original champions, Drs Gilling and Fraundorfer report on 120 patients with urodynamic obstruction who were randomized to either HoLRP or TURP. While HoLRP took significantly longer to perform, perioperative morbidity, catheter time, nursing time, and hospital stay were significantly less, and the efficacy parameters were equal, if not superior, in the HoLRP group. Symptom score improvements were realized from 22 points to 5 points in the HoLRP group and from 23 to 6.6 points in the TURP group.

In the second contribution, a multinational group reports on a randomized prospective trial in 200 patients comparing transurethral HoLEP and TURP in patients with a transrectal US prostate weight of less than 100 g. They found HoLEP superior to TURP in terms of catheter time, hospital stay, and blood loss, as measured by decrease in hemoglobin, but they also experienced a longer operating time.

Both the studies as well as a multitude of other contributions to the literature document the efficacy and safety of HoLEP and HoLRP, mostly for larger glands, when compared with traditional TURP. The learning curve is somewhat steep, particularly for HoLEP compared with TURP, and also compared to the GreenLight laser prostatectomy. However, the outcome data speak for themselves, and those familiar with the technology will likely continue to use it to the advantage of their patients.

C. G. Roehrborn, MD

The Natural History of Lower Urinary Tract Dysfunction in Men: The Influence of Detrusor Underactivity on the Outcome After Transurethral Resection of the Prostate With a Minimum 10-Year Urodynamic Follow-up

Thomas AW, Cannon A, Bartlett E, et al (Bristol Urological Inst, England)

BJU Int 93:745-750, 2004 11–25

Objectives.—To assess the long-term outcome of the efficacy of transurethral resection of the prostate (TURP) in men with detrusor underactivity (DUA), a cause of lower urinary tract symptoms (LUTS) in a significant minority of men.

Patients and Methods.—Neurologically intact men with LUTS, who were investigated in our department between 1972 and 1986, diagnosed with DUA and who underwent surgical intervention, were invited for a repeat symptomatic and urodynamic assessment. Identical methods were used, allowing direct comparison of the results.

Results.—In all, 224 men were initially diagnosed with DUA; 87 (39%) of these died in the interim and 22 followed had a TURP, with a mean follow-up since surgery of 11.3 years. There were no significantly sustained reductions in any symptoms. There was a small but significant reduction of questionable clinical significance in the bladder outlet obstruction index, but this did not translate into an improved flow rate. Comparison with 58 age-matched patients with DUA who remained untreated showed no significant advantage of surgical intervention in the long-term; on the contrary, there was more chronic retention in those who had had surgery.

Conclusions.—There are no long-term symptomatic or urodynamic gains from TURP in men shown to have DUA. The results of TURP in men with DUA are important, as urologists who surgically treat patients based on the symptoms and uroflowmetry alone will do so in a significant minority of men with DUA. These results strengthen the argument for a routine preoperative urodynamic assessment.

▶ While it is accepted dogma that TURP leads to significant improvement in symptoms, flow rate, and urodynamics, there is a paucity of long-term outcome studies. From Mr Abrams' department at the Bristol Urological Institute comes this most unusual and very attractive study that assesses the natural history of LUTS in those men diagnosed with DUA, and it analyzes the outcome in those who underwent TURP with a minimum of 10-year urodynamic follow-up. In all, between 1972 and 1986 224 men were diagnosed with DUA. Thirty-nine percent of them died in the interim. A significant number of these patients underwent TURP; however, there were no long-term symptomatic or urodynamic improvements realized from TURP in those patients originally diagnosed with DUA. This is important for surgeons and for physicians consulting with men with LUTS and benign prostatic hyperplasia. It is not uncommon by urodynamic testing that men are diagnosed with DUA but then are counseled to undergo TURP, as there is a paucity of other attractive treatment interventions. Realistically, if a patient is particularly bothered by his symptoms, perhaps related to high amounts of residual urine, clean intermittent catheterization and medical therapy might be the only treatment option available. Surgeons occasionally may be tempted to perform TURP even knowing that the outcomes may not be as good as they might be in patients who have a normally functioning detrusor. This study, which has an extremely long follow-up, suggests that, in fact, we do not do these patients a major favor when offering surgery. Indeed, patients with DUA are not likely to experience a sustained improvement in their symptoms and thus may be spared the surgical intervention to begin with. The authors also make the point that DUA is indistinguishable from bladder outlet obstruction on clinical criteria alone and emphasizes once more the importance of performing urodynamic studies to select those patients who truly would benefit from TURP in contrast to those with DUA who would not likely experience symptomatic improvement.

C. G. Roehrborn, MD

12 Male Incontinence

New Perineal Bone-Anchored Male Sling: Lessons Learned

Onur R, Rajpurkar A, Singla A (Wayne State Univ, Detroit)

Urology 64:58-61, 2004 12–1

Objectives.—To identify factors affecting outcome after the male sling procedure for stress urinary incontinence.

Methods.—A total of 46 incontinent men, with a mean age of 67 years, underwent perineal bone-anchored male sling placement. Three titanium bone screws with preattached pairs of No. 1 polypropylene sutures were placed directly into the medial aspect of each inferior ramus of the pubic bone. To compress the urethra, three different types of materials were used: absorbable biomaterial, silicone-coated polypropylene mesh, or a composite graft. Patient characteristics, incontinence etiology and severity before surgery, prior collagen injections, and type of material used were assessed, and the association with the outcome of the male sling procedure was determined.

Results.—The procedure was successful in 35 (76%) of 46 patients at a mean follow-up of 18 months (range 6 to 30). Nineteen patients were totally dry and 16 had improved 50% or more compared with before surgery. Failure occurred in 11 patients (24%). Patients who received a composite graft or mesh alone had a better outcome compared with the absorbable sling group (97% and 75% versus 0%, respectively, $P = 0.001$). The severity of pretreatment incontinence also had a negative impact on the outcome.

Conclusions.—Patients with mild-to-moderate incontinence and the use of a composite graft had the best outcomes after the perineal bone-anchored male sling.

The Male Perineal Sling: Comparison of Sling Materials

Dikranian AH, Chang JH, Rhee EY, et al (Kaiser Permanente Med Ctr, Los Angeles and San Diego, Calif)

J Urol 172:608-610, 2004 12–2

Purpose.—Urinary incontinence continues to be a significant problem for patients after radical prostatectomy. The male perineal sling is emerging as a safe and effective treatment option for postprostatectomy stress urinary incontinence. We compare the efficacy of porcine dermal collagen and silicone mesh as the sling material.

Materials and Methods.—Of 36 patients with postprostatectomy stress urinary incontinence a porcine dermal collagen sling was placed in 20 and a silicone mesh sling was placed in 16. The sling was placed at the bulbar urethra and secured to 3 titanium bone screws anchored into the medial aspect of bilateral inferior pubic rami.

Results.—Results at 12 months were compared. In the dermis group 9 (56%) patients were cured of incontinence (no pads daily), 5 (31%) had significant improvement (decrease of 50% or more in pads daily) and 2 (13%) had no change in symptoms. In the silicone mesh group 14 (87%) patients were cured of incontinence and 2 (13%) were significantly improved. Results showed that a previously placed artificial urinary sphincter led to poorer outcomes but a history of radiation therapy did not affect results. The most common complication was temporary urinary retention observed in 1 (5%) patient in the dermis group and 2 (12%) in the silicone mesh group.

Conclusions.—Early results demonstrate that the male sling is a safe and efficacious treatment option for postprostatectomy urinary incontinence. This study demonstrates superior outcomes with the synthetic silicone mesh sling compared to the porcine dermal collagen.

▶ The technique of male perineal slings for stress urinary incontinence has undergone several refinements in the last 2 years. Based on these 2 small studies (Abstracts 12–1 and 12–2), it appears that synthetic materials seem to do better in the long term than biologic materials and, furthermore, patients with less severe degrees of incontinence seem to do better, or at least are cured to a greater degree compared with those with more severe incontinence preoperatively. Obstruction and other complications related to the surgical technique appear to be minimal. This technique represents a reasonable alternative to artificial urinary sphincter in select patients.

E. S. Rovner, MD

13 Renal Tumors

Relation of Height, Body Mass, Energy Intake, and Physical Activity to Risk of Renal Cell Carcinoma: Results From the Netherlands Cohort Study

van Dijk BAC, Schouten LJ, Kiemeney LALM, et al (Maastricht Univ, The Netherlands; Univ Med Ctr Nijmegen, The Netherlands; TNO Nutrition and Food Research, Zeist, The Netherlands)

Am J Epidemiol 160:1159-1167, 2004 13–1

Introduction.—Data from the Netherlands Cohort Study on Diet and Cancer were used to investigate the association between anthropometry, energy intake, and physical activity and risk of renal cell carcinoma (RCC). The Netherlands Cohort Study on Diet and Cancer consists of 120,852 men and women aged 55-69 years who completed a self-administered questionnaire at baseline (1986). A case-cohort approach was used. After 9.3 years of follow-up, 275 microscopically confirmed incident cases were available for analysis. Incidence rate ratios for RCC were estimated using Cox proportional hazards models. Height was associated with RCC risk only in women (per 5-cm increment, rate ratio (RR) = 1.23, 95% confidence interval (CI): 1.03, 1.46). Body mass index (weight (kg)/height $(m)^2$) was associated with increased risk of RCC (per 1-kg/m(2)increment, RR = 1.07, 95% CI: 1.02, 1.12) for men and women, as was gain in body mass index from age 20 years to baseline (per 1-kg/m^2)increment, RR = 1.06, 95% CI: 1.01, 1.10). Energy intake was not related to RCC risk, while a possible protective effect was observed for physical activity in men. These results suggest that body mass index and gain in body mass index since age 20 are associated with increased risk of RCC.

Relation of Height and Body Mass Index to Renal Cell Carcinoma in Two Million Norwegian Men and Women

Bjørge T, Tretil S, Engeland A (Norwegian Radium Hosp, Oslo, Norway; Inst of Population-based Cancer Research, Oslo, Norway; Norwegian Inst of Public Health, Oslo, Norway)

Am J Epidemiol 160:1168-1176, 2004 13–2

Introduction.—A positive association between body mass index (BMI) and renal cell carcinoma (RCC) has been observed. The association between height and RCC has been less clear. The authors explored these relations in a very large Norwegian cohort. Height and weight were measured in two million Norwegian men and women aged 20-74 years during 1963-2001. During follow-up, 6,453 cases of RCC were registered in the national cancer database. Measurements were also performed in 227,000 adolescents aged 14-19 years, and 154 cases of RCC were registered. Relative risks for RCC were estimated using Cox proportional hazards regression. The risk of RCC increased with increasing BMI among both adults and adolescents. Among adults, the relative risk associated with a one-unit increase in BMI was 1.05 (95% confidence interval (CI): 1.04, 1.06) in both sexes. The relative risk associated with a 10-cm increase in height was 1.19 (95% CI: 1.13, 1.26) in men and 1.17 (95% CI: 1.09, 1.26) in women. In a subgroup analysis, the relation between BMI and RCC was most pronounced in men and women who were never smokers, and the relation between height and RCC was confined to ever smokers. The authors conclude that elevated BMIs are associated with RCC risk in both males and females across a wide age range.

▶ Obesity is a growing epidemic that greatly threatens the health of society. It has long been realized that obesity increases the risk of cardiovascular disease but there is now emerging evidence demonstrating that obesity is an important risk factor for cancer. In these 2 large epidemiologic studies (Abstracts 13–1 and 13–2) from The Netherlands and Norway, the risk of RCC increased with increasing BMI.

D. K. Ornstein, MD

Natural History of Small Renal Cell Carcinoma: Evaluation of Growth Rate, Histological Grade, Cell Proliferation and Apoptosis

Kato M, Suzuki T, Suzuki Y, et al (Tohoku Univ, Japan; Izumi Chuo Hosp, Sendai, Japan)

J Urol 172:863-866, 2004 13–3

Purpose.—We investigated the natural history of incidentally discovered small renal cell carcinomas (RCCs), and we evaluated growth rate, apoptosis, cell proliferation and histological grade.

Materials and Methods.—A total of 18 patients with RCCs extirpated after at least 12 months of observation were reviewed retrospectively. The period of observation ranged from 12 to 63 months (median 22.5). Median patient age was 56.5 years, ranging from 37 to 71. Annual tumor growth rate was calculated from diameter obtained from computerized tomography or ultrasound. Cell proliferation and apoptosis were assessed by immunostaining using Ki-67 and TUNEL.

Results.—Average tumor growth rate was 0.42 cm per year (standard error 0.09, 95% confidence interval 0.24 to 0.61). Of the 18 tumors 7 were grade 1, 8 were grade 2 and 3 were grade 3. Tumor growth rate and Ki-67 positive ratio were not correlated. In contrast, growth rate and positive ratio of TUNEL were significantly correlated. A significant difference in growth rate was observed between grade 2 and 3 tumors but not between grade 1 and 2 tumors.

Conclusions.—The growth rate of RCCs correlates with apoptosis and grade. Most incidentally found RCCs are slow growing. However, those with certain histopathological features can grow rapidly and have a poor prognosis. More attention should be given to the observation of small renal masses.

▶ Historically, all solid renal masses were thought to be RCC until proven otherwise and most were treated with surgical excision. However, since the widespread use of abdominal imaging has dramatically increased the incidental discovery of small renal masses, this practice must be reassessed. There is now mounting evidence in the literature suggesting that many of these small renal masses have a low malignant potential. This article specifically addresses the growth rate of small renal tumors and confirms that most small renal masses are slow growing. In fact, the average tumor growth rate was 0.42 cm per year and only 2 of 18 patients experienced growth rates greater than 1 cm. Because experience with von Hipple-Lindau disease suggests that metastasis is exceedingly rare in patients with renal tumors smaller than 3 cm, this information should be useful in counseling patients. These data support the conservative management of small renal masses in older patients with significant comorbidites and limited life expectancies. Because these patients were only monitored for 1 year without treatment, the applicability of these findings to younger patients is not clear. Although the article suggests that tumor grade and apoptosis index were predictors of rapid growth rates, there is no reliable method to predict tumor growth rate and most patients with small renal masses are treated with excision or ablative therapies. Hopefully in the future, molecular markers that identify slow-growing tumors will be found so that these patients can be spared unnecessary treatment-related morbidity.

D. K. Ornstein, MD

Guidelines for the Surveillance of Localized Renal Cell Carcinoma Based on the Patterns of Relapse After Nephrectomy

Stephenson AJ, Chetner MP, Rourke K, et al (McGill Univ, Montréal; Univ of Alberta, Edmonton, Canada; Univ of British Columbia, Vancouver, Canada; et al)

J Urol 172:58-62, 2004 13–4

Purpose.—We characterized relapse patterns in patients with sporadic renal cell carcinoma (RCC) following radical and partial nephrectomy, and developed surveillance guidelines.

Materials and Methods.—Between 1989 and 2000, 495 patients underwent nephrectomy for RCC at 1 of 5 Canadian referral centers. Median followup was 42 months.

Results.—The rate of relapse, time to relapse and site of relapse were associated with pathological stage. Five-year progression-free probability was

93% for pT1, 81% for pT2, 67% for pT3A and 57% for pT3B ($p < 0.001$). Compared to patients with pT1-2 those with pT3A-B lesions had earlier relapse after nephrectomy (median 12 vs 26 months, $p = 0.001$) and were at higher risk for relapse at abdominal sites (14% vs 1.8%, $p < 0.001$). Abdominal relapse was detected in the absence of symptoms, abnormal biochemical profile or thoracic metastases detectable by chest x-ray in 7 patients (1.4%) overall, including 3 (0.9%) with pT1, 3 (4%) with pT3A and 1 (3%) with pT3B.

Conclusions.—The risk and the pattern of relapse of RCC after nephrectomy are associated with pathological stage. For the surveillance of recurrent disease after nephrectomy we recommend annual clinical assessment and chest x-ray in pT1-2 cases. Patients with pT3A-B should be followed every 6 months for the first 3 years with clinical assessment and chest x-ray, and annual followup thereafter. The higher risk of abdominal relapse in patients with pT3A-B indicates that they should receive surveillance abdominal imaging. We recommend abdominal computerized tomography 6, 12, 24 and 36 months postoperatively.

► Despite several publications in the literature, there is no standardized protocol for follow-up care after total nephrectomy for renal cell cancer. Because, in most contemporary series, recurrence rates are less than 20%, intensive follow-up protocols for all patients are not appropriate. However, because some patients can be salvaged despite recurrence, it is essential to appropriately evaluate patients at risk for recurrence. Although molecular markers may have a prognostic role in the future, in current practice a patent's risk of recurrence is determined by tumor stage and Fuhrman grade. That is the progression-free rate for pT3B tumors was 57% compared with 93% for patients with pT1 tumors. Tumor stage can also provide helpful information regarding site of recurrences. Patients with pT3A-B tumors had a significantly higher risk of abdominal site recurrence than those with pT1-2 tumors (14% vs 1.8%). Because the risk of abdominal recurrence for pT1-2 tumors is less than 1%, the authors recommend foregoing routine abdominal CT scan, but because the risk of abdominal recurrence is 4% for pT3, they recommend abdominal pelvic CT scans at 6, 12, 24, and 36 months postoperatively. I agree in general with these recommendations but because of the 1% to 2% risk of bilateral disease, still obtain a CT scan at 1, 2, and 4 years postoperatively in patients after nephrectomy for T2 RCC.

D. K. Ornstein, MD

The Relationship Between Renal Tumor Size and Metastases in Patients With von Hippel-Lindau Disease

Duffey BG, Choyke PL, Glenn G, et al (NIH, Bethesda, Md)
J Urol 172:63-65, 2004 13–5

Purpose.—Patients with von Hippel-Lindau disease are at risk for multiple, bilateral, recurrent renal tumors and metastases. We previously evaluated the relationship between tumor size and metastases in families with hereditary renal cancer. We update our findings with about twice the number of patients with von Hippel-Lindau disease.

Materials and Methods.—Screening affected kindred or retrospective review of medical records identified 181 patients with von Hippel-Lindau disease and renal cell carcinoma. Patients with small tumors were followed with serial imaging until the largest tumor reached 3 cm, at which point surgery was recommended. Surgical resection was recommended to patients with tumors larger than 3 cm. Patients not undergoing screening often had large renal tumors.

Results.—A total of 108 patients with von Hippel-Lindau disease and solid renal tumors on computerized tomography imaging smaller than 3 cm (group 1) were followed a mean of 58 months (range 0 to 244). Metastatic disease did not develop in any of these patients. Renal tumors larger than 3 cm developed in 73 patients with von Hippel-Lindau disease (group 2). Mean followup of group 2 was 72.9 months (range 0 to 321). The proportion of procedures that were nephron sparing was higher in group 1 than in group 2 (120 of 125 [97%] compared to 85 of 125 [69%], Fisher's exact test $p < 0.0001$). Metastases developed in 20 of 73 (27.4%) patients in group 2. The frequency of renal tumor metastases increased with increasing tumor size.

Conclusions.—No renal tumor metastases were found in patients with renal tumors less than 3 cm in diameter. We advocate a 3 cm threshold for parenchymal sparing surgery in patients with von Hippel-Lindau disease to decrease the risk of metastatic disease while preserving renal function, avoiding or delaying the need for dialysis and/or renal transplant, and decreasing the number of operations which a patient may undergo. We stress the importance of early screening in the kindred of patients with von Hippel-Lindau disease and vigilant followup thereafter.

► Because patients with von Hippel-Lindau disease (vHL) have bilateral multifocal renal cell carcinomas, conservative management of small renal tumors has been advocated. The authors have an extensive experience with the evaluation and management of vHL families, and it has long been their practice to observe small renal tumors and only to perform nephron-sparing surgery once tumors were greater than 3 cm. After this strategy, none of the 108 patients had metastatic disease develop after a mean follow-up of 58 months. These data support the authors' recommendations to observe vHL patients with renal masses 3 cm or less. Although all the patients in the study were affected with vHL, the information can likely be extrapolated to other patients, especially those with multiple tumors smaller than 3 cm or with significant comorbidities.

D. K. Ornstein, MD

A Postoperative Prognostic Nomogram Predicting Recurrence for Patients With Conventional Clear Cell Renal Cell Carcinoma

Sorbellini M, Kattan MW, Snyder ME, et al (Mem Sloan-Kettering Cancer Ctr, New York; Columbia Univ, New York)

J Urol 173:48-51, 2005 13–6

Purpose.—Few published studies have simultaneously analyzed multiple prognostic factors to predict recurrence after surgery for conventional clear cell renal cortical carcinomas. We developed and performed external validation of a postoperative nomogram for this purpose. We used a prospectively updated database of more than 1,400 patients treated at a single institution.

Materials and Methods.—From January 1989 to August 2002, 833 nephrectomies (partial and radical) for renal cell carcinoma of conventional clear cell histology performed at Memorial Sloan-Kettering Cancer Center were reviewed from the center's kidney database. Patients with von Hippel-Lindau disease or familial syndromes, as well as patients presenting with synchronous bilateral renal masses, or distant metastases or metastatic regional lymph nodes before or at surgery were excluded from study. We modeled clinicopathological data and disease followup for 701 patients with conventional clear cell renal cell carcinoma. Prognostic variables for the nomogram included pathological stage, Fuhrman grade, tumor size, necrosis, vascular invasion and clinical presentation (ie incidental asymptomatic, locally symptomatic or systemically symptomatic).

Results.—Disease recurrence was noted in 72 of 701 patients. Those patients without evidence of disease had a median and maximum followup of 32 and 120 months, respectively. The 5-year probability of freedom from recurrence for the patient cohort was 80.9% (95% confidence interval 75.7% to 85.1%). A nomogram was designed based on a Cox proportional hazards regression model. Following external validation predictions by the nomogram appeared accurate and discriminating, and the concordance index was 0.82.

Conclusions.—A nomogram has been developed that can be used to predict the 5-year probability of freedom from recurrence for patients with conventional clear cell renal cell carcinoma. This nomogram may be useful for patient counseling, clinical trial design and effective patient followup strategies.

pT2 Classification for Renal Cell Carcinoma: Can Its Accuracy Be Improved?

Frank I, Blute ML, Leibovich BC, et al (Mayo Med School and Mayo Clinic, Rochester, Minn)

J Urol 173:380-384, 2005 13–7

Purpose.—The 2002 tumor classification for renal cell carcinoma (RCC) classifies pT2 tumors as more than 7 cm in greatest dimension, limited to the kidney. In this study we determined whether a size cutoff point exists within pT2 tumors and whether such subclassification would further improve the accuracy of the current tumor classification.

Materials and Methods.—We studied 544 patients with unilateral, sporadic pT2 RCC treated with radical nephrectomy or nephron sparing surgery between 1970 and 2000. The association of tumor size with death from RCC was examined using martingale residuals from a Cox proportional hazards regression model to determine the optimal size cutoff point.

Results.—There were 204 deaths from RCC a median of 3.8 years following nephrectomy. Univariately tumor size was significantly associated with death from RCC (risk ratio 1.08, 95% CI 1.04 to 1.13, $p < 0.001$). A scatterplot of tumor size vs expected risk of death per patient suggested that a cutoff point between 9 and 10 cm was appropriate. When adjusted for regional lymph node involvement and distant metastases, the 10 cm cutoff point performed better than the 9 cm point (risk ratio 1.42, 95% CI 1.07 to 1.90, $p = 0.017$ vs 1.22, 95% 0.86 to 1.72, $p = 0.268$). Therefore, we propose using a 10 cm cutoff point to subclassify patients into pT2a and pT2b.

Conclusions.—Our data suggest that the prognostic accuracy of the 2002 pT2 tumor classification can be further improved by subclassifying patients with tumors greater than 7 and less than 10 cm into a pT2a category, and those with tumors 10 cm or greater into a pT2b category.

Use of the University of California Los Angeles Integrated Staging System to Predict Survival in Renal Cell Carcinoma: An International Multicenter Study

Patard J-J, Kim HL, Lam JS, et al (Rennes Univ, France; CHU Henri Modor, Créteil, France; CHU Saint Etienne, France; et al)

J Clin Oncol 22:3316-3322, 2004 13–8

Purpose.—To evaluate ability of the University of California Los Angeles Integrated Staging System (UISS) to stratify patients with localized and metastatic renal cell carcinoma (RCC) into risk groups in an international multicenter study.

Patients and Methods.—4,202 patients from eight international academic centers were classified according to the UISS, which combines TNM stage, Fuhrman grade, and Eastern Cooperative Oncology Group performance status. Distribution of the UISS categories was assessed in the overall population and in each center.

Results.—The UISS stratified both localized and metastatic RCC into three different risk groups ($P < .001$). For localized RCC, the 5-year survival rates were 92%, 67%, and 44% for low-, intermediate-, and high-risk groups, respectively. A trend toward a higher risk of death was observed in all centers for increasing UISS risk category. For metastatic RCC, the 3-year survival rates were 37%, 23%, and 12% for low-, intermediate-, and high-risk groups, respectively; in 6 of 8 centers, a trend toward a higher risk of death was observed for increasing UISS risk category. A greater variability in survival rates among centers was observed for high-risk patients.

Conclusion.—This study defines the general applicability of the UISS for predicting survival in patients with RCC. The UISS is an accurate predictor of survival for patients with localized RCC applicable to external databases. Although the UISS may be useful for patients with metastatic RCC, it may be less accurate in this subset of patients due to the heterogeneity of patients and treatments.

▶ RCC has a wide spectrum of clinical behaviors and historically tumor stage has been believed to be the most important prognostic indicator. Until recently, accurate prognostic information is of limited importance because it is used primarily to counsel patients and direct follow-up care, but has not been used to direct therapy. The emergence of potentially beneficial adjuvant therapies (currently being evaluated in clinical trials) increases the importance of accurate prognostic information for patients with RCC. In 2002, the American Joint Committee on Cancer defined tumors larger than 7 cm in diameter to be pT2. Improved prognostic information can be achieved by subclassifying pT2 lesions into pT2a (7-10 cm) and pT2b (>10 cm). In the report by Frank et al (Abstract 13–7) of 544 patients with pT2 renal cell carcinoma, the 10-year cancer specific survival was 78% for tumors smaller than 10 cm compared with 65% for tumors 10 cm or larger. Although tumor stage remains an important prognostic factor, there is strong evidence that Fuhrman grade and performance status are important factors as well. The UISS provides prognostic information for patients with both localized and metastatic RCC. This report validates the predictive power of this staging system for localized renal cell carcinoma but not for metastatic renal cell carcinoma. Another predictive nomogram incorporates pathologic stage, Fuhrman grade, necrosis, vascular invasion, and clinical presentation. Sorbellini et al (Abstract 13–6) reported an accuracy of 82% for predicting recurrence with this nomogram. Interestingly, in multivariate analysis only Fuhrman grade and microvascular invasion were independently predictive. Collectively, these studies demonstrate that in addition to tumor stage, factors such as Fuhrman grade and other histologic features provide important prognostic information for patients with RCC.

D. K. Ornstein, MD

Prognostic Significance of Tumor Thrombus Level in Patients With Renal Cell Carcinoma and Venous Tumor Thrombus Extension: Is All T3b the Same?

Moinzadeh A, Libertino JA (Lahey Clinic, Burlington, Mass)
J Urol 171:598-601, 2004 13–9

Background.—Tumors of the kidney are responsible for about 31,900 new diagnoses per year and about 11,900 deaths in the United States. Of these cases, from 4% to 10% will have tumor thrombus extending into the inferior vena cava (IVC). In the absence of metastatic disease at surgery, survival has been reported even when tumor thrombus extends to the right atrium. Some studies have indicated that the cephalad extent of the tumor thrombus may be a negative prognostic factor, but other studies have not shown decreased survival in patients with tumor thrombus in the inferior vena cava (IVC). The prognostic significance of venous tumor thrombus extension in patients with renal cell carcinoma was investigated, with particular emphasis on determining whether the level of thrombus in the IVC has an effect on long-term survival, and whether there is a difference in long-term survival when tumor thrombus is in the renal vein versus the IVC for patients classified a T3b by the 1997 TNM classification.

Methods.—From July 1970 to July 2000, 153 patients (101 men, 52 women), 39 to 82 years old (median age, 61 years), with renal cell carcinoma with venous vascular extension were treated with radical nephrectomy and tumor thrombus extraction at 1 institution, mainly by 1 surgeon. Venous extension in these cases was defined as gross involvement. The tumor size ranged from 2.2 to 20 cm (median, 8 cm). Cancer-specific survival was determined retrospectively for different levels of tumor thrombus.

Results.—The follow-up ranged from 12 to 221 months (mean, 60 months). The level of tumor thrombus was the renal vein (n = 46), level I (n = 68), level II (n = 17), and level III (n = 22). No differences were noted between the levels in age, sex, perinephric extension, Fuhrman grade, percentage of metastatic disease, and tumor size (Fisher's exact test). Patients with evidence of nodal disease or metastasis at surgery were eliminated from cancer-specific survival analysis. The overall 10-year cancer-specific survival for patients at levels I, II, and III was 30%, 19%, and 29%, respectively. Patient survival at 5 and 10 years was not significantly different between the 3 IVC levels. A significant difference was noted in 10-year survival between patients with renal vein involvement and those with level I involvement (66% vs 29%; $P = .0001$).

Conclusions.—Long-term survival in patients with renal cell carcinoma and venous tumor thrombus extension is not significantly affected by the level of tumor thrombus in the IVC.

Prognostic Significance of Venous Thrombus in Renal Cell Carcinoma: Are Renal Vein and Inferior Vena Cava Involvement Different?

Kim HL, Zisman A, Han K-R, et al (Univ of California, Los Angeles)

J Urol 171:588-591, 2004 13–10

Background.—Several studies have examined the prognostic significance of the level of venous extension in renal cell carcinoma. Most of these studies have found no difference in survival based on the level of involvement of the inferior vena cava (IVC) or on the basis of involvement of the renal vein (RV) versus the IVC. However, it has been suggested that long-term survival may be significantly better in patients with RV involvement than in those with IVC involvement in renal cell carcinoma.

It has also been suggested that the 1997 TNM classification be revised so that tumors involving the IVC and those involving the RC are not grouped together as stage T3b. The experience of 1 center with renal cell carcinoma involving the venous system was reviewed, and the implications of these findings for prognosis was assessed.

Methods.—A retrospective review was conducted of the records of 226 patients who underwent a nephrectomy and tumor thrombectomy for RV (117 patients) and IVC (109 patients) involvement between 1998 and 2001. Findings for these patients were compared with those of 654 patients who underwent nephrectomy without venous involvement.

Results.—Among patients with localized renal cell carcinoma (N0M0), the risk of recurrence after nephrectomy was significantly increased for patients with venous thrombus compared with patients without venous thrombus. However, the significance of this difference did not persist in multivariate analysis. In patients with localized renal cell carcinoma, disease-specific survival was similar in patients with RV and IVC involvement below the diaphragm (T3b). However, survival was significantly worse on multivariate analysis for patients with IVC involvement above the diaphragm. All patients treated for metastatic renal cell carcinoma had a similar prognosis, regardless of the level of venous involvement.

Conclusion.—For patients with stage pT3b renal cell carcinoma, local tumor stage and grade are better predictors of prognosis than the extent of venous involvement. These findings support the current TNM classification of venous involvement with RV and IVC invasion.

► Renal carcinoma is well known to invade into the RV and up the IVC. Controversy exists as to whether the level of the thrombus influences survival. Both of these groups attempted to determine if the extent of the thrombus predicts the risk of recurrence. The group from UCLA (Abstract 13–10) found that patients with thrombus had higher recurrence rates than those without and that patients with thrombus above the diaphragm had higher recurrence rates than patients with thrombus below the diaphragm. The group from the Lahey Clinic (Abstract 13–9) found that survival (not recurrence) was better for patients with RV thrombus than IVC thrombus and that the level of thrombus in the IVC made no difference.

While the conclusions drawn by the 2 groups are slightly different, I believe this is due more to analysis of the data than fundamental differences in patient outcome. First and foremost, as in all retrospective analysis, selection is the silent partner of the surgeon. As a result, while on paper the patients being operated on at UCLA and at the Lahey Clinic appear to be a similar cohort, in point of fact they may be quite different.

Second, the differences may simply be a result of sample size. For example, the UCLA group's Kaplan Meier curves demonstrate that extent of thrombus influences disease-specific survival, but since the sample size is small, the differences are not statistically significant. Interestingly, the UCLA group also did multivariant analysis and found that grade, T stage, and performance status were much more important than the presence of a thrombus.

The bottom line is that no matter what the thrombus extent, these patients' only chance for cure is surgical excision. For that reason, I believe all tumors that are surgically resectable in patients with adequate performance status should be offered surgical excision. The alternative is either death from metastatic disease as the disease progresses or fatal pulmonary embolism when the thrombus breaks free.

A. S. Kibel, MD

Long-term Survival of Patients With Unilateral Sporadic Multifocal Renal Cell Carcinoma According to Histologic Subtype Compared With Patients With Solitary Tumors After Radical Nephrectomy

DiMarco DS, Lohse CM, Zincke H, et al (Mayo Clinic, Rochester, Minn)
Urology 64:462-467, 2004 13–11

Objectives.—To determine the pathologic features, including histologic subtype and tumor size, associated with multifocal renal cell carcinoma (RCC) and the impact of multifocality on survival after radical nephrectomy, about which controversy exists.

Methods.—We studied 2373 patients who underwent radical nephrectomy for RCC from 1970 to 2000. Histologic subtype, stage (2003 TNM), nuclear grade, tumor size, and multifocality, defined as the presence of more than one ipsilateral RCC tumor of the same histologic subtype, were evaluated. Associations of multifocality with ipsilateral and contralateral recurrence and death from RCC were evaluated using Cox proportional hazards models.

Results.—The incidence of sporadic histologically concordant multifocality was greater in papillary RCC (29 of 266; 10.9%) compared with clear cell RCC (40 of 1934; 2.0%; $P < 0.001$) and chromophobe RCC (2 of 104; 1.9%; $P = 0.005$). Patients with solitary clear cell and papillary RCC had larger tumors compared with multifocal clear cell and papillary RCC ($P < 0.001$ and $P = 0.024$, respectively). Patients with multifocal clear cell RCC were more likely to have a contralateral recurrence than were patients with solitary clear cell RCC (risk ratio 2.91, $P = 0.142$). Multifocality was not significantly associated with ipsilateral recurrence or death from RCC in patients with clear cell or papillary RCC.

Conclusions.—The incidence of multifocality was significantly greater among patients with papillary RCC than among patients with clear cell or chromophobe RCC. Patients with multifocal clear cell RCC were more likely to experience a contralateral recurrence. Multifocality was not significantly associated with ipsilateral recurrence or death from RCC. In addition, multifocality was not associated with larger and higher stage tumors, as previously reported.

▶ There are emerging data demonstrating that different histologic subtypes of RCC are associated with different clinical behaviors. For instance, papillary RCC is more likely to be multifocal compared with clear cell renal carcinoma (10% vs 2%). This has important implications in regard to clinical decision making. Because papillary RCCs are more likely associated with multifocal disease, some might argue that these tumors are best treated with total nephrectomy. Alternatively, as I believe, the increased risk of multifocality is associated with increased risk of bilateral tumors and it is exactly these patients who should undergo partial nephrectomy. In fact, in this report, patients with multifocal tumors were more likely to experience a contralateral recurrence than those with a solitary tumor but were not more likely to experience a local recurrence or death from RCC. Thus, I believe that when technically feasible, patients with multiple renal tumors should undergo nephron-sparing surgery rather than total nephrectomy, particularly for papillary tumors.

D. K. Ornstein, MD

Early Onset Hereditary Papillary Renal Carcinoma: Germline Missense Mutations in the Tyrosine Kinase Domain of the Met Proto-Oncogene

Schmidt LS, Nickerson ML, Angeloni D, et al (NIH, Bethesda, Md; Natl Cancer Inst, Rockville, Md; et al)

J Urol 172:1256-1261, 2004 13–12

Purpose.—Hereditary papillary renal carcinoma (HPRC) is characterized by a predisposition to multiple, bilateral papillary type 1 renal tumors caused by inherited activating missense mutations in the tyrosine kinase domain of the *MET* proto-oncogene. In the current study we evaluated the clinical phenotype and germline *MET* mutation of 3 new HPRC families. We describe the early onset clinical features of HPRC.

Materials and Methods.—We identified new HPRC families of Italian (family 177), Spanish (family 223) and Cuban (family 268) descent. We evaluated their clinical features, performed *MET* mutation analysis by denaturing high performance liquid chromatography and DNA sequencing, and estimated age dependent penetrance and survival using Kaplan-Meier analysis. We characterized renal tumors by histology and fluorescence in situ hybridization.

Results.—Identical germline *MET* c.3522G→A mutations (V1110I) were identified in families 177 and 268 but no evidence of a founder effect was found. Affected members of family 223 carried a germline c.3906G→C.3522G→A *MET* mutation (V1238I). Age dependent penetrance but not survival was significantly earlier for the c.3522G→A mutation than for the c.3906G→A mutation in these HPRC families. Trisomy of chromosome 7 and papillary renal carcinoma type 1 histology were detected in papillary renal tumors.

Conclusions.—HPRC can occur in an early onset form. The median age for renal tumor development in these 3 HPRC families was 46 to 63 years. HPRC associated papillary renal tumors may be aggressive and metastasize, leading to mortality. Median survival age was 60 to 70 years. Families with identical germline mutations in *MET* do not always share a common ancestor. HPRC is characterized by germline mutations in *MET* and papillary type 1 renal tumor histology.

▶ Renal cell carcinoma is associated with 4 different hereditary syndromes: von Hippel-Lindau disease, hereditary leiomyomatosis and renal cell carcinoma, Birt-Hogg-Dube syndrome, and HPRC. Each of these symdrones is the result of different genetic defects and each are associated with renal tumors of different histologic subtypes. HPRC is a form of inherited kidney cancer characterized by bilateral multifocal renal tumors of papillary histology. Mutations in the tyrosine kinase domain of the *MET* proto-oncogene are the inherited genetic defect responsible for HPRC. Similar to other inherited cancer syndromes, not all mutations result in the same clinical phenotype. In this report it is shown that a specific mutation c.3522G-A is associated with an earlier age of unset of papillary renal cell carcinomas. Although this specific mutation is a rare cause of renal cell carcinoma, this report demonstrates an important concept related to the molecular cause of renal cancer. That is mutations in the *MET* proto-oncogene are not an "all or nothing" event but rather the specific mutations lead to renal cancers with unique clinical phenotypes. In the future, molecular information could be used to help tailor follow-up and treatment strategies for affected families with specific mutations.

D. K. Ornstein, MD

Polymorphisms of the *CYP1B1* Gene as Risk Factors for Human Renal Cell Cancer

Sasaki M, Tanaka Y, Okino ST, et al (Univ of California, San Francisco; Kagoshima Univ, Japan; Kagoshima Univ, Japan; et al)

Clin Cancer Res 10:2015-2019, 2004 13–13

Purpose.—*CYP1B1* activates various environmental carcinogens in human tissues, including renal tissues. We hypothesize that certain polymorphisms of the *CYP1B1* gene are risk factors for renal cell cancer. The rationale for this hypothesis is that chemical procarcinogenic compounds require metabolic activation by oxidative enzymes such as *CYP1B1* to be transformed into potentially carcinogenic forms. To test this hypothesis, we investigated the genotypic distributions of six different loci on the *CYP1B1* gene and their association with renal cell cancer.

Experimental Design.—DNA from 211 cases of human renal cell cancer and 200 healthy controls was analyzed by sequence-specific PCR and direct DNA sequencing to determine the genotypic frequencies of six different polymorphic loci on the *CYP1B1* gene.

Results.—The results of this study demonstrate that the frequencies of genotype *119T/T* and genotype *432G/G* were significantly higher in renal cell cancer patients compared with healthy normal controls. The relative risks were calculated as 3.01 and 2.17 for genotypes *119T/T* and *432G/G*, respectively, in renal cell carcinoma patients. These genotypic distributions were also significantly different between male and female patients. The relative risks of genotype *119T/T* were calculated as 3.95 in males and 1.92 in females, and the relative risks of genotype *432G/G* were calculated as 2.81 in males and 1.35 in females.

Conclusions.—The present study demonstrates for the first time that the polymorphisms at codons 119 and 432 may be risk factors for renal cancer, especially in the male population.

► Polymorphisms are single base-pair changes that can result in an amino acid change but does not prevent translation of the full length protein. There is emerging evidence that specific genetic polymorphisms are associated with increased risk of disease. The *CYP1B1* gene encodes for an oxidative enzyme that activates procarcinogenic compounds. Cell culture studies have demonstrated that certain polymorphisms of the *CYP1B1* gene are associated with increased enzymatic activity. This report demonstrates that 2 specific polymorphisms (*432G/G* and *119T/T*) are associated with a 2- to 3-fold increased risk to develop renal cell carcinoma. Because this study was conducted in Japan, these findings may not be widely applicable. Despite this caveat, this is an important example of the potential predictive value of genetic polymorphisms. It is likely in the future, cancer screening will be individualized based on a person's unique genetic makeup.

D. K. Ornstein, MD

Quantitative Detection of Promoter Hypermethylation of Multiple Genes in the Tumor, Urine, and Serum DNA of Patients With Renal Cancer

Hoque MO, Begum S, Topaloglu O, et al (Johns Hopkins School of Medicine, Baltimore, Md)

Cancer Res 64:5511-5517, 2004 13–14

Introduction.—Aberrant promoter hypermethylation of several known or putative tumor suppressor genes occurs frequently during the pathogenesis of human cancers and is a promising marker for cancer detection. We investigated the feasibility of detecting aberrant DNA methylation in the urine and serum samples of renal cancer patients. We examined the tumor and the matched urine and serum DNA for aberrant methylation of 9 gene promoters (CDH1, APC, MGMT, RASSF1A, GSTP1, p16, RAR-beta2, and ARF) from 17 patients with primary kidney cancer by quantitative fluorogenic real-time PCR. An additional 9 urine samples (total, 26) and 1 serum sample (total, 18) also were tested from renal cancer patients. Urine from 91 patients without genitourinary cancer and serum from 30 age-matched noncancer individuals were used as controls. Promoter hypermethylation of at least two of the genes studied was detected in 16 (94%) of 17 primary tumors. Aberrant methylation in urine and serum DNA generally was accompanied by methylation in the matched tumor samples. Urine samples from 91 control subjects without evidence of genitourinary cancer revealed no methylation of the *MGMT*, *GSTP1*, *p16*, and *ARF* genes, whereas methylation of *RAR-β2*, *RASSF1A*, *CDH1*, *APC*, and *TIMP3* was detected at low levels in a few control subjects. Overall, 23 (88%) of 26 urine samples and 12 (67%) of 18 serum samples from cancer patients were methylation positive for at least one of the genes tested. By combination of urine or serum analysis of renal cancer patients, hypermethylation was detected in 16 of 17 patients (94% sensitivity) with high specificity. Our findings suggest that promoter hypermethylation in urine or serum can be detected in the majority of renal cancer patients. This noninvasive high-throughput approach needs to be evaluated in large studies to assess its value in the early detection and surveillance of renal cancer.

► In addition to gene mutations and deletions, DNA hypermethylation is a common mechanism to silence tumor suppressor genes in cancer. In fact, aberrant promoter hypermethylation is a common finding in most human cancers. This fact is now being exploited in an attempt to develop better noninvasive cancer diagnostic tests. It has been reported that a series of specific genes are commonly hypermethylated in kidney cancers. In this report 94% of tumors displayed hypermethylation of at least 2 of 9 genes. Most importantly there was a strong collection between detection of promoter hypermethylation in serum and/or urine from patients with renal cell carcinomas in promoter hypermethylation was detected. Combining methylation of serum and urine yielded a 94% sensitivity for the detection of renal cell cancer. More importantly promoter methylation is highly specific for malignancy because it was not detected (except for the *TIMP1* gene) in any of the 91 control patients. Molecular analysis of human body fluids (urine and serum) holds great promise as a useful noninvasive diagnostic tool for human cancers.

D. K. Ornstein, MD

Molecular Profiling and Classification of Sporadic Renal Cell Carcinoma by Quantitative Methylation Analysis

Gonzalgo ML, Yegnasubramanian S, Yan G, et al (Johns Hopkins Med Institutions, Baltimore, Md)

Clin Cancer Res 10:7276-7283, 2004 13–15

Purpose.—Preoperative histologic classification of solid renal masses remains limited with current technology. We determine the utility of molecular profiling based on quantitative methylation analysis for characterization of sporadic renal cell carcinoma.

Experimental Design.—Primary renal cell carcinomas representing three different histologic subtypes were obtained from a total of 38 patients who underwent radical nephrectomy for suspected malignant disease. Genomic DNA was isolated from tumors and was subjected to sodium bisulfite modification. The normalized index of methylation (NIM) for each sample was determined by quantitative real-time methylation-specific PCR at 17 different gene promoters. Hierarchical cluster analysis was performed by using an unsupervised neural network with binary tree topology.

Results.—The majority of gene promoters that were analyzed in this study demonstrated very low levels of methylation (NIM <1.0). The *RASSF1A* gene promoter, however, was methylated in 30 of 38 (79%) cases. The frequency of *RASSF1A* methylation in papillary, clear-cell, and oncocytoma subtypes was 100, 90, and 25%, respectively. The highest levels of *RASSF1A* methylation were observed in the papillary (mean NIM = 78.9) and clear-cell (mean NIM = 13.4) subtypes. The vast majority of oncocytomas were completely unmethylated, and none demonstrated >1% methylation (mean NIM = 0.11). Hierarchical cluster analysis based on quantitative methylation levels resulted in stratification of sporadic renal cell carcinomas into their discrete histologic subtypes.

Conclusions.—Classification of sporadic renal cell carcinomas into histologic subtypes can be accomplished via multigene quantitative methylation profiling. Validation of this approach and selection of appropriate methylation markers may ultimately lead to use of this technology in the preoperative assessment of suspicious renal masses.

▶ There is emerging data demonstrating that different histologic subtypes of renal cell carcinoma are associated with different genetic alterations. The most common and best characterized subtype, clear cell, is commonly associated with an alteration in the *VHL* gene. Most commonly *VHL* is inactivated by a mutation and/or deletion, but gene silencing by promoter methylation has also been observed. It has been suggested that in addition to *VHL*, promoter methylation of several other genes occurs commonly in renal cell carcinoma. In this study the methylation status of 17 different genes was evaluated. Only the *RASSF1A* gene was commonly methylated (in 79% of cases). Interestingly, *RASSF1A* was methylated in 100% of papillary and 90% of clear cells, but was not methylated in benign oncocytomas. These findings suggest that the methylation status of *RASSF1A* may be a useful molecular marker to help discriminate malignant from benign renal masses but will not help histologic classification. If it is possible to accurately determine the *RASSF1A* methylation status from a fine needle aspirate, this test may have important clinical relevance in regard to the management of patients with small indeterminant renal masses.

D. K. Ornstein, MD

Phase II Trial of Bortezomib for Patients With Advanced Renal Cell Carcinoma

Kondagunta GV, Drucker B, Schwartz L, et al (Mem Sloan-Kettering Cancer Ctr, New York; Cornell Univ, New York)
J Clin Oncol 22:3720-3725, 2004 13–16

Purpose.—To assess the efficacy and toxicity of bortezomib (Velcade; Millennium Pharmaceuticals Inc, Cambridge, MA; formerly PS-341) in patients with metastatic renal cell carcinoma (RCC).

Patients and Methods.—Thirty-seven patients with metastatic RCC were treated with bortezomib. The first 25 patients enrolled onto the trial were treated with a dose of 1.5 mg/m^2. The dose was decreased to 1.3 mg/m^2 for the subsequent 12 patients, because more than 50% of the patients treated at the higher dose required dose reductions. Bortezomib was given by intravenous administration on a twice-weekly schedule for 2 weeks followed by 1 week without treatment until progression or unacceptable toxicity occurred. Twenty-three patients (62%) previously had undergone nephrectomy, and 19 patients (51%) had previously been treated with cytokine therapy.

Results.—Of the 37 assessable patients, the best response was a partial response in four patients (11%; 95% CI, 3% to 25%) and stable disease in 14 patients (38%; 95% CI, 23% to 55%). The four patients with partial response experienced response durations of 8, 8+, 15+, and 20+ months. Grade 2 or 3 sensory neuropathy was present in 10 patients (53%) overall. One patient in the 1.5 mg/m² group had grade 3 sensory neuropathy; no grade 3 sensory neuropathy was seen in the 1.3 mg/m² group.

Conclusion.—The results of this trial suggest that bortezomib has an antitumor effect in individual patients with metastatic RCC. The small proportion of patients who achieved a partial response does not support routine use in metastatic RCC. Efforts to identify the molecular profile associated with clinical response or combination therapy with interferon α or other novel agents, may be considered.

► Proteosomes are enzymatic systems that normally degrade proteins tagged for destruction by ubiquitin. Dysregulation of the proteosome system may play a role in cancer progression and chemotherapy residence. Bortezomib is a proteosome inhibitor that has been shown to have some activity against malignant melanoma. In this trial of patients with metastatic RCC that was refractory to cytokine therapy, only 11% experienced a partial response and 38% stabilization of disease. More than 50% of the patients experienced sensory neuropathies. Although these results do not support the use of bortezomib as a single agent for the treatment of metastatic RCC, further study into the role of proteosome inhibitors is warranted. In particular, there is theoretical evidence to suggest that bortezomib may potentiate an antitumor effect for cytokine or chemotherapy. An interesting trial design would combine bortezomib with interferon and/or chemotherapy.

D. K. Ornstein, MD

Adjuvant Autologous Renal Tumour Cell Vaccine and Risk of Tumour Progression in Patients With Renal-Cell Carcinoma After Radical Nephrectomy: Phase III, Randomised Controlled Trial

Jocham D, Richter A, Hoffmann L, et al (Univ of Lübeck, Germany; Klinikum St Georg, Leipzig, Germany; Wald-Klinikum Gera, Meiningen, Germany; et al)

Lancet 363:594-599, 2004 13–17

Background.—Organ-confined renal-cell carcinoma is associated with tumor progression in nearly half of patients after radical nephrectomy. Currently, no effective adjuvant treatment is available to reduce the risk of tumor progression after nephrectomy for these patients. The effect of an autologous renal tumor cell vaccine on the risk of tumor progression in patients with stage pT2-3b pN0-3 MO renal cell carcinoma was determined.

Methods.—This multicenter study included 558 patients with a renal tumor scheduled for radical nephrectomy between January 1997 and September 1998 at 55 centers in Germany. All of the patients were centrally selected randomly before surgery to receive either autologous renal tumor cell vaccine (vaccine group) or no adjuvant treatment (control group). The main outcome measure was the reduction in risk of tumor progression, which was defined as progression or death. All of the patients were assessed after standardized diagnostic investigations at 6-month intervals for a minimum of 4 to 5 years.

Results.—Of the 558 patients enrolled, 379 were assessable for the intention-to-treat analysis. At 5-year and 70-month follow-up, the hazard ratios for tumor progression were 1.58 and 1.59, respectively, in favor of the vaccine group. The 5-year and 70-month progression-free survival rates were 77.4% and 72%, respectively, in the control group. The vaccine was well tolerated, and only 12 adverse events associated with receipt of the vaccine occurred.

Conclusions.—Adjuvant autologous renal tumor cell vaccine is beneficial in patients with renal cell carcinoma who have undergone radical nephrectomy. This therapy should be considered in such patients with organ-confirmed renal-cell carcinoma of greater than 2.5 cm in diameter.

▶ The management of the locally advanced renal carcinoma is difficult. We know that many patients will fail and once they have metastatic disease, the likelihood of cure is remote. For this reason, several groups have begun using immunotherapy in the adjuvant setting to improve cure rates. This multi-institutional study from Germany gave patients with T2 and T3, N0-3, M0 renal cell carcinoma an autologous tumor vaccine. The endpoint was progression-free survival, not disease-specific or overall survival. The authors found, in an intent-to-treat analysis, the treatment group was less likely to progress, and the benefit was most notable in patients with T3 disease. In addition, while no data were presented, they did state in the discussion that patients with other risk factors, such as high tumor grade and larger tumor size, derived greater benefit than the group as a whole.

I hope with additional follow-up, we will see a disease specific or overall survival benefit. If other adjuvant immunotherapy trials demonstrate similar results, we will finally have a treatment that improves patients' outcome with high-risk renal cell carcinoma.

A. S. Kibel, MD

Is Frozen Section Analysis in Nephron Sparing Surgery Necessary? A Clinicopathological Study of 301 Cases

Duvdevani M, Laufer M, Kastin A, et al (Chaim Sheba Med Ctr, Ramat-Gan, Israel; Bnei Zion Med Ctr, Haifa, Israel)

J Urol 173:385-387, 2005 13–18

Purpose.—One of the basic principles of nephron sparing surgery for renal cell carcinoma is resection of the tumor with normal tissue margins verified by frozen section analysis. In cases of positive tumor margins the surgeon is committed to complete the local resection or to perform radical nephrectomy. In this study we retrospectively evaluated the yield of frozen section analysis performed during nephron sparing surgeries, especially concerning compatibility with the final histological report and the long-term oncological outcome.

Materials and Methods.—Between 1988 and 2003, 172 men and 129 women with a mean age of 59 years (range 16 to 83) underwent nephron sparing surgery due to suspected renal tumors. Mean tumor size was 3.56 cm (range 1 to 12.5). Frozen section analysis was routinely performed during surgery.

Results.—Positive tumor margins in frozen section analysis were found in 2 cases (0.7%). In both cases the tumor was centrally located. Those 2 patients underwent immediate radical nephrectomy but no residual tumor was subsequently found in the radical nephrectomy specimens. Paraffin sections disclosed positive tumor margins in 4 other cases (1.3%) in whom the frozen section analysis had shown tumor negative margins. Of the 4 patients 1 underwent radical nephrectomy for tumor recurrence after 9 months. The other 3 patients showed no evidence of disease recurrence after 26, 59 and 120 months of followup.

Conclusions.—Our results suggest that frozen section analysis during nephron sparing surgery has minimal clinical significance and hence routine incorporation in urological practice should be reconsidered.

▶ It is common practice to perform intraoperative frozen sections during nephron-sparing surgery to assure negative margins. Although this practice is commonly accepted, it has not been proven to be beneficial. This report specifically questions the use of routing intraoperative frozen sections. In a series of 301 patients undergoing partial nephrectomy for renal cell carcinoma, frozen sections were positive in only 2 cases. Disturbingly, both of these patients underwent radical nephrectomy and no residual tumor was found. Furthermore, 4 cases had positive margins on permanent sections, despite a negative frozen section. These findings suggest that information derived from intraoperative frozen sections at the time of partial nephrectomy is probably not helpful and may even be misleading. The routine use of frozen sections during nephron-sparing surgery should be reexamined.

D. K. Ornstein, MD

14 Urothelial Cancer

Detection of Bladder Cancer Using a Point-of-Care Proteomic Assay

Grossman HB, Messing E, Soloway M, et al (MD Anderson Cancer Ctr, Houston; Univ of Rochester, NY; Univ of Miami, Fla; et al)

JAMA 293:810-816, 2005 14–1

Context.—A combination of methods is used for diagnosis of bladder cancer because no single procedure detects all malignancies. Urine tests are frequently part of an evaluation, but have either been nonspecific for cancer or required specialized analysis at a laboratory.

Objective.—To investigate whether a point-of-care proteomic test that measures the nuclear matrix protein NMP22 in voided urine could enhance detection of malignancy in patients with risk factors or symptoms of bladder cancer.

Design, Setting, and Patients.—Twenty-three academic, private practice, and veterans' facilities in 10 states prospectively enrolled consecutive patients from September 2001 to May 2002. Participants included 1331 patients at elevated risk for bladder cancer due to factors such as history of smoking or symptoms including hematuria and dysuria. Patients at risk for malignancy of the urinary tract provided a voided urine sample for analysis of NMP22 protein and cytology prior to cystoscopy.

Main Outcome Measures.—The diagnosis of bladder cancer, based on cystoscopy with biopsy, was accepted as the reference standard. The performance of the NMP22 test was compared with voided urine cytology as an aid to cancer detection. Testing for the NMP22 tumor marker was conducted in a blinded manner.

Results.—Bladder cancer was diagnosed in 79 patients. The NMP22 assay was positive in 44 of 79 patients with cancer (sensitivity, 55.7%; 95% confidence interval [CI], 44.1%-66.7%), whereas cytology test results were positive in 12 of 76 patients (sensitivity, 15.8%; 95% CI, 7.6%-24.0%). The specificity of the NMP22 assay was 85.7% (95% CI, 83.8%-87.6%) compared with 99.2% (95% CI, 98.7%-99.7%) for cytology. The proteomic marker detected 4 cancers that were not visualized during initial endoscopy, including 3 that were muscle invasive and 1 carcinoma in situ.

Conclusion.—The noninvasive point-of-care assay for elevated urinary NMP22 protein can increase the accuracy of cystoscopy, with test results available during the patient visit.

▶ There are 2 possible uses for a urine-based bladder cancer screening test. The first is to replace cystoscopy, and the second is to act as an adjunct to cystoscopy. Cytology, the most common urine based test, is used only as an adjunct to cystoscopy because it fails to identify many tumors. Newer urine tests attempt to fill both voids and in most cases come up short.

While the results of the NMP22 test are clearly impressive, the fact that it missed 35 tumors and had a sensitivity of only 55.7% would indicate that it is not ready to replace cystoscopy. Whether the NMP22 test can replace cytology as an adjunct to cystoscopy is a more difficult question. The receiver/operator characteristics are clearly better for the NMP22 test than cytology. In addition, 1) this office based test provides a rapid result, 2) it is not dependent on the ability of the pathologist, and 3) it has significantly lower cost than cytology. Still on the negative side, the specificity of the NMP22 test was 85.7% compared to 99.2% for cytology. What does this mean in clinical practice? We all know that some of the most difficult patients to manage are those with positive cytologies and no evidence of carcinoma. My concern is that routine use of the NMP22 test will result in a larger population of patients in a very similar position: a positive test but no evidence of any malignancy. Are these patients a ticking time bomb or is it simply a false positive?

This test has shown a great deal of promise, and this study supports its use in clinical practice. It will simply be a matter of time and physician experience to determine how useful the test will be.

A. S. Kibel, MD

Alkylaniline–Hemoglobin Adducts and Risk of Non–Smoking-Related Bladder Cancer

Gan J, Skipper PL, Gago-Dominguez, et al (Massachusetts Inst of Technology, Cambridge; Univ of Southern California, Los Angeles)

J Natl Cancer Inst 96:1425-1431, 2004 14–2

Background.—Some members of the arylamine family of compounds, specifically 4-aminobiphenyl (ABP), 2-naphthylamine, and benzidine, are established human bladder carcinogens. Cigarette smoking and use of permanent hair dye contribute substantially to current arylamine exposure. Low levels of 4-ABP exposure have been associated with non-smoking-related bladder cancer. Other arylamine compounds coming from as yet unidentified environmental sources may also be human bladder carcinogens.

Methods.—We conducted a population-based case-control study in Los Angeles County, California, involving 298 case subjects with bladder cancer and 308 control subjects, who were matched on age, sex, race/ethnicity, and neighborhood of residence. In-person interviews provided information on tobacco smoking and other potential risk factors for bladder cancer. To assess arylamine exposure, levels of arylamine-hemoglobin adducts of nine selected alkylanilines (2,3-dimethylaniline [2,3-DMA], 2,4-DMA, 2,5-DMA, 2,6-DMA, 3,4-DMA, 3,5-DMA, 2-ethylaniline [2-EA], 3-EA, 4-EA) were measured in peripheral blood collected from study subjects. Analysis of covariance and conditional logistic regression methods were used to analyze the relationship between arylamine-hemoglobin adducts and bladder cancer risk. All statistical tests were two-sided.

Results.—Levels of all arylamine-hemoglobin adducts, with the exception of 2,6-DMA, were higher in smokers than in nonsmokers, and levels of all arylamine-hemoglobin adducts were higher in case subjects than in control subjects. Arylamine-hemoglobin adducts of 2,6-DMA, 3,5-DMA, and 3-EA were all independently, statistically significantly (all $P<.001$) associated with bladder cancer risk after adjusting for cigarette smoking at the time of blood collection, lifetime smoking history, and other potential risk factors. These adducts were also independently associated with bladder cancer risk when only nonsmokers at time of blood draw were considered (highest quartile versus lowest quartile: 2,6-DMA, relative risk [RR] of bladder cancer = 8.1, 95% confidence interval [CI] = 3.6 to 18.0; 3,5-DMA, RR = 2.7, 95% CI = 1.2 to 6.0; 3-EA, RR = 4.3, 95% CI = 1.6 to 11.6).

Conclusions.—Diverse arylamine exposures are strongly associated with bladder cancer risk among nonsmokers. Because arylamines may account for a substantial proportion of bladder cancers among the general population, identification of environmental sources of these compounds is needed.

▶ One of the most striking statistics about bladder cancer is that approximately 50% of the disease is attributable to cigarette smoking. One of the most clinically intriguing aspects of this statistic is that means that 50% of bladder cancer is not attributable to smoking. This rather nice study demonstrates that arylamines may account for a substantial portion of the bladder cancer risk. The authors examined 298 case subjects with bladder cancer and 308 controls and found that the arylamine hemoglobin adducts were significantly higher in the patients than in the controls. The risk associated with adducts was particularly strong when analysis was limited to nonsmokers.

One of the key aspects of this study is that the controls were matched by race, age, and geographic location. This would imply that both patients and controls were exposed to similar environmental carcinogens. While this study did not attempt to identify the source of the arylamines, future work identify the environmental sources of these carcinogenic compounds is clearly warranted.

A. S. Kibel, MD

Bladder Cancer as a Prognostic Factor for Upper Tract Transitional Cell Carcinoma

Mullerad M, Russo P, Golijanin D, et al (Mem Sloan-Kettering Cancer Ctr, New York)

J Urol 172:2177-2181, 2004 14–3

Purpose.—Upper tract transitional cell carcinoma (UTTCC) is a relatively rare tumor. Overall 5-year disease specific survival is in the range of 16.5% to 95% depending on stage. In this study we evaluated predictors associated with disease recurrence and disease specific survival.

Materials and Methods.—We report on 129 patients with a median age of 68 years who underwent nephroureterectomy for UTTCC between July 1989 and June 2002. A total of 67 patients had primary UTTCC and 62 had previous (52) or synchronous (10) transitional cell carcinoma of the bladder (BTCC). Medical records were reviewed and analyzed for possible prognostic predictors (primary tumor stage, grade, multifocality, carcinoma in situ, symptoms and signs at presentation, sex, and history of smoking). Disease specific survival and freedom from bladder recurrence were assessed with the Kaplan-Meier method, and differences between the groups were compared using the log rank test. The Cox proportional hazards regression model was used to assess the significance of each predictor.

Results.—Disease specific death was reported for 44 patients. In a multivariate analysis using previous BTCC as a predictor (categorized as superficial, invasive or none), primary disease stage and history of BTCC were associated with disease specific survival ($p = 0.001$ and $p = 0.018$). History of BTCC grouped the patients into distinct populations in terms of disease specific survival and freedom from bladder recurrence.

Conclusions.—This study demonstrates that a history of BTCC (invasive or superficial) has an adverse effect on the prognosis of patients diagnosed with UTTCC independent of primary tumor stage.

▶ This rather nice study from Memorial Sloan-Kettering demonstrates an association between history of bladder carcinoma and disease-specific survival for UTTCC. All the patients examined underwent nephroureterectomy for UTTCC. Multivariant analysis demonstrated that history of bladder disease along with stage of the upper tract tumor were the primary determinants of disease-specific survival. Kaplan-Meier curves demonstrated a convincing separation of the curves which was statistically significant. It is important to emphasize that the bladder cancer was not necessarily synchronous with the upper tract disease.

The question is what to do with this information. If this result is replicated in other studies, it *may* provide an additional variable to choose patients for adjuvant chemotherapy.

A. S. Kibel, MD

Primary T1G3 Bladder Cancer: Organ Preserving Approach or Immediate Cystectomy

Thalmann GN, Markwalder R, Shahin O, et al (Univ of Bern, Switzerland)
J Urol 172:70-75, 2004 14–4

Introduction.—When treated with transurethral resection of the bladder (TURB) alone, transitional cell carcinoma invading the lamina propria of the bladder wall (stage T1) is linked with a high recurrence rate (69%-80%) and high progression rate (33%-48%) that impacts patient survival. Optimal treatment for primary T1G3 bladder cancer is under debate. The long-term outcome of patients with newly diagnosed stage T1G3 bladder cancer treated with TURB and bacillus Calmette-Guérin or immediate cystectomy was examined in a retrospective, nonrandomized investigation.

Methods.—The median age of 121 patients with a diagnosis of primary T1G3 bladder cancer given between 1976 and 1999 was 67 years (range, 36-88 years). Of these, 92 underwent TURB with additional bacillus Calmette-Guerin and 29 underwent immediate cystectomy.

Results.—Of 92 patients who underwent TURB, 29 remained disease free; 33 (36%) had local recurrence and 30 (33%) had progression at a median follow-up of 6.9 years (range, 0.6-16.5 years). Among these 92 patients, 27 (29%) underwent deferred cystectomy at a median of 12.9 months (range, 4.8-136 months). Ten (37%) with a median postoperative follow-up of 19 months (range, 2-173 months) died of progressive disease (median survival, 13 months; range, 3-34 months) post cystectomy.

Most patients who died of progressive disease refused cystectomy, were referred too late for cystectomy, were inoperable, or had upper urinary tract disease. Six of the 29 patients (21%) who underwent immediate cystectomy had progression at a median of 13.2 months (range, 5.5-37 months). The overall and tumor-specific survivals at 5 years for patients who underwent an organ-preserving approach were 69% and 80%, respectively. For those treated with immediate cystectomy, they were 54% and 69%, respectively.

Conclusion.—An organ-preserving approach is acceptable and spares the bladder in about half of patients with primary T1G3 bladder cancer. Of these, 30% need deferred cystectomy, which necessitates meticulous, close follow-up mandatory.

► Stage T1 high grade bladder cancer is a challenging problem. Managing patients with this stage of disease is often confounded by understaging. In this report, the authors show that meticulous and aggressive local care with TURB and intravesical bacillus Calmette-Guérin therapy can salvage the bladder in up to 50% of patients with high-grade T1 disease. Of their patients who initially underwent bladder-sparing salvage, cystectomy was equivalently effective as to those who underwent immediate cystectomy. This, however, is testimony to the aggressive follow-up regimen used by the authors. Clinicians who are applying this approach to high-grade T1 bladder cancer must realize that the onus of close follow-up is on them and their patients.

G. L. Andriole, Jr, MD

Microscopic and Gross Extravesical Extension in Pathological Staging of Bladder Cancer

Quek ML, Stein JP, Clark PE, et al (Univ of Southern California, Los Angeles)
J Urol 171:640-645, 2004 14–5

Background.—The standard treatment for high-grade, muscle-invasive bladder cancer is radical cystectomy. The long-term clinical outcomes of this treatment are directly related to pathologic stage and lymph node status. The 1997 revised TNM classification has stratified extravesical involvement, which was previously defined as pT3b, into microscopic (PTA) and gross (pT3b) extravesical tumor extension. Also, muscle-invasive, organ-confined tumors are stratified into superficial (PTA) and deep muscle (pT2b) involvement. There have been few studies of the TNM staging for bladder cancer in terms of predicting clinical outcomes. Clinical outcomes were evaluated for patients with pathologic microscopic (PTA) and gross (pT3b) extravesical tumor extension with transitional cell carcinoma of the bladder after radical cystectomy.

Methods.—Radical cystectomy for pathologic primary bladder transitional cell carcinoma with extravesical extension was performed in 236 patients (173 men and 63 women). Of these patients, 69 (29%) had PTA and 167 (71%) had pT3b disease. The main outcome measures were lymph node involvement, local and distant recurrences, and clinical outcomes at a median follow-up of 8.9 years (range, 0 to 19.4 years).

Results.—The 10-year recurrence-free survival rate was 48% for patients with PTA tumors and 47% for patients with pT3b disease. Recurrence-free survival was significantly better for patients with lymph node–negative disease than for patients with positive lymph nodes, regardless of the extent of extravesical involvement. Local pelvic recurrence developed in 13 of the 236 patients (6%), while 84 patients (36%) had distant metastatic disease. Of the patients with recurrence, the type of recurrence—whether local or distant—was not associated with tumor stage. Lymph node involvement was a significant risk factor for distant recurrence of tumor.

Conclusion.—There is no evidence of a prognostic significance to the differentiation between PTA and pT3b extravesical tumor involvement of transitional cell carcinoma as outlined in the revised 1997 TNM staging system.

► A common problem faced in management of bladder cancer is who needs adjuvant chemotherapy following cystectomy. By and large, most medical oncologists and urologic oncologists believe that extravesical extension is a key pathologic variable for predicting risk of recurrence. However, often there is the perception that a small amount of extravesical extension is not as significant and, for that reason, the current TNM staging system separates extravesical extension into T3a disease (microscopic fat involvement) and T3b disease (extensive extravesical involvement).

This group from UCLA found that the 10-year recurrence-free survival rate was practically identical at 48% for PT3a and 47% for PT3b. For this reason, I believe that patients who even have microscopic extension into the perivesical fat have tumors and should be referred to a medical oncologist to at least discuss whether or not adjuvant chemotherapy is of any utility.

A. S. Kibel, MD

Nodal Involvement in Bladder Cancer Cases Treated With Radical Cystectomy: Incidence and Prognosis

Abdel-Latif M, Abol-Enein H, El-Baz M, et al (Urology-Nephrology Ctr, Mansoura, Egypt)

J Urol 172:85-89, 2004 14–6

Introduction.—Regional lymph node status is an important predictor of survival in patients with bladder cancer who undergo cystectomy. The superiority of radical versus simple cystectomy has yet to be established by a randomized trial. Several retrospective trials have indicated that radical cystectomy can be curative in a subpopulation of patients with bladder cancer and nodal disease. Factors that promote the incidence of nodal metastasis were examined and survival predictors were characterized.

Methods.—A total of 418 bladder cancer patients treated with radical cystectomy and bilateral endopelvic lymphadenectomy were retrospectively examined. The incidence of nodal involvement was correlated with various patient and tumor characteristics. The number of involved nodes was additionally correlated with the number of retrieved nodes. Survival in node-positive cases was correlated with some select pathologic characteristics.

Results.—Nodal involvement was observed in 110 cases (26.3%). The mean number of harvested nodes per patient was 17.9 and the mean number of positive nodes per involved case was 4.1. A weak correlation was observed between the number of retrieved nodes and the number of positive nodes ($r = 0.4$). The tumor pT stage and grade and the lymphovascular invasion were independent factors fostering the rate of nodal involvement. The mean incidence of 3-year disease-free survival of patients who were node-positive was 37.8%. The pT stage and the number of positive nodes had an independent impact on survival among patients who were node-positive.

Conclusion.—Tumor pT stage and grade and lymphovascular invasion independently impact the incidence of lymph node involvement in patients with bladder cancer and nodal disease. A weak correlation was observed between the number of nodes retrieved and the number of positive nodes. The survival probability in cases of pT N+ cases depends on pT stage and the number of involved nodes.

► In this nice series of over 400 cases of invasive bladder cancer, 46% had pathologically confirmed positive nodes. The authors have attempted to correlate pathological T-stage, grade, lymphovascular invasion, and the number and proportion of positive lymph nodes with outcome. The 2 most important factors are pathologic T-stage and the number of positive nodes. This confirms earlier studies suggesting that node-positive disease can be cured in selected patients if the surgeon performs a meticulous and complete lymphadenectomy.

G. L. Andriole, Jr, MD

Surgical Factors Influence Bladder Cancer Outcomes: A Cooperative Group Report

Herr HW, Faulkner JR, Grossman HB, et al (Mem Sloan-Kettering Cancer Ctr, New York; Southwest Oncology Group Statistical Ctr, Seattle; Univ of Texas MD Anderson Cancer Ctr, Houston; et al)

J Clin Oncol 22:2781-2789, 2004 14–7

Purpose.—A randomized, cooperative group trial (Southwest Oncology Group 8710, Intergroup 0080) reported that neoadjuvant chemotherapy improved the survival of patients with locally advanced bladder cancer who were treated with radical cystectomy. We evaluated whether surgical factors from patients enrolled onto the study predicted bladder cancer outcomes.

Patients and Methods.—Surgical and tumor factors were recorded from surgical and pathologic reports from 268 patients with muscle-invasive bladder cancer who received radical cystectomy. Cystectomies were performed by 106 surgeons in 109 institutions. Half of the patients received neoadjuvant methotrexate, vinblastine, doxorubicin, and cisplatin (MVAC) chemotherapy. Variables were tested in univariate and multivariate analyses for associations with postcystectomy survival (PCS) and local recurrence (LR) in all patients receiving cystectomy.

Results.—Five-year PCS and LR rates were 54% and 15%, respectively. A multivariate model adjusted for MVAC (P =.97), age (P =.03), pathologic stage (P =.0002), and node status (P =.04) showed that surgical variables associated with longer PCS were negative margins (v positive; hazard ratio [HR], 0.37; P =.0007), and ≥ 10 nodes removed (v < 10; HR, 0.51; P =.0001). These associations did not differ by treatment arms (P > .21 for all tests of interactions between treatment and surgical variables). Predictors of LR in a multivariate model adjusted for MVAC (P =.16), pathologic stage (P =.02), and node status (P =.37) were positive margins (v negative; odds ratio [OR], 11.2; P =.0001) and fewer than 10 nodes removed (v ≤ 10; OR, 5.1; P =.002).

Conclusion.—Surgical factors influence bladder cancer outcomes after cystectomy, after adjustment for pathologic factors and neoadjuvant chemotherapy usage.

► The bottom line is that surgical quality matters. SWOG-8710 examined the role of neoadjuvant chemotherapy in the treatment of bladder carcinoma. This study examines surgical factors to determine if they predict survival and LR rates. The authors found that survival was related factors that are beyond the control of the surgeon (ie, age), and factors that are at least in part within the control of the surgeon (ie, margin rates and number of nodes removed).

For example, survival was improved if 10 lymph nodes or more were removed irrespective of whether they were positive or not. To put this another way: If the patient had lymph node-negative disease, he benefited from an aggressive lymph node dissection *and* if the patient has positive lymph nodes, he benefited from a more aggressive dissection. In fact, if you simply broke patients down into those who received no lymph node dissection versus limited lymph node dissection versus standard lymph node dissection, patients who received the standard lymph node dissection did best followed by those who received a limited lymph node dissection followed by those who received none.

The author's analysis was not limited to quality of lymph node dissection. For example, they found that operative setting affected survival with survival being highest in academic institutions. A second example is that they found that surgeons who describe themselves as urologic oncologists have better survival rates than general urologists. I think the most striking thing about this paper.

The bottom line is surgical quality matters. We should all continue to strive to perform the best possible operation. While chemotherapy is very useful in the adjuvant and neoadjuvant setting, we cure patients with good operations and should continue to strive for perfection.

A. S. Kibel, MD

Partial Cystectomy: A Contemporary Review of the Memorial Sloan-Kettering Cancer Center Experience and Recommendations for Patient Selection

Holzbeierlein JM, Lopez-Corona E, Bochner BH, et al (Mem Sloan-Kettering Cancer Ctr, New York)

J Urol 172:878-881, 2004 14–8

Background.—In highly selected patients, partial cystectomy is a reasonable alternative to radical resection for the treatment of invasive bladder cancer. Authors from the Memorial Sloan-Kettering Cancer Center review their recent experience with partial cystectomy for invasive bladder cancer, and identify selection criteria for maximizing outcomes.

Methods.—The medical records of 58 patients (81% men, mean age 65.5 years) with primary bladder cancer who underwent partial cystectomy from 1995 to 2001 were reviewed. Patients were followed a mean of 33 months to identify demographic and clinical characteristics most closely associated with outcomes.

Results.—Most of the patients (79%) had transitional cell carcinoma, and most had clinical stage Ta (7%), T1 (22%), or T2 (59%) disease. The most common tumor location was the dome (41%). During follow-up, 12 patients (21%) died of disease and 2 patients (3%) died of other causes. Of the remaining 44 patients, 40 (69% of total) had no evidence of disease at last follow-up, and 4 patients (7%) were alive with disease at last follow-up. The Kaplan-Meier estimate for 5-year overall survival was 69%. At last follow-up, all but 1 of the survivors had an intact bladder; 39 of these patients (67% of total) were currently disease-free, including 32 (55%) who had been continuously disease-free since the partial cystectomy. Recurrence in the bladder developed in 11 patients (19%). In 7 of these 11 patients (12% of total), the recurrence was superficial (Ta-T1), and treatment with transurethral resection of bladder tumor (TURBT) alone or with bacillus Calmette-Guérin was successful. One patient with a focal muscle-invasive recurrence underwent cystectomy and had been recurrence-free for 20 months. The other 3 patients with recurrence had locally advanced cancer that was either unresectable (2 cases) or recurred in the pelvis shortly after surgery (1 case). In all, 12 patients (21%) had recurrence with metastatic disease. Five patients had positive margins after partial cystectomy; 4 of them developed advanced recurrence. Similarly, 5 patients had positive lymph nodes after partial cystectomy; 4 of them developed advanced recurrence. Univariate regression analyses indicated concomitant carcinoma in situ (CIS), and multifocality before surgery significantly increased the risk of superficial recurrence. Multivariate regression analyses indicated that concomitant CIS (odds ratio 7.05) and lymph node involvement at partial cystectomy (odds ratio 4.38) were significant independent predictors of advanced recurrence.

Conclusion.—Partial cystectomy provides good long-term results in highly selected patients with invasive bladder cancer. Patients with concomitant CIS or multifocal disease before surgery are at increased risk of superficial recurrence and, thus, are poor candidates for partial cystectomy. Similarly, patients with concomitant CIS or metastasis to lymph nodes at partial cystectomy are at increased risk of developing advanced disease. Also, patients with positive margins after partial cystectomy are more likely to develop advanced recurrence, and should be considered for radical cystectomy.

► Partial cystectomy is an underutilized treatment for bladder cancer. This retrospective review of the partial cystectomy experience at Memorial Sloan Kettering supports the conclusion that in well-selected patients, excellent outcomes can be achieved. The authors identified 58 patients treated with partial cystectomy between 1995 and 2001 and calculated a 5-year overall survival rate of 69%. Twenty-six patients (45%) had a local recurrence, and 12 patients (21%) developed metastatic disease. These results should not be extrapolated to all patients with bladder cancer since this was a highly selected population. Eighty-eight percent of patients had clinical T2 or less, and 41% of tumors were located in the dome.

The most important data from this article are the clinical characteristics that predicted local and advanced recurrence. On multivariate analysis, not surprisingly, CIS and multifocality predicted local recurrence. Also not surprisingly, positive nodes and positive margins predicted risk of advanced disease. On multivariate analysis, the presence of CIS increased the risk of progression to advanced disease 7-fold, and positive lymph nodes increased the risk 4-fold.

How should this impact patient care? The first thing is to recognize that partial cystectomy is an effective treatment option for selected patients. Tumor location is a critical issue, not because the cancer behaves differently in different locations, but because the ability to achieve a negative margin is more difficult in locations other than the dome. Importantly, patients with multifocal tissue and carcinoma in situ are not good candidates for partial cystectomy, and for this reason, any patient in whom partial cystectomy is being considered must have random bladder biopsies. Lastly, I think if one encounters a positive margin, one should proceed with a radical cystectomy; in this study of the 5 patients with 5 margins, 3 required a subsequent cystectomy for a muscle-invasive recurrence, and another developed metastatic disease.

A. S. Kibel, MD

Neoadjuvant Chemotherapy in Invasive Bladder Cancer: A Systematic Review and Meta-analysis

Vale C, for the Advanced Bladder Cancer (ABC) Meta-analysis Collaboration (MRC Clinical Trials Unit, London)

Lancet 361:1927-1934, 2003 14–9

Background.—Controversy exists as to whether neoadjuvant chemotherapy improves survival in patients with invasive bladder cancer, despite randomised controlled trials of more than 3000 patients. We undertook a systematic review and meta-analysis to assess the effect of such treatment on survival in patients with this disease.

Methods.—We analysed updated data for 2688 individual patients from ten available randomised trials.

Findings.—Platinum-based combination chemotherapy showed a significant benefit to overall survival (combined hazard ratio [HR] 0.87 [95% CI 0.78-0.98, p=0.016]; 13% reduction in risk of death; 5% absolute benefit at 5 years [1-7]; overall survival increased from 45% to 50%). This effect was observed irrespective of the type of local treatment, and did not vary between subgroups of patients. The HR for all trials, including those using single-agent cisplatin, tended to favour neoadjuvant chemotherapy (HR=0.91, 95% CI 0.83-1.01) although this tendency was not significant (p=0.084). Although platinum based combination chemotherapy was beneficial, there was no evidence to support the use of single-agent platinum; indeed, there was a significant difference in the effect between these groups of trials (p=0.044).

Interpretation.—This improvement in survival encourages the use of platinum-based combination chemotherapy for patients with invasive bladder cancer.

► A problem with all studies examining neoadjuvant chemotherapy prior to cystectomy is that the studies have been underpowered. A solution is to perform a meta-analysis. This rather nice meta-analysis demonstrated an approximately 5% improvement in overall survival from neoadjuvant chemotherapy. Subset analysis was hampered by the small number of patients in each treatment and clinical category. The only thing that could be said with any certainty from this study is that cisplatin-based combination therapy was more effective than single-agent platinum therapy.

In my opinion, data have clearly demonstrated that chemotherapy is effective in patients with clinically localized disease. The questions that remain to be answered are: (1) whether this should given as a neoadjuvant or as an adjuvant treatment and (2) if all patients would benefit from chemotherapy or if treatment should be limited to those with the highest-risk disease. My personal opinion is that adjuvant chemotherapy in the long run will turn out to be more effective than neoadjuvant chemotherapy for the vast majority of patients. This is based on the fact that staging is more accurate following radical cystectomy, and chemotherapy is only going to be useful in the highest risk patients, ie, those with a high likelihood of having occult metastatic disease.

A. S. Kibel, MD

A Single Immediate Postoperative Instillation of Chemotherapy Decreases the Risk of Recurrence in Patients With Stage Ta T1 Bladder Cancer: A Meta-Analysis of Published Results of Randomized Clinical Trials

Sylvester RJ, Oosterlinck W, van der Meijden APM (European Organization for the Research and Treatment of Cancer Data Ctr, Brussels, Belgium; Universitair Ziekenhuis Ghent, Belgium; Jeroen Bosch Hosp, 's-Hertogenbosch, The Netherlands)

J Urol 171:2186-2190, 2004 14–10

Background.—Among patients with bladder cancer, 70% to 80% are initially seen with superficial disease. After transurethral resection (TUR), chemotherapy is the treatment of choice for patients with high-risk tumors. However, chemotherapy is considered overtreatment in patients with low-risk tumors. Under investigation was whether 1 instillation of chemotherapy after TUR will decrease the risk of recurrence in patients with stage Ta T1 single and multiple bladder cancer overall and separately.

Methods.—A meta-analysis was conducted of the published results of randomized clinical trials that compared TUR alone with TUR plus 1 immediate instillation of chemotherapy.

Results.—The analysis included 7 randomized trials with recurrence information on 1476 patients. The median follow-up was 3.4 years, with a maximum of 14.5 years. On the basis of this follow-up, 267 of 728 patients (36.7%) receiving 1 postoperative instillation of epirubicin, mitomycin C, thiopeta, or pirarubicin had recurrence, compared with 363 of 728 patients (48.4%) with TUR alone.

This difference represents a 39% reduction in the odds of recurrence with chemotherapy. Patients with a single tumor and those with multiple tumors benefited. However, after 1 instillation, 65% of patients with multiple tumors had recurrence compared with 35.8% of patients with single tumors. This finding indicated that 1 instillation alone is not sufficient for patients with multiple tumors.

Conclusion.—One intravesical instillation of chemotherapy immediately after TUR can significantly decrease the risk of recurrence in patients with stage Ta T1 single and multiple bladder cancer. This is the treatment of choice for patients with a single, low-risk papillary tumor and is recommended as the initial treatment for patients with high-risk tumors.

▶ This article reviews 7 randomized trials of TUR alone versus TUR plus 1 immediate instillation of postoperative chemotherapy. With a median follow-up of 3.4 years, there was a 39% decrease in the odds of recurrence for patients who received intravesical chemotherapy. This result was consistent over most of the trials. The mechanism by which this treatment exerts its beneficial effects is not known. It could relate to incomplete TUR or to destroying tumor cells floating within the bladder that could have just implanted at the site of resection. Mitomycin C seems to be the preferable agent.

G. L. Andriole, Jr, MD

Treatment of Urethral Recurrence Following Radical Cystectomy and Ileal Bladder Substitution

Varol C, Thalmann GN, Burkhard FC, et al (Univ of Bern, Switzerland)

J Urol 172:937-942, 2004 14–11

Introduction.—With the introduction of orthotopic bladder substitution after radical cystectomy for patients with bladder cancer, recurrent urethral disease has become challenging to treat. The use of a novel transurethral bacillus Galmette-Guerin (BCG) treatment technique that has provided good local effect was described.

Methods.—Patients with urethral recurrences treated with a urethra-sparing approach after orthotopic bladder substitution were reviewed retrospectively. Depending on the extension of recurrence and eventual concomitant metastases, patients were given either urethrectomy, no treatment, systemic chemotherapy, or intrauethral BCG. Three times the usual dose of BCG in 150 mL NaCl 0.9% was used for intraurethral perfusion therapy according to an institutional protocol using a modified Foley catheter. This regimen was administered weekly for 6 weeks. Patients were followed up prospectively.

Results.—Between 1985 and 2001, 15 of 371 patients (4%) who received orthotopic bladder substitute experienced urethral recurrence. Two patients were treated with systemic chemotherapy (methotrexate, vinblastine, doxorubicin, and cisplatin) alone due to metastatic disease and 10 underwent intraurethral BCG therapy. Five of the 6 patients (83%) with carcinoma in situ remained free of recurrent disease after BCG treatment. Four with papillary or invasive disease failed treatment. Three patients underwent urethrectomy, including 2 after failed BCG therapy for papillary disease.

Conclusion.—Carcinoma in situ urethral recurrence after orthotopic bladder substitution can be successfully treated with intraurethral BCG perfusion for about 80% of patients. It is recommended that papillary and invasive transition cell recurrence be treated with urethrectomy.

▶ This nice paper looks at management options for the relatively small proportion (4%) of patients who receive an orthotopic neobladder who experienced a urethral recurrence. The authors demonstrate that carcinoma in situ can be treated successfully with intraurethral BCG perfusion in most cases. However, gross papillary and other recurrences should be treated with urethrectomy. This is a reminder that urologists performing orthotopic neobladders should monitor the urethra regularly at 6 month intervals for the first 2 years and annually thereafter.

G. L. Andriole, Jr, MD

Urethral Recurrence in Patients Following Orthotopic Urinary Diversion

Hassan JM, Cookson MS, Smith JA Jr, et al (Vanderbilt Univ, Nashville, Tenn)

J Urol 172:1338-1341, 2004 14–12

Purpose.—We present our experience with urethral recurrence of transitional cell carcinoma following cystectomy and orthotopic urinary diversion in a contemporary series.

Materials and Methods.—Between June 1995 and December 2001, 415 patients underwent radical cystectomy for transitional cell carcinoma. Of those patients 196 (47.2%) received an orthotopic urinary diversion. Demographics, clinical characteristics, pathological stage and patient outcomes were reviewed.

Results.—Mean followup was 34.1 months (range 0.3 to 97.3). Of the 196 patients who underwent orthotopic diversion, 59 (30.1%) had T3 or greater disease on final pathological evaluation. Thirteen patients (6.6%) were found to have prostatic urethral involvement while 83 (42.3%) had elements of carcinoma in situ. No patient with prostatic urethral involvement had subsequent urethral recurrence. Overall only 1 patient (0.5%) had urethral recurrence of transitional cell carcinoma following orthotopic urinary diversion. The urethral recurrence rate in patients with orthotopic diversion was less than in patients with ileal conduit creation during the same period (2.1%). The overall disease recurrence rate following orthotopic diversion was 31.6% (62 of 196).

Conclusions.—Urethral recurrence following orthotopic neobladder was rare in this series despite using selection criteria that were less stringent than those of other comparable series. Overall disease recurrence was relatively high in patients with high-risk pathological features, but urethral recurrence in this group with orthotopic urinary diversion remained low.

▶ Orthotopic urinary diversions are increasingly being used in the management of bladder carcinoma. The ability to create an artificial bladder not only improves that quality of life of properly selected patients, but may also encourage patients who abhor the idea of an ileal loop to undergo definitive treatment. A major concern in performing an orthotopic diversion is the risk of urethral recurrence. In general, the risk of urethral recurrence is believed to be approximately 10% in patients undergoing ileal loop diversion and approximately 2% in patients undergoing orthotopic bladder construction. This study from Vanderbilt demonstrates that the risk of urethral recurrence may be dropping in general, and particularly for patients undergoing orthotopic diversion. They found that only 2.1% of patients undergoing ileal conduit diversion and 0.5% of patients undergoing an orthotopic urinary diversion developed a urethral recurrence.

While the risk of urethral recurrence appears to be decreasing, particularly among patients undergoing orthotopic diversion, the unanswered question is why? Possible explanations range from secretion of DNA repair enzymes by the ileal segments to continued exposure to urine flow, preventing implantation and/or growth in the urethra. In addition, I (and the authors) believe that an element of patient selection is at work here. Clearly, with improved imaging and heightened awareness of cancer in general, patients undergoing surgical treatment probably have less aggressive disease than they did 10, 20, or 30 years ago, and this translates to a decrease in urethral recurrence. As a result, I do not believe that this manuscript is an invitation to broaden our criteria for orthotopic bladder reconstruction, but a reminder of how careful patient selection can improve outcomes.

A. S. Kibel, MD

The Management of Urethral Transitional Cell Carcinoma After Radical Cystectomy for Invasive Bladder Cancer

Clark PE, Stein JP, Groshen SG, et al (Univ of Southern California, Los Angeles; Wake Forest Univ, Winston-Salem, NC)

J Urol 172:1342-1347, 2004 14–13

Purpose.—Previous reports have identified risk factors for urethral recurrence following radical cystectomy for transitional cell carcinoma (TCC). However, reports of the clinical presentation, treatment and outcome in these patients are lacking. We report our experience with the diagnosis, management and outcome of urethral TCC after radical cystectomy for bladder cancer.

Materials and Methods.—A database of 1,054 patients who underwent radical cystectomy and urinary diversion for TCC from 1971 to 1997 was retrospectively reviewed. All patients with urethral TCC after surgery were identified.

Results.—Urethral TCC was diagnosed in 47 men a median of 18.5 months (range 2 to 116) after cystectomy with 20 (42%) diagnosed within 1 year. Symptomatic recurrence developed in 24 of 42 evaluable patients (57%), 21 had bloody urethral discharge and 7 had pain or a palpable mass. A total of 13 patients (31%) were asymptomatic with abnormal cytology. The remaining 5 patients underwent prophylactic urethrectomy based on cystectomy pathology. Overall 41 patients underwent urethrectomy, which was total in 36 and distal with perineal urethrostomy in 5, including later conversion to total urethrectomy in 2. Overall at a median followup of 26 months (range 3 to 275) since diagnosis 36 of 47 patients (76%) were dead, including 25 of metastatic disease. Only 10 patients (21%) remained disease-free. Median overall survival in patients with urethral TCC after radical cystectomy was only 28 months after the diagnosis of urethral TCC. Urethral stage (superficial vs invasive disease) at diagnosis was the most import predictor of overall survival in this cohort of patients.

Conclusions.—Most patients with urethral recurrence present with symptoms. However, screening cytology alone still detects a significant proportion. The median survival of patients with urethral TCC after radical cystectomy is only 28 months after diagnosis. Urethral stage (superficial vs invasive disease) at diagnosis is the most important predictor of overall survival in this cohort of patients.

▶ The bottom line from this study is that urethral recurrences are a poor prognostic sign. Patients who undergo cystectomy with either neobladder or conduit need to be monitored closely for recurrence. If recurrences occur, we should have a low threshold for an aggressive surgical intervention because the likelihood of them progressing to metastatic disease is quite high.

A. S. Kibel, MD

15 Prostate Cancer

Epidemiology/Outcomes

Natural History of Early, Localized Prostate Cancer

Johansson J-E, Andrén O, Andersson S-O, et al (Örebro Univ Hosp, Sweden; Karolinska Inst, Stockholm; Univ Hosp, Uppsala, Sweden; et al)

JAMA 291:2713-2719, 2004 15–1

Introduction.—Without understanding the natural history of prostate cancer diagnosed at an early, localized stage, patient counseling and clinical management are challenging. Little is known concerning disease progression and mortality beyond 10 to 15 years of watchful waiting. The long-term natural history of untreated, early stage prostate cancer was evaluated in a population-based, cohort investigation with a mean observation period of 21 years.

Methods.—A consecutive sample of 223 patients with early stage (T0-T2 NX MO classification), initially untreated prostate cancer was monitored. Patients with tumor progression underwent hormonal treatment with either orchiectomy or estrogens if they were symptomatic. The primary outcome measure was progression-free, cause-specific, and overall survival.

Results.—After complete follow-up, 39 (17%) patients had generalized disease. The course for most cancers was indolent during the initial 10 to 15 years. Further follow-up from 15 years (49 patients were still alive) to 20 years showed a marked reduction in cumulative progression-free survival (45.0%-36.0%), survival without metastases (76.9%-51.2%), and prostate cancer–specific survival (78.7%-54.4%). The incidence of prostate cancer mortality rose from 15 of 1000 person-years (95% confidence interval [CI], 10-21) during the initial 15 years to 44 of 1000 person-years (95% CI, 22-88) beyond 15 years of follow-up (P = .01).

Conclusion.—Most prostate cancers diagnosed at an early stage have an indolent course. Local tumor progression and aggressive metastatic disease can develop during the long term. These findings support early radical treatment, particularly among patients with an estimated life expectancy of more than 15 years.

▶ Dr Johansson has now been following this cohort of prostate cancer patients for over 2 decades. When his series was originally published, it was often cited by those who believed that watchful waiting was the best approach for the majority of patients with prostate cancer. It is interesting that now the patients have been followed for an extended period of time, the mortality from prostate cancer has increased dramatically. Prostate cancer was the ultimate cause of death in 16% of the patients, and in those patients who were younger than 70 years of age at diagnosis, fully 22% died of prostate carcinoma.

Of particular interest was the fact that on multivariant analysis, the authors found that mortality appeared to accelerate over the years, ie, the mortality rate from prostate cancer was higher 15 years after enrollment than during the first 5 years. This study appropriately concludes that patients with a life expectancy exceeding 15 years should be treated with early radical treatment.

I think the findings of this article are not surprising to most clinicians. We all know that patients with early localized prostate cancer do remarkably well for the first 5 to 10 years, even with no treatment, but once it metastasizes, it can be very difficult to manage. It is important to recognize that these patients were enrolled in the pre-PSA era. It is therefore unclear if the timeline presented in the article accurately reflects practice in the United States in 2004. It is entirely possible (though by no means certain) that the acceleration in prostate mortality seen at 15 years and beyond would be seen even later following the diagnosis in the United States in 2004.

A. S. Kibel, MD

▶ This Scandinavian study reports on the outcome of slightly more than 200 men undergoing watchful waiting for clinically localized prostate cancer. The patients were followed for a mean observation period of 2 decades. The rate of progression to metastatic disease was 18 per 1000 life-years, and the prostate cancer mortality rate was 15 per 1000 person-years.

These data indicate that prostate cancer is not always a "toothless lion," and these findings argue persuasively for early radical treatment of patients with a prolonged life expectancy.

G. L. Andriole, Jr, MD

Survival in Prostate Carcinoma—Outcomes From a Prospective, Population-Based Cohort of 8887 Men With up to 15 Years of Follow-up: Results From Three Counties in the Population-Based National Prostate Cancer Registry of Sweden

Aus G, for the South-East Region Prostate Cancer Group (Sahlgrens Univ, Göteborg, Sweden)

Cancer 103:943-951, 2005 15–2

Background.—To decide on screening strategies and curative treatments for prostate carcinoma, it is necessary to determine the incidence and survival in a population that is not screened.

Methods.—The 15-year projected survival data were analyzed from a prospective, complete, population-based registry of 8887 patients with newly diagnosed prostate carcinoma from 1987 to 1999.

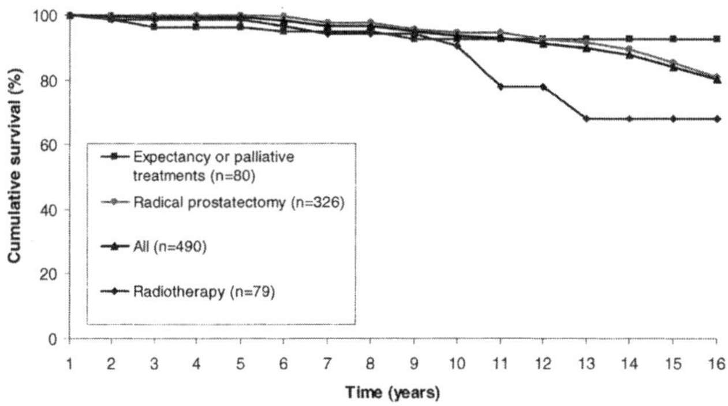

FIGURE 9.—Disease-specific survival for patients age < 75 years with low-risk prostate carcinoma (T1-T2, N0, M0; Grade 1-2; prostate-specific antigen [PSA] concentration either missing or < 20 ng/mL; n = 490 men). Tumors in these men had the following characteristics: TNM classification: T1 in 131 men (26.8%) and T2 in 359 men (73.3%); N0 in 490 men (100.0%), and M0 in 490 men (100.0%); tumor grade: Grade 1 in 128 men (26.1%) and Grade 2 in 362 men (73.9%); PSA concentration: 0-4 ng/mL in 39 men (8.0%), 4-10 ng/mL in 106 men (21.6%), 10-20 ng/mL in 80 men (16.3%), and missing in 265 men (54.1%). (Courtesy of Aus G, for the South-East Region Prostate Cancer Group: Survival in prostate carcinoma—outcomes from a prospective, population-based cohort of 8887 men with up to 15 years of follow-up: Results from three counties in the population-based national prostate cancer registry of Sweden. *Cancer* 103: 943-951, 2005. Copyright 2005 American Cancer Society. Reprinted by permission of Wiley-Liss, Inc, a subsidiary of John Wiley & Sons, Inc.)

Results.—The median patient age at diagnosis was 75 years (range, 40-96 years), and 12% of patients were diagnosed before the age 65 years. The median follow-up was 80 months for patients who remained alive. In total, 5873 of 8887 patients (66.1%) had died, and 2595 of those patients (44.2%) died directly due to prostate carcinoma. The overall median age at death was 80 years (range, 41-100 years). The projected 15-year disease-specific survival rate was 44% for the whole population. In total, 18% of patients had metastases at diagnosis (M1), and their median survival was 2.5 years. Patients with nonmetastatic T1-T3 prostate carcinoma (age < 75 years at diagnosis; n=2098 patients) had a 15-year projected disease-specific survival rate of 66%. Patients who underwent radical prostatectomy had a significantly lower risk of dying from prostate carcinoma (relative risk, 0.40) compared with patients who were treated with noncurative therapies or radiotherapy.

Conclusions.—The disease-specific mortality was comparatively high, but it took 15 years to reach a disease-specific mortality rate of 56%. These data form a truly population-based baseline on how prostate carcinoma will affect a population when screening is not applied and can be used for comparison with other health care strategies (Fig 9).

▶ This paper provides long-term follow-up on cohort of patients with clinically localized prostate cancer. In this study, the 15 year projected disease specific survival rate was 66% and men who underwent a radical prostatectomy had a significantly lower risk of dying of prostate cancer (relative risk was about 40%) in comparison to patients treated non-curatively. This is illustrated in Fig 9.

Also reported in this paper is that men treated with radiation therapy had a worse outcome, although these data are not convincing enough to eliminate radiation therapy as a viable treatment option for men with localized prostate cancer.

G. L. Andriole, Jr, MD

Comorbidity Independently Predicted Death in Older Prostate Cancer Patients, More of Whom Died With Than From Their Disease

Fouad MN, Mayo CP, Funkhouser EM, et al (Univ of Alabama, Birmingham; Ctrs for Disease Control and Prevention, Atlanta, Ga; Birmingham VAMC, Ala)

J Clin Endocrinol Metab 57:721-729, 2004 15–3

Background.—Diagnosis of prostate cancer at an earlier stage of tumor development should provide for earlier treatment and prolonged survival However, many prostate tumors are slow growing, and autopsy and cystoprostatectomy studies have suggested that a large number of these slow-growing, undetected tumors may be present in the population. Thus, many men may die of other causes before dying of or experiencing significant morbidity from prostate cancer. The number of men who died *from* prostate cancer compared to *with* prostate cancer were investigated, and the comorbid conditions associated with other-cause deaths were assessed.

Methods.—All male decedents in 1 county in Alabama from 1993 to 1995 were identified. Crosslinking of 3 databases was used to identify men whose deaths might have been caused by prostate cancer. Medical records were used to rate comorbid conditions and determine whether death was caused by prostate cancer.

Results.—Of the 561 men with a premortem diagnosis of prostate cancer, 42% died from prostate cancer and 53% died with prostate cancer. The mortality rate from prostate cancer was higher among African Americans (502%) than among whites (36.9%). Other factors related to dying with prostate cancer included older age at death and a serious or very serious comorbid condition. Treatment had no independent effect on the cause of death.

Conclusions.—Comorbidity was an independent predictor of dying with prostate cancer even after adjustment for ethnicity, age, and treatment. Among the men who die with a diagnosis of prostate cancer, only one third to one half died from the disease. These findings have provided new information for use in prostate cancer screening decisions.

▶ For urologists treating localized prostate cancer, the nagging question is always whether the patient will "die with" or "die of" prostate cancer. To date, disease-based prognostication has been investigated with demonstration of higher disease-free survival for those with less-aggressive, lower stage disease. However, the mortality scale is balanced by competing causes of mortality, particularly among older patients.

In this population-based study, deceased men who were aged at least 65 years at the time of death were identified from decedent records in the Jefferson County Alabama Department of Public Health. Through crosslinking of databases and individual record abstraction, 561 men with a confirmed premortem diagnosis of prostate cancer were identified. The analyses then determined which factors were associated with likelihood of dying with or dying from prostate cancer. Significantly, a nontrivial 42% of men died from prostate cancer, suggesting that prostate cancer is not an uncommon cause of death among men who died with a prostate cancer diagnosis. Moreover, white race, older age, and more comorbid conditions were significant predictors of dying from prostate cancer.

Using the validated Index of Disease Severity, the investigators found that comorbid scores of 3 and 4 were associated with a 2.8 and 5.2 times the likelihood of dying with prostate cancer than from prostate cancer, respectively. These data provide important validation for the current practice of recommending expectant management for localized prostate cancer among elderly men and men in poor health. Although more work will be required, this well-designed population-based study provides necessary evidence to support clinical guidelines and policy.

J. T. Wei, MD, MSc

Impact of Surgical Delay on Long-term Cancer Control for Clinically Localized Prostate Cancer

Khan MA, Mangold LA, Epstein JI, et al (Johns Hopkins Univ, Baltimore, Md)

J Urol 172:1835-1839, 2004 15–4

Purpose.—Radical retropubic prostatectomy (RRP) as definitive management for clinically localized prostate cancer is commonly performed within months of diagnosis. Despite patient anxiety there is little evidence to suggest that a delay of several months from diagnosis to RRP is associated with a worse cancer control rate. However, a recent study cast doubt on the safety of such a delay with respect to cancer control. Therefore, in a contemporary series we determined long-term cancer control in men who underwent RRP for clinically localized prostate cancer with some treated early and others treated after a longer delay.

Materials and Methods.—We analyzed data on 926 men who underwent RRP between January 1989 and December 1994. Age, preoperative serum prostate specific antigen (PSA), biopsy Gleason score, clinical and pathological stage, and biochemical recurrence were compared between 162 men who underwent RRP 60 days or less from biopsy and 764 who underwent RRP after a greater delay. Disease-free (PSA less than 0.2 ng/ml) survival rates were compared using Kaplan-Meier analysis. Pathological staging was compared using logistic regression.

Results.—The different groups were well matched for age, serum PSA, pathological stage and followup. However, significantly more men who underwent RRP between 121 and 150 days, and 151 days or greater had T1c disease (48% and 57% vs 35%, p<0.04 and <0.0001, respectively). In addition, significantly more men operated on at 151 days or greater had biopsy Gleason scores 2 to 6 (86% vs 65%, p<0.0001) and significantly fewer had Gleason score 7 disease (13% vs 30%, p<0.002). Men who underwent RRP after 60 or less days had 5- and 10-year biochemical disease-free survival rates comparable to those in men who underwent RRP after 61 to 90, 91 to 120 and 121 to 150 days after diagnosis (82% and 78%, 86% and 78%, 86% and 75%, and 86% and 82%, respectively). Those operated on at 151 days or greater had significantly greater 5- and 10-year biochemical disease-free survival rates (89% and 87%, p<0.04). However, when patients were stratified into different subgroups based on clinical stage, serum PSA and biopsy Gleason score, a delay of 150 days or greater no longer impacted differently on long-term cancer control rates.

Conclusions.—Delays of up to several months from prostate cancer diagnosis to RRP do not appear to impact long-term biochemical cancer control rates. Therefore, patients can be reassured that there is no immediate urgency to perform RRP after prostate cancer diagnosis, especially in those with T1c disease and biopsy Gleason scores less than 7.

► A common concern of patients undergoing radical prostatectomy is whether a delay in treatment will alter prognosis. This study from Johns Hopkins basically boils down to a "no." Patients were stratified by time between diagnosis and surgery, and there was absolutely no difference in PSA-free survival. In fact, patients who delayed the longest appeared to do the best. This raises an important question of whether clinical parameters influenced the interval until surgery, and if they did, was that a potential confounding variable in this study. The authors attempt to answer this by dividing the patients into higher- and lower-risk groups. Once they do this, there still appears to be no difference in PSA-free survival.

I have always believed that there is an element of chance as to whether the majority of individuals' prostate cancer is diagnosed this year, next year, or last year. For these patients, a delay of weeks to months will make no difference. However, I also believe that there is a subset of patients in whom delay of surgery does influence outcome. Unfortunately, in 2004 we have limited means to identify these high-risk patients. So while I agree that waiting a month or two will have minimal to no impact on outcome, I personally would be very concerned about waiting much longer than that to provide definitive treatment. My concern is based on the simple fact that some of these patients will fail, and they (and you) will always wonder whether earlier treatment would have cured their disease.

A. S. Kibel, MD

Geographic Variation Across Veterans Affairs Medical Centers in the Treatment of Early Stage Prostate Cancer

Spencer BA, Fung CH, Wang M, et al (Univ of California, Los Angeles; RAND Health Science Program, Santa Monica, Calif)

J Urol 172:2362-2365, 2004 15–5

Purpose.—We investigated geographic variation in the treatment of early stage prostate cancer in a national sample of veterans after widespread adoption of the prostate specific antigen test.

Materials and Methods.—Our sample consisted of 16,352 cases from the Veterans Affairs Central Cancer Registry that were diagnosed between January 1997 and December 1999 with stage I or II prostate cancer. We used a 2-stage nested logit model to compare surgery, radiation therapy and noncurative treatment among 4 geographic regions of the United States.

Results.—Multivariate analysis showed that patients in the West (referent group) had a higher OR of undergoing surgery than radiation compared with the Northeast, South or Midwest (OR 0.77, 95% CI 0.67 to 0.87, OR 0.86, 95% CI 0.76 to 0.98 and OR 0.75, 95% CI 0.64 to 0.87, respectively. Black men, men with lower grade and higher stage tumors, and unmarried men were less likely to undergo curative treatment and less likely to undergo surgery than radiation.

Conclusions.—Geographic variation persists in patterns of care in men with early stage prostate cancer. However, this variation is limited to the choice between surgery and radiation rather than to the choice between curative and noncurative treatment.

► Variations in care are evident across all medical disciplines and have been classified into 2 categories—warranted and unwarranted. Warranted variation is that which can be explained by differences in the distribution of established risk factors or indications for a specific treatment at the population level. Unwarranted variation is therefore variation caused by factors that are not supported by evidence and, in fact, may be due to factors deemed inappropriate by societal standards. A source of unwarranted variation is insurance status. One can postulate that populations with limited or no health insurance may have care dictated not by informed choice but rather by ability to pay.

The Veterans Affairs Health System has often been cited as a large clinical population that is unfettered by medical access. The study by Spencer and colleagues demonstrates that even with relatively equal medical access in the Veterans Affairs Health System, broad geographic, racial and ethnic variations can still be demonstrated. It is interesting to note that, while the odds of undergoing a curative treatment did not vary by geography, the type of active treatment received did vary, so that that men in the West were more likely to undergo surgery. One plausible population level explanation is differences in racial/ethnic distribution among the geographic regions. It has been demonstrated in the Surveillance Epidemiology and End Results program of the National Cancer Institute (SEER) and other datasets that Hispanic men are more likely to undergo surgery (in and of itself, a known source of unwarranted variation) and that there are more Hispanic men living in the Western and Southern regions. While the investigators did adjust for Hispanic ethnicity, it was a variable that was more often missing than others, and an explicit interaction of treatment geography with ethnicity was not discussed.

The significant contribution of this study is that the authors demonstrated a persistent effect of Hispanic ethnicity on utilization of radical prostatectomy in a health system with fairly equal medical access and that this may potentially be seen at a geographic level. Further research is clearly needed in examining racial and ethnic differences in decision making for prostate cancer care.

J. T. Wei, MD, MSc

Ejaculation Frequency and Subsequent Risk of Prostate Cancer

Leitzmann MF, Platz EA, Stampfer MJ, et al (NIH, Bethesda, Md; Johns Hopkins Univ, Baltimore, Md; Harvard Univ, Boston; et al)

JAMA 291:1578-1586, 2004 15–6

Context.—Sexual activity has been hypothesized to play a role in the development of prostate cancer, but epidemiological data are virtually limited to case-control studies, which may be prone to bias because recall among individuals with prostate cancer could be distorted as a consequence of prostate malignancy or ongoing therapy.

Objective.—To examine the association between ejaculation frequency, which includes sexual intercourse, nocturnal emission, and masturbation and risk of prostate cancer.

Design, Setting, and Participants.—Prospective study using follow-up data from the Health Professionals Follow-up Study (February 1, 1992, through January 31, 2000) of 29 342 US men aged 46 to 81 years, who provided information on history of ejaculation frequency on a self-administered questionnaire in 1992 and responded to follow-up questionnaires every 2 years to 2000. Ejaculation frequency was assessed by asking participants to report the average number of ejaculations they had per month during the ages of 20 to 29 years, 40 to 49 years, and during the past year (1991).

Main Outcome Measure.—Incidence of total prostate cancer.

Results.—During 222 426 person-years of follow-up, there were 1449 new cases of total prostate cancer, 953 organ-confined cases, and 147 advanced cases of prostate cancer. Most categories of ejaculation frequency were unrelated to risk of prostate cancer. However, high ejaculation frequency was related to decreased risk of total prostate cancer. The multivariate relative risks for men reporting 21 or more ejaculations per month compared with men reporting 4 to 7 ejaculations per month at ages 20 to 29 years were 0.89 (95% confidence interval [CI], 0.73-1.10); ages 40 to 49 years, 0.68 (95% CI, 0.53-0.86); previous year, 0.49 (95% CI, 0.27-0.88); and averaged across a lifetime, 0.67 (95% CI, 0.51-0.89). Similar associations were observed for organ-confined prostate cancer. Ejaculation frequency was not statistically significantly associated with risk of advanced prostate cancer.

Conclusions.—Our results suggest that ejaculation frequency is not related to increased risk of prostate cancer.

► The Physicians Health Study has provided a treasure trove of epidemiologic data. In this study, the authors sought to determine if increased sexual activity was associated with an increased risk of prostate cancer. The authors found that the exact opposite was true; increased ejaculatory frequency was associated with a decreased risk of developing prostate cancer. One of the problems with a study such as this one is that multiple confounding variables exist. To give a few examples: (1) age is clearly related to both ejaculatory frequency and risk of prostate cancer; (2) ejaculation affects prostate-specific antigen levels and may therefore influence the decision to perform a biopsy and indirectly increase the risk of being diagnosed with prostate cancer; and (3) diet and exercise may influence both ejaculatory frequency and risk of prostate cancer. The authors did their best to control for factors using multivariate analysis and did demonstrate that it was indeed the ejaculatory frequency that was responsible for the decreased risk. Does this mean we should be advising our patients to ejaculate more frequently and thereby prevent prostate cancer? I think not. However, I do think it will reassure patients that a high level of sexual activity may not necessarily increase their risk of disease.

A. S. Kibel, MD

Impact of the Percentage of Positive Prostate Cores on Prostate Cancer—Specific Mortality for Patients With Low or Favorable Intermediate-Risk Disease

D'Amico AV, Renshaw AA, Cote K, et al (Dana-Farber Cancer Inst, Boston; Univ of Connecticut, Storrs)

J Clin Oncol 22:3726-3732, 2004 15–7

Purpose.—We investigated whether pretreatment factors predicted time to prostate cancer-specific mortality (PCSM) after conventional-dose and conformal radiation therapy (CRT).

Patients and Methods.—Between 1988 and 2002, 421 patients with low (prostate-specific antigen [PSA] level ≤ 10 ng/mL and biopsy Gleason score ≤ 6) or favorable intermediate-risk (PSA > 10 to 15 ng/mL or biopsy Gleason score 3 + 4, but not both factors) disease underwent CRT (median dose, 70.4 Gy). Cox regression multivariable analysis was performed to determine whether the PSA level, Gleason score, T category, or the percentage of positive cores (% PC) predicted time to PCSM after CRT. After a median follow-up of 4.5 years, 117 (28%) patients have died.

Results.—The % PC was the only significant predictor (Cox $P \leq .03$). The relative risk of PCSM after CRT for patients with ≥ 50% as compared with less than 50% PC was 10.4 (95% CI, 1.2 to 87; Cox $P = .03$), 6.1 (95% CI, 1.3 to 28.6; Cox $P = .02$), and 12.5 (95% CI, 1.5 to 107; Cox $P = .02$) in men with a PSA ≤ 10 and Gleason score ≤ 6, PSA ≤ 10 and Gleason score ≤ 7, and PSA ≤ 15 and Gleason score ≤ 6, respectively. By 5 years after CRT, 5%

to 9% compared with less than 1% (log-rank $P \leq .01$) of these patients experienced PCSM if they had ≥ 50% compared with less than 50% PC, respectively.

Conclusion.—CRT dose-escalation techniques, the addition of hormonal therapy, or both should be considered in the management of patients with low or favorable intermediate-risk disease and ≥ 50% PC.

▶ This well done study documents that among low and intermediate risk men with prostate cancer that those individuals with more than 50% prostate cancer on core biopsy have approximately a 10-fold relative risk of disease failure. Based on this, the authors advocate use of a contemporary dose escalation techniques and/or the addition of neoadjuvant and adjuvant hormonal therapy.

G. L. Andriole, Jr, MD

Prognostic Significance of High Grade Prostatic Intraepithelial Neoplasia and Atypical Small Acinar Proliferation in the Contemporary Era

Moore CK, Karikehalli S, Nazeer T, et al (Albany Med College, NY)

J Urol 173:70-72, 2005 15–8

Purpose.—High grade prostatic intraepithelial neoplasia (HGPIN) and atypical small acinar proliferation (ASAP) in the sextant biopsy had been associated with a high risk of prostate cancer. We determined whether the extended biopsy schemes used in the contemporary era have altered the prognostic value of these lesions at repeat biopsies.

Materials and Methods.—From 1998 to 2003, 105 of 1,188 men had at least 1 repeat extended biopsy due to the presence of HGPIN (33 men) or ASAP (72 men) in a previous extended biopsy. Median biopsy interval for HGPIN and ASAP was 15 and 10 weeks ($p < 0.05$), respectively. Differences in cancer detection rates were analyzed using the Pearson chi-square test.

Results.—In the HGPIN group only 1 of 22 (4.5%) men had cancer on 1st repeat biopsy and 0 of 11 men had cancer on 2nd repeat biopsy. In men with ASAP 19 of 53 (36%, $p < 0.005$) had cancer on 1st repeat biopsy, and 3 of 19 (16%) had cancer on 2nd repeat biopsy. Cancer was confined to a single core in 16 of 22 (73%) men. Median Gleason score was 6. Patient age, digital rectal examination status, prostate specific antigen, free prostate specific antigen, number of cores and biopsy interval were not independent predictors of cancer in men with ASAP.

Conclusions.—HGPIN found in the contemporary extended biopsy does not warrant repeat biopsy. ASAP continues to be associated with a high risk of cancer and requires at least 1 repeat biopsy using the extended biopsy scheme.

▶ In 2005, is high-grade PIN as important a prognostic variable as it was a decade ago? This study would emphatically state that it is not. Only 4.5% of the patients had cancer on a repeat biopsy, but none of the patients had cancer on the second repeat biopsy. In contrast, ASAP, which has only recently come into the clinical arena, was found in 36% of the patients on first repeat biopsy and 16% of the patients on a second repeat biopsy.

What has led to the change of prognostic significance of HGPIN? It is unclear. Possibly pathologists are doing a better job of diagnosing carcinoma. This may not only be a product of experience but new immunohistochemical stains aid in difficult cases. A second possibly is that the increased number of biopsies at each session has resulted in patients essentially getting their repeat biopsy at the same time as the initial biopsy. Lastly, it is simply due to stage migration in the PSA era. Numerous studies have demonstrated changes in prostate carcinoma in radical prostatectomy specimens, and it is entirely possible that the same pathologic migration is occurring with HGPIN. The bottom line is that while I continue to recommend repeat biopsy on patients who are diagnosed with HGPIN, I am no longer certain that a large fraction of these patients truly harbor prostate carcinoma.

A. S. Kibel, MD

Immediate Versus Deferred Hormonal Treatment for Patients With Prostate Cancer Who Are Not Suitable for Curative Local Treatment: Results of the Randomized Trial SAKK 08/88

Studer UE, Hauri D, Hanselmann S, et al (Swiss Group for Clinical Cancer Research, Bern, Swizterland; Univ of Bern, Switzerland)

J Clin Oncol 22:4109-4118, 2004 15–9

Purpose.—To determine if immediate hormonal therapy is advantageous compared with deferred treatment in newly diagnosed asymptomatic prostate cancer patients who, for any reason, were not candidates for curative local treatment.

Patients and Methods.—Between February 1988 and February 1992, 197 patients with a median age of 76 years (range, 56 to 86 years) were randomly assigned to receive either immediate or deferred orchiectomy on symptomatic progression. The two groups did not differ significantly in clinical or laboratory parameters; 67% had T3-4 tumors and 20% had lymph node metastases. Patient accrual was stopped prematurely because of a similar competing trial. Therefore, observation time was prolonged to achieve the desired number of events and statistical power.

Results.—Deferred orchiectomy was necessary in 58% of the patients. Median time to disease progression was 2.8 years less than for patients with immediate orchiectomy. However, overall pain-free time from random assignment to symptomatic progression after immediate or deferred orchiectomy, and performance status, were identical in both groups. Cancer-specific survival tended to be longer in the immediate group ($P = .09$) but there was no difference in overall survival between the two groups ($P = .96$). The median hemoglobin value decreased significantly after immediate orchiectomy ($P < .001$).

Conclusion.—For elderly, asymptomatic patients not undergoing curative local treatment, we were unable to show any major advantage of immediate compared with deferred hormonal treatment regarding quality of life or overall survival in our limited number of patients. Disabling complications were prevented in the deferred-treatment arm by careful follow-up; 42% of these patients never required any tumor-specific treatment.

▶ When does one begin hormone ablation? The early versus late treatment debate rages on. This study by Studer and colleagues provides evidence for delaying hormone ablation. This study enrolled patients who were not candidates for radiation therapy or surgery and randomized them to orchiectomy immediately versus orchiectomy at the time of progression. Progression was defined as symptomatic metastasis, ureteric obstruction, or new asymptomatic metastases which were believed to potentially cause severe complications (pathologic fractures, spinal compression, etc). They specifically did not institute hormone ablation for biochemical progression. What they found was that cancer-specific survival favored the immediate treatment group in a non-statistically significant manner ($P = 0.09$), but there was absolutely no difference in overall survival. Why the difference in progression-free survival but no difference in overall survival? Clearly, the patients who received early hormone ablation died of other causes. This begs the question were these early deaths due to hormone ablation and its sequela? This possibility should give food for thought to those advocating very early hormone ablation.

How do we interpret this study? Well, first of all, the study it very similar to the MRC Study randomizing patients with advanced local disease to immediate versus delayed hormone ablation.[1] That study was faulted because many of the patients never received any hormone ablation. Since all the patients in this study received orchiectomy and were followed very closely, there is no concern about patients never receiving treatment in this trial.

Does this study settle the debate? Of course not. But for those physicians who believe in delayed hormone ablation, this study clearly provides sound experimental data in order to justify their position.

A. S. Kibel, MD

Reference

1. Immediate vs. deferred treatment for advanced prostate cancer: Initial results of the medical research council trial. *Br Journal of Urology* 79:235-246, 1997.

Five-Year Outcomes After Prostatectomy or Radiotherapy for Prostate Cancer: The Prostate Cancer Outcomes Study

Potosky AL, Davis WW, Hoffman RM, et al (Natl Cancer Inst, Bethesda, Md; New Mexico VA Health Care Sysytem, Albuquerque, NM, Fred Hutchinson Cancer Research Ctr, Seattle; et al)

J Natl Cancer Inst 96:1358-1367, 2004 15–10

Background.—Men treated for clinically localized prostate cancer with either radical prostatectomy or external beam radiotherapy usually survive many years with the side effects of these treatments. We present treatment-specific quality-of-life outcomes for prostate cancer patients 5 years after initial diagnosis.

Methods.—The cohort consisted of men aged 55–74 years who were newly diagnosed with clinically localized prostate cancer in 1994–1995 and were treated with radical prostatectomy (n = 901) or external beam radiotherapy (n = 286). We used clinical and quality-of-life data previously collected at the time of diagnosis (i.e., baseline) and at the 2-year follow-up and data newly collected at 5 years after diagnosis to compare urinary, bowel, and sexual function and to examine temporal changes in those functions. Odds ratios (ORs) and adjusted percentages were calculated by logistic regression. All statistical tests were two-sided.

Results.—At 5 years after diagnosis, overall sexual function declined in both groups to approximately the same level. However, at 5 years after diagnosis, erectile dysfunction was more prevalent in the radical prostatectomy group than in the external beam radiotherapy group (79.3% versus 63.5%; OR = 2.5, 95% confidence interval [CI] = 1.6 to 3.8). Approximately 14%–16% of radical prostatectomy and 4% of external beam radiotherapy patients were incontinent at 5 years (OR = 4.4, 95% CI = 2.2 to 8.6). Bowel urgency and painful hemorrhoids were more common in the external beam radiotherapy group than in the radical prostatectomy group. All of these differences remained statistically significant after adjustment for confounders and for differences between treatment groups in some baseline characteristics.

Conclusions.—At 5 years after diagnosis, men treated with radical prostatectomy for localized prostate cancer continue to experience worse urinary incontinence than men treated with external beam radiotherapy. However, the two treatment groups were more similar to each other with respect to overall sexual function, mostly because of a continuing decline in erectile function among the external beam radiotherapy patients between years 2 and 5.

▶ The side effects of prostate cancer treatment are not far from the minds of both physician and patient as they decide between surgery, radiation therapy, and observation. The Prostate Cancer Outcomes Study is a study designed to prospectively evaluate men who have undergone treatment for prostate carcinoma. The primary symptoms reviewed in this paper are urinary, bowel, and sexual. Worsening symptoms are likely related to the treatment, though progression could simply be a result of age.

Five years after surgery, problems with urinary incontinence clearly are more prevalent in the radical prostatectomy group. However, obstructive symptoms were much more common in the external beam radiation therapy group. Bowel symptomatology tended to be higher in the external beam radiation therapy cohort, however, not as dramatically as one might expect. Lastly, sexual function did not appear to dramatically favor one group or the other. While erections insufficient for intercourse were slightly more common in the radical prostatectomy cohort, prevalence overall in both cohorts was rather high, approximately 60% to 70%, and the bother was identical in both groups.

What does this mean? It is actually hard to say. Since men chose their own therapy in consultation with the physician (ie, it is not a randomized study), it is entirely likely that some bias has entered the Prostate Cancer Outcomes Study. With that said, I think it is clear that all treatment alternatives for prostate cancer result in some level of complications/side effects. Essentially the patient has to choose his poison. We need to strive to refine both techniques and choose our patients very carefully for treatment to ensure that our patients receive the best quality of life.

A. S. Kibel, MD

Testosterone Replacement Therapy After Primary Treatment for Prostate Cancer

Agarwal PK, Oefelein MG (Case Western Reserve Univ, Cleveland; Univ Hosps of Cleveland, Ohio)

J Urol 173:533-536, 2005 15–11

Purpose.—A history of prostate cancer has been an absolute contraindication for testosterone supplementation. We studied a cohort of hypogonadal patients treated with radical retropubic prostatectomy (RRP) for organ confined prostate cancer to determine if testosterone replacement therapy (TRT) could be efficacious and administered safely without causing recurrent prostate tumor.

Materials and Methods.—Ten hypogonadal patients previously treated with RRP for organ confined prostate cancer were identified. They presented with low serum total testosterone (TT) and symptoms of hypogonadism after RRP. Patients had baseline serum determinations of prostate specific antigen (PSA) and TT, and were started on testosterone supplementation. They were assessed periodically for changes in PSA and TT, and for symptomatic improvement using the hormone domain of the Extended Prostate Inventory Composite Health Related Quality of Life questionnaire.

Results.—At a median followup of 19 months no patient had detectable (greater than 0.1 ng/ml) PSA. TT increased significantly after starting TRT from a mean ± SD of 197 ± 67 to 591 ± 180 ng/dl ($P = 0.0002$). The Hormone Domain of the Extended Prostate Inventory Composite Health Related Quality of Life questionnaire increased significantly from 38 ± 5 to 49 ± 3 ($P = 0.00005$), primarily due to a decrease in hot flashes and an increase in energy level.

Conclusions.—At a median of 19 months of TRT hypogonadal patients with a history of prostate cancer had no PSA recurrence and had statistically significant improvements in TT and hypogonadal symptoms. In highly select patients after RRP TRT can be administered carefully and with benefit to hypogonadal patients with prostate cancer.

► Hypogonadism is a known clinical entity that is bothersome to many men following curative treatment for localized prostate cancer. Clinicians have long been reluctant to replace testosterone, given a theoretical concern that this may contribute to treatment failures. This question is clearly controversial with some evidence, as demonstrated by Agarwal and Oefelein, that TRT may be feasible in select patients. However, the evidence for the proper selection of patients and timing of TRT are limited. The authors conclude that a randomized trial to measure the potential benefits of TRT on health function and quality of life balanced by the potential harms on promoting cancer recurrence is necessary. Such a study is simplified as the primary end point can be serologic, using PSA. The potential findings from such a study would potentially affect treatment and quality of life for the evergrowing population of prostate cancer survivors.

J. T. Wei, MD, MSc

Screening/Diagnosis

Prevalence of Prostate Cancer Among Men With a Prostate-Specific Antigen Level ≤4.0 ng Per Milliliter

Thompson IM, Pauler DK, Goodman PJ, et al (Univ of Texas, San Antonio; Fred Hutchinson Cancer Research Center, Seattle; Univ of Colorado, Denver; et al)
N Engl J Med 350:2239-2246, 2004 15–12

Introduction.—The optimal upper limit of the normal range for prostate-specific antigen (PSA) has not been determined. The prevalence of prostate cancer was examined in the Prostate Cancer Prevention Trial among men who had a PSA level of 4.0 ng/mL or less.

Methods.—Of 18,882 men enrolled in this phase III, double-blind, placebo-controlled trial, 9459 were randomly assigned to receive a placebo and underwent annual measurement of PSA and digital examination and prostate biopsy after being in the trial for 7 years. It was this cohort that was followed for prevalence of prostate cancer among participants with PSA levels below 4.0 ng/mL. Of the 9459 who received placebo rather than active treatment (which was 5 mg finasteride daily), 2950 never had a PSA level above 4.0 ng/mL or an abnormal digital rectal examination.

Results.—The age range of the 2950 men evaluated was 62 to 91 years. Prostate cancer was diagnosed in 449 (15.2%). Of these, 67 (14.9%) had a Gleason score of 7 or more. The incidence of prostate cancer was 6.6% in men with a PSA level of up to 0.5 ng/mL, 10.1% among those with values of 1.1 to 2.0 ng/mL, 23.9% in those with values of 2.1 to 3.0 ng/mL, and 26.9% in those with values of 3.1 to 4.0 ng/mL. The incidence of high-grade cancers rose from 12.5% of cancers associated with a PSA level of 0.5 ng/mL or less to 25.0% of cancers linked with a PSA level of 3.1 to 4.0 ng/mL.

Conclusion.—Biopsy-identified prostate cancer, including high-grade cancers, is not rare among men with PSA levels of 4.0 ng/mL or lower, levels that are generally regarded as being in the normal range.

► Since the advent of PSA screening, we have tried to use it as a dichotomous variable. The test is either positive or negative and the patient is or is not at risk for prostate cancer. The study proves what we have all known: Patients with mildly elevated PSAs are at significant risk for prostate cancer. Even at PSA levels less than 4, the higher the PSA the more likely one is to have prostate cancer. Importantly, as the PSA rises, so does the patient's risk of having high-grade prostate carcinoma.

While the patient's risk of prostate cancer for a PSA of less than 0.5 ng/mL is 6.6% and the risk of high-grade disease is approximately 0.8%, the risk gradually increases as the PSA rises until for a PSA between 3.1 and 4.0 ng/mL, the risk of having prostate cancer is approximately 27%, and the risk of having high-grade disease is approximately 7%.

How should this study affect our practice? Should our threshold for biopsy be a risk 10%, 15%, 20%? I am not sure. We will clearly diagnose many patients with clinically insignificant disease. Maybe we should have a threshold geared more to the diagnosis of aggressive cancer. Again, what should be our threshold: 6%, 5%, 4% I don't have the answer. The key question is whether patients with prostate cancer with these low PSA levels require treatment, and this will require further study.

A. S. Kibel, MD

Results of a Randomized, Population-Based Study of Biennial Screening Using Serum Prostate-Specific Antigen Measurement to Detect Prostate Carcinoma

Hugosson J, Aus G, Lilja H, et al (Sahlrenska Univ, Gothenburg, Sweden; Lund Univ, Malmö, Sweden)

Cancer 100:1397-1405, 2004 15–13

Background.—The purpose of the current study was to evaluate the effectiveness of a prostate carcinoma screening program in which serum prostate-specific antigen (PSA) levels were measured.

Methods.—From a group of 20,000 men born between January 1, 1930, and December 31, 1944, 10,000 men were randomized into a screening group and 10,000 were randomized into a control group. Patients in the screening group were invited to undergo initial PSA testing between 1995 and 1996 and then were invited to receive testing every second year thereafter for 8 years (for a total of 4 PSA tests). Men with PSA levels ≥3 ng/mL (or ≥2.54 ng/mL, in the third and fourth screening rounds) were invited to undergo clinical investigation, which included sextant biopsy of the prostate. By linking to the regional cancer registry, the authors were able to obtain the true and expected incidence rates for the screening and control groups.

Results.—The screening participation rate was high (73%). A total of 884 malignancies have been detected to date, with 640 having been detected in the screening group. There was an early and marked shift toward more favorable disease stage and grade for malignancies detected on repeat screening. In the fourth screening round, only 2 of 82 detected malignancies were classified as advanced disease. Of the 227 screen-detected tumors on which surgery was performed, only 20 (8.8%) had small volume (<0.2 cm^3). Forty-three interval malignancies were detected, but only 5 were accompanied by symptoms. At 8 years, the cumulative disease incidence rate among screening participants was 7.3%, compared with 2.4% in the control arm. The incidence rate observed in the screening population corresponds to the cumulative incidence rate observed in the Swedish male population at age 72 years.

Conclusions.—Biennial PSA screening was very successful in diagnosing prostate carcinoma at an early stage, when curative treatment typically is effective. In addition, the results regarding interval malignancies were favorable. Thus, decreased mortality should be observed on long-term follow-up. The lead time associated with screening appears to fall within the range described in earlier studies involving frozen sera (i.e., 5-9 years).

► There is an increasing push to screen patients for prostate cancer less frequently. The hope is that this will result in significant cost savings while not altering the cancer detection rate or, ultimately, prostate cancer survival. This study from the European Randomized Screening For Prostate Cancer Study provides data that every-other-year screening will be as effective as annual screening. I'm not sure whether patients can remember to return to their urologist once every 2 years. However, as the majority of screening is done by internists, they may be able to integrate this more cost-effective approach into their clinical practice.

A. S. Kibel, MD

The Prostate Specific Antigen Era in the United States Is Over for Prostate Cancer: What Happened in the Last 20 Years?

Stamey TA, Caldwell M, McNeal JE, et al (Stanford Univ, Calif)

J Urol 172:1297-1301, 2004 15–14

Purpose.—We assessed how well preoperative serum prostate specific antigen (PSA) reflects the largest cancer in consecutive untreated radical prostatectomies during the last 20 years at Stanford University.

Materials and Methods.—A total of 1,317 consecutive radical prostatectomies were divided into 4, 5-year periods between August 1983 and July 2003, and examined sequentially in 3 mm step sections by 1 pathologist. The largest cancer and 5 other histological variables in each prostate were measured. Preoperative clinical stages were tabulated for each 5-year period. Means, Pearson correlation coefficients, % change and multiple regression were used to compare selected variables.

Results.—Most parameters decreased linearly during the 20 years, including palpable nodules on digital rectal examination from 91% to 17%, mean age from 64 to 59 years, mean serum PSA from 25 to 8 ng/ml, and index (largest) cancer volume from 5.3 to 2.4 cc. Percent Gleason grade 4/5 of the largest cancer averaged 27% to 35% and prostate weight 44 to 53 gm. Contrasting August 1983 to December 1988 with January 1999 to July 2003, 6 histological cancer parameters had statistically significant relationships to serum PSA in the first period. In the last 5 years serum PSA was related only to prostate size.

Conclusions.—Serum PSA was related to prostate cancer 20 years ago. In the last 5 years serum PSA has only been related to benign prostatic hyperplasia. There is an urgent need for serum markers that reflect the size and grade of this ubiquitous cancer.

▶ This article received significant amounts of attention in the lay press. Essentially, if one was to believe the local media, PSA was no longer useful. Not surprisingly, that is not what the article concluded. The authors found that in a population of patients operated on from 1983 to 1988, PSA correlated with important pathological variables such as volume of the largest cancer, presence of capsular penetration, positive lymph nodes, percent seminal vesicle invasion, percent Gleason 4 and 5, clinical stage, and prostate weight. However, in the period from 1999 to 2003, the only parameter that still correlated with PSA was prostate weight.

I think it is important to remember several things in evaluating this article. First, it is important to recognize that the pathological variables Stamey et al are evaluating are surrogate endpoints. The authors have not proven that PSA no longer correlates with survival, but that it no longer correlates with adverse pathology. This may simply reflect that fact that PSA is an effective screening tool. Since the goal of PSA screening is to diagnose patients early, when they are still treatable, the fact that these terrible pathologic variables no longer correlate with PSA screening may simply indicate that we are succeeding in diagnosing patients earlier, when they still have treatable cancer. A second, equally plausible possibility is that PSA diagnoses clinically unimportant as well as clinically important cancers. Clearly, PSA screening over-diagnoses prostate carcinoma, and more than 50% of patients may have clinically insignificant disease. Dr Stamey and colleagues recognize the potential for over-diagnosis and are not calling for the end of PSA screening, but for improved markers. These markers would not be used to predict the presence of prostate cancer but the presence of clinically significant prostate cancer.

A. S. Kibel, MD

Relationship Between Initial Prostate Specific Antigen Level and Subsequent Prostate Cancer Detection in a Longitudinal Screening Study

Antenor JAV, Han M, Roehl KA, et al (Washington Univ, St Louis; Northwestern Univ, Chicago)

J Urol 172:90-93, 2004 15–15

Purpose.—Previous studies of archived blood samples from nonscreened populations have shown an association between the prostate specific antigen (PSA) and the subsequent detection of prostate cancer. In the current study we evaluated the relationship between the initial screening PSA and the subsequent risk of prostate cancer detected in a prospective, longitudinal screening study. We also examined the relationship between initial PSA and the clinicopathological features of the cancers detected.

Materials and Methods.—Between May 1991 and November 2001 we enrolled 26,111 volunteers in our PSA and digital rectal examination based prostate cancer screening study. The men were followed biannually or annually depending on the results of previous screening tests. The chi-square and Kruskal-Wallis tests were used to compare the clinical stage, pathological stage and Gleason score of subsequently detected prostate cancers as well as the time to cancer detection in different initial screening PSA strata.

Results.—The initial screening PSA stratum was strongly associated with the subsequent detection of prostate cancer as well as the clinicopathological stage and grade of the cancers detected.

Conclusions.—Even in the lower PSA ranges initial screening serum PSA can help identify men at increased risk for subsequent prostate cancer detected in a longitudinal screening study.

▶ This study demonstrates the rather striking association between even slight elevations in PSA and subsequent risk for developing prostate cancer. Individuals who had PSAs between 4 and 10 had a relative risk of 38.7 of eventually developing prostate cancer. Even for lower PSAs the relative risks were relatively high. This highlights the fact that there is no "normal" PSA.

Another striking statistic from this paper is the high likelihood of a PSA increasing to greater than 4 ng/mL as the patient is followed. To put it another way, how likely was it that a PSA would remain within the normal range? If the initial PSA is between 0 and 1, the likelihood of the PSA increasing to greater than 4 was a relatively low 2%. However, for PSA between 1 and 2.5, the likelihood was 12% and for a PSA between 2.6 and 4.0, the likelihood was 42%.

A very similar study was done early in the PSA era by Gann et al.[1] This study demonstrates that in the mature PSA era, marginally elevated PSAs should continue to be of concern. Particularly patients with PSAs of greater than 2.5 ng/mL should be monitored closely for 2 reasons. First, there is an almost 50% chance that the patient's PSA will increase to greater than 4 ng/mL in the near future and second, the patient's relative risk is 15 to 25 times that of a patient with a PSA of less than 1.

One of the interesting aspects of this study that is not addressed is whether patients with very low PSAs (ie, < 1) could be screened less vigorously, say once every 5 years. The likelihood of developing prostate cancer and of the PSA increasing to greater than 4 are both so low in this patient population that a significant cost savings could be obtained in this population without failing to diagnose disease.

A. S. Kibel, MD

Reference

1. Gann PH, Hennekens CH, Stampfer MJ: A prospective evaluation of plasma prostate-specific antigen for detection of prostatic cancer. *JAMA* 273:289-94, 1995.

An Ecologic Study of Prostate-Specific Antigen Screening and Prostate Cancer Mortality in Nine Geographic Areas of the United States

Shaw PA, Etzioni R, Zeliadt SB, et al (Fred Hutchinson Cancer Research Ctr, Seattle)

Am J Epidemiol 160:1059-1069, 2004 15–16

Introduction.—Ecologic studies of cancer screening examine cancer mortality rates in relation to use of population screening. These studies can be confounded by treatment patterns or influenced by choice of outcome and time horizon. Interpretation can be complicated by uncertainty about when mortality differences might be expected. The authors examined these issues in an ecologic analysis of prostate-specific antigen (PSA) screening and prostate cancer mortality across nine cancer registries in the United States. Results suggested a weak trend for areas with greater PSA screening rates to have greater declines in prostate cancer mortality; however, the magnitude of this trend varied considerably with the time horizon and outcome measure. A computer model was used to determine whether divergence of mortality declines would be expected under an assumption of a clinically significant survival benefit due to screening. Given a mean lead time of 5 years, the model projected that differences in mortality between high- and low-use areas should be apparent by 1999 in the absence of other factors affecting mortality. The authors concluded that modest differences in PSA screening rates across areas, together with additional sources of variation, could have produced a negative ecologic result. Ecologic analyses of the effectiveness of PSA testing should be interpreted with caution (Figs 4 and 5).

▶ This population-based study of 9 SEER registries analyzed intensity of PSA screening use, practice patterns and prostate cancer mortality outcomes. One interesting finding is shown in the attached Fig 4 showing an association between use of hormonal therapy and magnitude of prostate cancer mortality declines. An analysis looking at the intensity of PSA testing (Fig 5) did not show much mortality reduction in high PSA usage groups.

The authors of this paper correctly point out that their results do not prove that PSA-based screening does not save lives. On the other hand, the mortality benefits we have been observing in the past several years may well be attributable to more intensive use of hormonal therapy. Knowledge about the ability of PSA-based screening to reduce prostate cancer death rates must await the results of randomized screening trials such as the PLCO Cancer Screening Study.

G. L. Andriole, Jr, MD

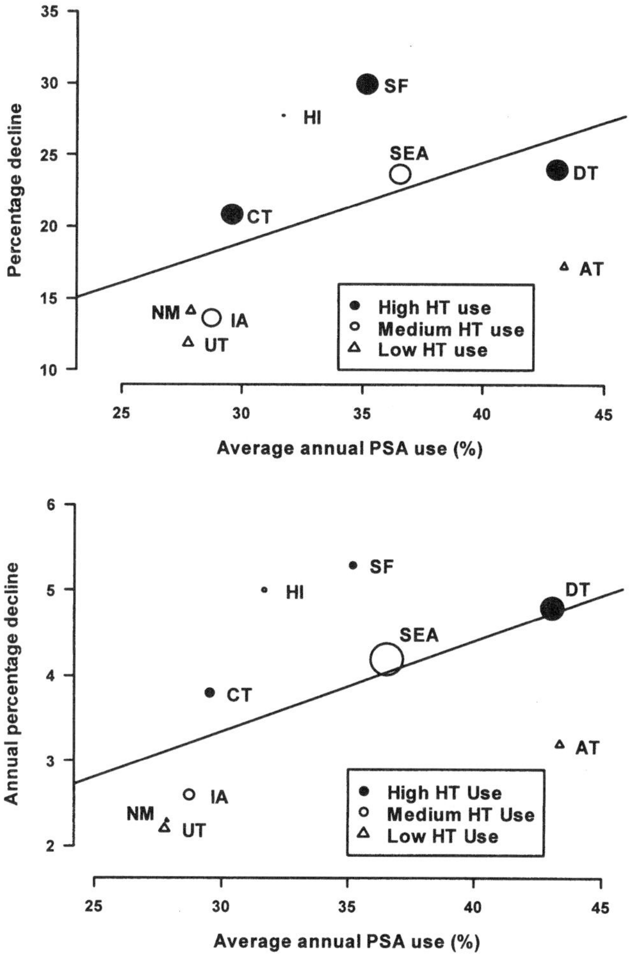

FIGURE 4.—Decline in age-adjusted prostate cancer mortality rates vs average prostate-specific antigen (PSA) screening use. Rates were age adjusted to the 2000 US Census population. **Top**, Percentage decline in prostate cancer mortality from 1991 to 1993 to 1997 to 1999. **Bottom**, Annual percentage decline estimated for 1991 to 1999. The size of the plotting character is inversely related to the variance within a particular registry of the Surveillance, Epidemiology, and End Results Program of the National Cancer Institute for percentage decline (**top**) and average percentage decline (**bottom**). *Abbreviations: HT*, hormone; *AT*, Atlanta, Georgia; *CT*, Connecticut; *DT*, Detroit, Michigan; *HI*, Hawaii; *IA*, Iowa; *NM*, New Mexico; *SEA*, Seattle, Washington; *SF*, San Francisco, California; *UT*, Utah. (Courtesy of Shaw PA, Etzioni R, Zeliadt SB, et al: An ecologic study of prostate-specific antigen screening and prostate cancer mortality in nine geographic areas of the United States. *Am J Epidemiol* 160:1059-1069, 2004. Reprinted by permission of Oxford University Press.)

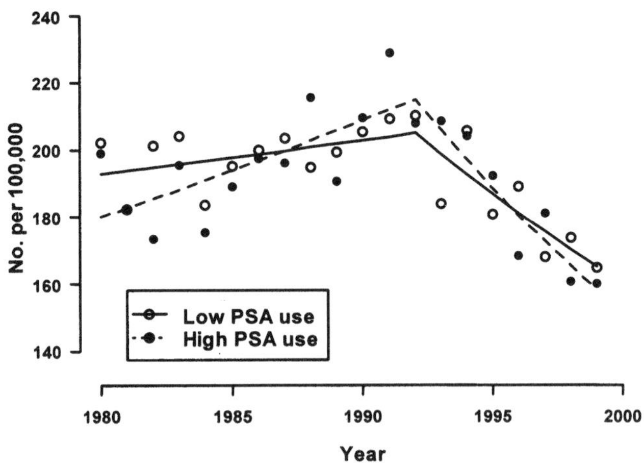

FIGURE 5.—Age-adjusted prostate cancer mortality rates by registry of the Surveillance, Epidemiology, and End Results Program of the National Cancer Institute for White men aged 65 to 84 years, grouped by high vs low use of prostate-specific antigen (PSA) screening. Rates were age adjusted to the 2000 US Census population. Joinpoint regression was used to summarize the trends within each group. Low PSA screening use: Connecticut, Hawaii, Iowa, New Mexico, and Utah; high PSA screening use: Detroit, Michigan, and Atlanta, Georgia. (Courtesy of Shaw PA, Etzioni R, Zeliadt SB, et al: An ecologic study of prostate-specific antigen screening and prostate cancer mortality in nine geographic areas of the United States. *Am J Epidemiol* 160:1059-1069, 2004. Reprinted by permission of Oxford University Press.)

Clinical Utility of proPSA and "Benign" PSA When Percent Free PSA is Less Than 15%

Khan MA, Sokoll LJ, Chan DW, et al (Johns Hopkins Univ, Baltimore, Md; Hybritech Incorp, San Diego, Calif)

Urology 64:1160-1164, 2004 15–17

Objectives.—To investigate the clinical utility of the subforms of free prostate-specific antigen (PSA), namely proPSA and "benign" PSA (BPSA), to improve cancer detection when the percent free PSA level is less than 15%. Percent free PSA, while maintaining sensitivity, has greatly improved the specificity of PSA for the early detection of prostate cancer. A low percent free PSA value indicates a greater risk of cancer, but only 30% to 50% of men with percent free PSA levels of less than 15% actually have cancer at biopsy.

Methods.—Archived sera from 161 consecutive men who were prospectively enrolled in our Early Detection Research Network prostate cancer early detection biomarker program with a percent free PSA value of less than 15% were included in the study. Total PSA, free PSA, proPSA, and BPSA were measured for each sample.

Results.—The mean total PSA was 6.1 ng/mL (range 1.8 to 24.0). The mean age of the study group was 62 ± 7 years. Prostate cancer was detected in 66 (41%) of 161 men. The area under the curve-receiver operating characteristic for total and percent free PSA was 0.51 and 0.54, respectively. BPSA and proPSA/BPSA both improved cancer detection compared with percent free PSA alone; the improvement was statistically significant (P <0.001). The area under the curve-receiver operating characteristic for proPSA/BPSA was 0.72, giving a sensitivity and specificity of 90% and 46%, respectively.

Conclusions.—The results of our preliminary studies have suggested that the ratio of proPSA and BPSA can distinguish cancer with greater accuracy when the percent free PSA value is very low (less than 15%), and may, therefore, provide better clinical utility in this lower range of percent free PSA.

▶ This study evaluates 2 relatively new markers for prostate diseases: proPSA and BPSA. In this analysis, the authors suggest that the ratio of proPSA divided by BPSA provides a statistically significant improvement in the ability to identify prostate cancer. Larger studies, however, are necessary to truly confirm this relationship.

G. L. Andriole, Jr, MD

The Association of Body Mass Index and Prostate-Specific Antigen in a Population-Based Study

Baillargeon J, Pollock BH, Kristal AR, et al (Univ of Texas, San Antonio)

Cancer 103:1092-1095, 2005 15–18

Background.—Recent studies of men with prostate carcinoma suggest that obesity may be associated with more advanced-stage disease and lower overall survival rates. One possible link between body mass index (BMI) and prostate carcinoma prognosis may be disease ascertainment. Prostate-specific antigen (PSA) is widely used to screen for prostate carcinoma.

Methods.—The authors examined the association between BMI and PSA in a population-based study of 2779 men without prostate carcinoma. Between 2001 and 2004, these men were enrolled in a study sponsored by the

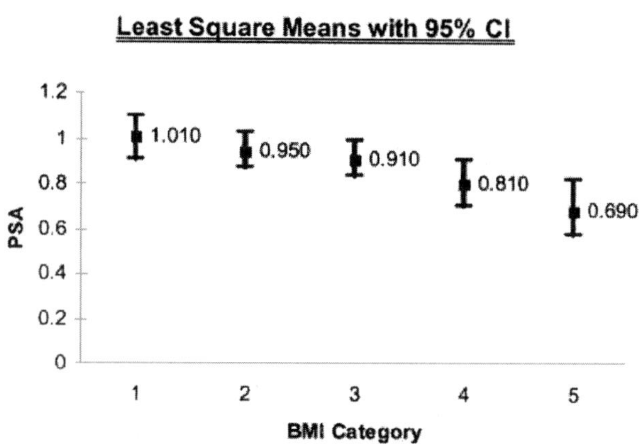

FIGURE 1.—Adjusted least-squares mean prostate-specific antigen (PSA) according to body mass index (BMI) category. 95% CI: 95% confidence interval. (Courtesy of Baillargeon J, Pollock BH, Kristal AR, et al: The associated of body mass index and prostate-specific antigen in a population-based study. *Cancer* 103:1092-1095, 2005. Copyright 2005 American Cancer Society. Reprinted by permission of Wiley-Liss, Inc, a subsidiary of John Wiley & Sons, Inc.)

San Antonio Center of Biomarkers of Risk, a clinical and epidemiologic center of the Early Detection Research Network of the National Cancer Institute.

Results.—The mean PSA value decreased in a linear fashion with an increase in BMI category, from 1.01 ng/mL in normal weight men to 0.69 ng/mL in obese (Class III) men, after adjusting for race/ethnicity and age.

Conclusions.—Lower levels of PSA in obese and overweight men could mask biologically consequential prostate carcinoma (Fig 1).

▶ Obesity may be associated with more advanced stages of prostate cancer and lower overall survival. This study examined the association between BMI and PSA in approximately 3000 men without prostate cancer. The finding that the mean PSA value decreased in linear fashion with increased BMI even after adjusting for race and age (as shown in Fig 1). It is important information as it calls into question whether recent reports of inferior outcomes of prostate cancer treatment in obese men may reflect more of a delay in diagnosis rather than some underlying aggressiveness of the disease.

G. L. Andriole, Jr, MD

Validation of a Nomogram for Predicting Positive Repeat Biopsy for Prostate Cancer

Yanke BV, Gonen M, Scardino PT, et al (State Univ of New York; Mem Sloan-Kettering Cancer Ctr, New York)

J Urol 173:421-424, 2005 15–19

Purpose.—We reported a nomogram and subsequently a corrected version for predicting the probability of positive biopsy in men with 1 or more prior negative biopsies. In this study we assessed the validity of this nomogram when applied to an external dataset.

Materials and Methods.—There were 230 patients from the Brooklyn Veterans Administration Medical Center who underwent 1 or more repeat biopsies after initial negative biopsy from January 1993 to June 2003. Predictor variables studied in the nomogram were patient age, family history of prostate cancer, digital rectal examination, serum prostate specific antigen, prostate specific antigen slope, months from initial negative biopsy session, months from previous negative biopsy session, cumulative number of negative cores previously taken and history of high grade intraepithelial neoplasm or atypical small acinar proliferation. We calculated the nomogram predicted probability in each patient. These predicted outcomes were compared with actual biopsy results. Area under the ROC curve was calculated as a measure of discrimination. Calibration was assessed graphically.

Results.—We evaluated a total of 356 repeat biopsies in 230 patients (mean 2.56 total biopsies per patient). The mean number of total cores per patient was 17.9. There were 78 positive biopsies. The area under the ROC curve was 0.71, which was greater than any single risk factor. Nomogram calibration appeared to be good.

Conclusions.—Our corrected nomogram for predicting positive repeat biopsy performed well when applied to a sample of men at the Brooklyn Veterans Administration Medical Center. This nomogram can provide important additional information to aid the urologist and patient with a negative biopsy in evaluating clinical options.

► A prostate biopsy is typically the final common pathway between prostate cancer risk evaluation and the diagnosis of prostate cancer. Unfortunately, our ability to predict who will have prostate cancer detected on a biopsy remains poor. Historically, a number of well-founded concepts for risk stratification have been developed, including prostate specific antigen, percent-free prostate specific antigen, prostate-specific antigen density, high-grade prostatic intraepithelial neoplasia, and atypical small acinar proliferation, but, given the plethora of potentially relevant pieces of data for any given patient, how is the clinician to decide? As in most situations where there is information overload, decision making is often defaulted to inaction and in the case of prostate biopsy, this translates into biopsying everyone at risk without consideration of stratification.

In this study, Kattan and colleagues apply their rigorous nomogram methodology to prognosticating prostate cancer detection among men with 1 or more prior negative biopsy. They incorporate no less than 10 factors in this nomogram and demonstrate that their nomogram predicts better than single-factor models. While this is an important step forward, it is still cumbersome to use this nomogram without a computer, and it requires that all factors be available for any given patient. Ultimately, software must be developed that will allow for entry of limited data to provide risk estimates in all clinical scenarios (first biopsy, repeat biopsy, etc). However, to do so will require that we continue efforts to collect outcomes data on which to power these and other prognostic models. In the future, we ought to be able to inform our patients, with a reasonably narrow confidence limit, of their personal risk of prostate cancer.

J. T. Wei, MD, MSc

Monofocal and Plurifocal High-grade Prostatic Intraepithelial Neoplasia on Extended Prostate Biopsies: Factors Predicting Cancer Detection on Extended Repeat Biopsy

Roscigno M, Scattoni V, Freschi M, et al (San Raffaele Hosp, Milan, Italy)

Urology 63:1105-1110, 2004 15–20

Objectives.—To evaluate factors predicting cancer detection by extended repeat prostate biopsies in patients with an initial, isolated, monofocal or plurifocal, high-grade prostatic intraepithelial neoplasia (HGPIN) diagnosis.

Methods.—From 1995 to 2002, after a first set of 10 to 12 systematic biopsy cores, 47 patients with an initial HGPIN diagnosis underwent repeat biopsy using the same technique (mean repeat biopsy cores 11.5) after a median follow-up of 11.4 months (range 3 to 24).

Results.—Cancer was detected at the second biopsy in 21 patients (44.6%). Cancer detection was significantly greater in patients with plurifocal HGPIN than in those with monofocal HGPIN (70% vs. 10%, respectively; $P < 0.005$) and in patients who underwent repeat biopsy more than 6 months after the first biopsy set (65%) compared with patients who underwent repeat biopsy within 6 months (25%; $P < 0.01$; mean follow-up 15.5 and 3.8 months, respectively). Multivariate analysis showed that prostate-specific antigen, prostate-specific antigen density, digital rectal examination, and transrectal ultrasound findings were not statistically significant predictors of prostate cancer, and HGPIN multifocality and interval between biopsies (more than a 6-month follow-up interval) were independent prognostic factors (odds ratio 4.65 and 2.65, respectively). After radical prostatectomy (14 patients), no statistically significant differences were found in the pathologic stage between patient groups stratified by repeat biopsy interval (within or after 6 months).

Conclusions.—After a 10 to 12-core biopsy, patients with initial, isolated monofocal or plurifocal HGPIN diagnoses had an overall cancer detection rate of 45% on repeat extended biopsies. Plurifocal HGPIN on the first biopsy set was the strongest independent predictive factor in cancer detection. A 12 to 18-month interval before repeat biopsy could permit a significantly greater cancer detection rate, with no apparent likelihood of clinical cancer progression.

► This paper reports that close to 50% of men with plurifocal HGPIN were found to have prostate cancer on subsequent biopsy. The authors advocate waiting 12 to 18 months before the repeat biopsy to enhance prostate cancer discovery. Interestingly, about 15% of all cancers occurred in the contralateral lobe of the prostate.

In some recent series, a HGPIN was shown not to be an independent predictor of later prostate cancer detection especially if one considered the ascertainment biopsy in this group of patients in comparison to similarly matched patients without a history of HGPIN. However, I think many patients who carry this diagnosis deserve very close follow-up and annual rebiopsy would seem beneficial to them.

G. L. Andriole, Jr, MD

Quantitative GSTP1 Methylation Levels Correlate With Gleason Grade and Tumor Volume in Prostate Needle Biopsies

Zhou M, Tokumaru Y, Sidransky D, et al (Johns Hopkins Med Institutions, Baltimore, Md)

J Urol 171:2195-2198, 2004 15–21

Background.—Prostate needle biopsy is the gold standard for the diagnosis of prostate cancer. However, the small size of the cancer present in some biopsies and benign mimickers can present significant diagnostic challenges. In response, objective molecular markers with high sensitivity have been proposed to supplement routine histologic evaluation to increase the sensitivity and specificity of prostate needle biopsies. Methylation of the *GSTP1* gene promoter region is the most common epigenetic change in prostate cancer. The recently developed quantitative *GSTP1* methylation assay facilitates the accurate discrimination between benign prostate tissue and prostate cancer, even in small, formalin-fixed prostate needle biopsies.

Whether *GSTP1* methylation correlated with Gleason grade and tumor volume in prostate biopsies was investigated. In addition, the study compared quantitative *GSTP1* methylation with the histologic diagnosis in each biopsy.

Methods.—The *GSTP1* methylation study used formalin-fixed, paraffin-embedded prostate needle cores. A total of 109 biopsies from 40 patients with prostate cancer of various Gleason grades and tumor volume, along with benign prostate tissue, were tested for *GSTP1* methylation with the use of quantitative fluorogenic real-time methylation-specific polymerase chain reaction.

Results.—The 109 biopsy specimens included 13 benign and 96 cancer biopsy parts. *GSTP1* methylation was positive in 83 to 96 cancer parts (86.5%). All 13 benign parts (100%) were negative for *GSTP1* methylation, with a methylation level of 0 in 12 biopsies and 1 in 1 biopsy. The sensitivity and specificity of quantitative *GSTP1* methylation correlated with Gleason grade, with higher *GSTP1* methylation in higher Gleason grade tumors. *GSTP1* also correlated with the cancer percentage per biopsy. Multiple linear regression analysis was predictive of a greater contribution of cancer percentage than Gleason grade to quantitative *GSTP1* methylation levels.

Conclusion.—The quantitative *GSTP1* methylation assay will reliably discriminate between benign and malignant prostate tissues and thus augment the routine histologic evaluation of prostate needle biopsies. Quantitative *GSTP1* methylation was also correlated with prostate cancer Gleason grade and cancer volume, which suggests that quantitative *GSTP1* methylation may be of prognostic significance in prostate needle biopsies.

▶ This is another piece of evidence suggesting that glutathione-S-transferase-π (*GSTP1*), an enzyme involved in the metabolism of genotoxic molecules, is a reliable marker for prostate cancer. This study confirms that *GSTP1* methylation reliably discriminates between benign and malignant prostate tissues and that quantitative methylation correlates with prostate cancer grade and tumor volume. A remaining challenge is to harvest an adequate amount of tissue via biopsy for the assay that presently requires approximately 100 μg of tissue.

G. L. Andriole, Jr, MD

Validity of Primary Care Patient Self-Report of Abnormal (But Not Cancer) Prostate Biopsy Results

McNaughton-Collins M, Barry MJ, Caubet J-F, et al (Univ of Massachusetts, Boston)

J Urol 172:2366-2368, 2004 15–22

Purpose.—We assessed the validity of patient self-report of abnormal (but not cancer) prostate biopsy results, ie, atypical cells or prostatic intraepithelial neoplasia.

Materials and Methods.—We compared survey responses and pathology records for 156 men from a multicenter, prospective cohort study, which was designed to evaluate the impact of a suspicious prostate cancer screening test followed by benign prostate biopsy.

Results.—Of the 156 subjects 45 (29%) reported having had atypical cells or prostatic intraepithelial neoplasia and 38 (24%) had a pathology report with atypia or prostate intraepithelial neoplasia. The sensitivity of the self-report was 87%, specificity was 90%, positive predictive value was 73% and negative predictive value was 95%. The kappa statistic was 0.7.

Conclusions.—Men in this study reported this complex result accurately. However, it was concerning that 5 men (13%) appeared unaware of an abnormal prostate biopsy result, especially given the substantial residual risk of prostate cancer conferred by this result.

► By and large, clinicians base medical care decisions on a patient's medical history and physical examination often relying on laboratory and radiologic tests as confirmation. The fidelity of patient self-reported health information has been questioned. When it comes to prostate biopsy, knowledge of prior prostate biopsy abnormalities, such as high-grade prostatic intraepithelial neoplasia, and atypical small acinar proliferation are critical and likely to influence decision making toward a repeat biopsy.

In this study, the authors evaluated the ability of men to recall complex pathologic details 4 to 6 weeks after their prostate biopsy. They found a good level of agreement between patient self-report and the actual pathology report with a κ (agreement beyond chance alone) of 0.7. While this is encouraging to see, the study population was largely college-educated men who underwent recent biopsy. It is plausible that literacy and education level, time since biopsy, and patient age will each affect the recall of such information. This brings to mind the old maxim that the decisions you make as a physician are only as good as the information you have in hand. It follows that if all patients "owned" their health information and brought it with them to their office visit, quality of care and efficiency would improve. At our center, we routinely give patients their results verbally and as a hard copy. In this day and age where patients switch physicians and insurance companies almost at a whim, the greatest beneficiary of providing patients with hard copies of their health information are likely to be the physicians themselves.

J. T. Wei, MD, MSc

Radical Prostatectomy

Radical Retropubic Prostatectomy: How Often Do Experienced Surgeons Have Positive Surgical Margins When There Is Extraprostatic Extension in the Region of the Neurovascular Bundle?

Hernandez DJ, Epstein JI, Trock BJ, et al (Johns Hopkins Med Institutions, Baltimore, Md)

J Urol 173:446-449, 2005 15–23

Purpose.—We determined the frequency of positive surgical margins (PSMs) in patients with extraprostatic extension (EPE) in the region of the neurovascular bundle (NVB) who underwent open radical retropubic prostatectomy by 2 experienced surgeons.

Materials and Methods.—A total of 204 men with EPE in the region of the NVB underwent surgery by 2 experienced surgeons. The frequency of PSMs in the area of the NVB as well as the nerve sparing status of each lobe of the prostate were determined through a retrospective investigation of the pathology database as well as the physician's database. The recovery of sexual function was determined and compared to controls.

Results.—The age, clinical stage, biopsy Gleason sum and serum prostate specific antigen of the patients operated on by surgeons 1 and 2 were similar. Surgeon 1 widely excised at least 1 neurovascular bundle in 16% of the patients and surgeon 2 in 63%. The overall frequency of PSMs at the NVB was 5.9% for surgeon 1 and 5.8% for surgeon 2. Of the evaluable patients followed for 12 months or longer 83.5% of those operated on by surgeon 1 were potent compared to 63.8% of those operated on by surgeon 2.

Conclusions.—Visual and tactile assessment during open surgery by an experienced surgeon provides valuable information on when and where it is safe to preserve the neurovascular bundle in patients with EPE in the region of the NVB. Surgical approaches in which tactile sensation is muted or absent, laparoscopic and robotic, need to undergo a similar evaluation to determine whether magnification of the operative field is sufficient to overcome the lack of haptic feedback and ability to palpate the tissue.

▶ This report by an experienced group of prostatic surgeons may provide some practical guidance for less experienced practitioners. These findings suggest that visual and in some cases, tactile, assessment provides valuable information on when and where it is safe to preserve or resect the NVB. The authors point out that when prostate cancer merely extends through the capsule, it rarely penetrates by more than 1 to 2 mm and that often this much tissue is present even if the neurovascular bundles are preserved ipsilaterally.

This is a nice paper that surgeons should study to enhance their ability to both cure prostate cancer and preserve sexual function.

G. L. Andriole, Jr, MD

Residual Benign Prostatic Glands at the Urethrovesical Anastomosis After Radical Retropubic Prostatectomy: Prediction and Impact on Disease Outcome

Paul R, Hoppmann M, van Randenborgh H, et al (Technische Universität Munich)

Eur Urol 46:321-326, 2004 15–24

Introduction.—Benign prostatic glands left behind after radical prostatectomy (RP) may impact prostate-specific antigen (PSA)–free survival and may therefore affect metastases-free, disease-specific, and overall survival and could explain PSA failure in patients with prostate cancer. The prediction and impact on disease outcome of residual benign glands at the urethrovesical anastomosis were evaluated.

Methods.—A total of 802 patients who underwent RP were retrospectively evaluated. A special focus was placed on residual benign glands (B+) at the urethrovesical anastomosis. B-status was determined from a biopsy of the urethral stump at the 9, 12, and 3 o'clock position.

Results.—A total of 73.6% of patients were classified as B+ and 26.4% were BO; 92.0% of B+ patients showed only isolated glands (B1) and 8.0% showed abundant glands (B2). No difference was observed in disease outcome for BO and B+ patients. Patients with early prostate cancer who are candidates for nerve-sparing procedures are more likely to have B+ status.

Conclusion.—Benign prostatic glands at the apical margin of the RP specimen are often found. Neither isolated nor abundant glands have an impact on disease outcome. It may be that a precise apical dissection to improve continence rates is possible. These patients are at risk for residual benign tissue at the apex.

▶ This retrospective study examined the impact of a positive "benign" margin on PSA-free survival defined as a PSA greater than 0.5 ng/mL. This team of investigators systematically examined the apical dissection margin in over 800 cases and found that nearly three quarters of their patients had evidence of benign prostatic hyperplasia (BPH) being left behind at the surgical margin. Their sobering finding of frequent prostate incursions during a "radical" prostatectomy clearly illustrate that an RP is often not so radical after all. Fortunately, unlike with positive cancer margins, there is no evidence that leaving benign tissue behind results in poorer cancer control.

A significant limitation of this work is that the investigators used a high threshold for biochemical recurrence, and use of a lower threshold is more likely to have demonstrated an effect. This study is also exclusive of bladder neck margins where a surgeon is apt to cut across BPH tissue posteriorly when there is a median lobe present.

Nevertheless, this pathologic study neatly documents that BPH tissue is often left behind and may account for low levels of postoperative PSA. Surgeons need to be aware of these findings, and studies examining doubling time in external beam–treated patients suggest that PSA velocity in the posttherapeutic setting may be a better discriminant of cancer recurrence than a simple PSA threshold.

J. T. Wei, MD, MSc

'Vanishing' Prostate Cancer in Radical Prostatectomy Specimens: Incidence and Long-term Follow-up in 38 Cases

Bostwick DG, Bostwick KC (Mayo Clinic, Rochester, Minn)

BJU Int 94:57-58, 2004 15–25

Objective.—To determine the incidence and long-term follow-up of the 'vanishing cancer' phenomenon, as complete sampling of some radical prostatectomy (RP) specimens reveals no residual cancer.

Materials and Methods.—The Mayo Clinic prostate cancer RP database for 1966-1995 was searched for all cases in which there was no residual adenocarcinoma (pathological stage pT0). Each case was confirmed by a review of all tissue specimen slides. Various clinical and pathological features were evaluated, and the follow-up obtained for all patients.

Results.—Among 6843 RPs there were 38 in which no residual cancer was identified despite careful sampling. There was a 10-fold decline in the incidence of this finding, from 2.1% before 1980 to 0.2% in 1993-95; this decline appeared to be caused by a decrease in the frequency of diagnosis of cancer by transurethral resection from > 10% before 1990 to < 2% in 1993-95. The mean (range) age of the patients was 63 (38-75) years. All cancers on biopsy or transurethral resection were well or moderately differentiated; clinical stages included T1a (42% of cases), T1b (45%) and T2 (13%). Six patients had a nerve-sparing RP, all after 1990. The mean follow-up was 9.6 (1.0-28.5) years, and there were no recurrences of cancer; the serum prostate specific antigen concentration remained at < 0.2 ng/mL in surviving patients. Six patients (16%) died from intercurrent disease.

Conclusions.—The incidence of 'vanishing cancer' declined between 1966 and 1995, probably as a result of the decline in the use of transurethral resection, occurring in 0.2% of RPs. The prognosis in such patients is excellent, indicating that there is no apparent clinical significance to microscopic foci of cancer that remain undetected after reasonably complete pathological sampling. The inability to identify cancer in a prostate removed for biopsy-confirmed carcinoma does not indicate technical failure.

► This interesting study looked at about 6000 radical prostatectomies of which in 38 there was no residual cancer identified despite careful sampling. While in the pre-PSA era it was relatively more common to find no residual tumor in the prostate (because of TURP detected tumors). This study shows that this occasionally occurs even in the modern era. However, the authors correctly point out that relatively high rates of "vanishing" cancer may indicate some quality of care issues worth closer scrutiny.

G. L. Andriole, Jr, MD

Prognosis of Patients With Lymph Node Positive Prostate Cancer Following Radical Prostatectomy: Long-term Results

Daneshmand S, Quek ML, Stein JP, et al (Univ of Southern California, Los Angeles)

J Urol 172:2252-2255, 2004 15–26

Purpose.—We determined the prognostic factors that affect recurrence and survival in patients with lymph node positive prostate cancer.

Materials and Methods.—Between 1972 and 1999, 1,936 patients underwent radical retropubic prostatectomy and pelvic lymph node dissection for clinically organ confined prostate cancer. A total of 235 patients (12.1%) were found to have disease metastatic to the lymph nodes (stage D1). Of the patients 69% received no adjuvant treatment. We reviewed the tumor stage (TNM), Gleason score, number and percent of involved lymph nodes (lymph node density), preoperative prostate specific antigen when available and adjuvant treatment. Overall survival and recurrence-free survival were estimated using Kaplan-Meier plots.

Results.—Followup was 1 to 24 years (median 11.4). Overall median survival was 15 years. Overall clinical recurrence-free survival at 5, 10 and 15 years was 80%, 65% and 58%, respectively. Patients who had 1 or 2 positive lymph nodes had a clinical recurrence-free survival of 70% and 73% at 10 years, respectively, vs 49% in those who had 5 or more involved lymph nodes ($p = 0.0031$). When stratified by lymph node density, patients with a lymph node density of 20% or greater were at higher risk for clinical recurrence compared to those with a density of less than 20% (relative risk = 2.32, $p < 0.0001$). On stratified log rank test only prostate cancer T stage, and the number and percent of positive lymph nodes correlated with recurrence-free and overall survival.

Conclusions.—Local tumor bulk and the number/percent of involved lymph nodes significantly affect disease progression and the survival rate. Radical prostatectomy may offer long-term survival in patients who have limited tumor bulk and nodal involvement.

► This relatively large series of close to 2000 patients undergoing radical prostatectomy with a median follow-up of 11 years showed that radical prostatectomy and lymphadenectomy may offer survival advantages to patients who have limited local disease and limited lymph node involvement.

In my own practice, I have expanded the template for standard lymph node dissection. Wider node dissections identify a slightly higher rate of positive lymph nodes. My personal series confirms that close to one third of men with a minimal lymph node metastases are cured even with prolonged follow-up.

G. L. Andriole, Jr, MD

Is Hispanic Race an Important Predictor of Treatment Failure Following Radical Prostatectomy for Prostate Cancer?

Lam JS, Sclar JD, Desai M, et al (Columbia Univ, New York)

J Urol 172:1856-1859, 2004 15–27

Introduction.—Prostate cancer is the most commonly diagnosed cancer and the second leading cause of cancer death among Hispanic men. Compared with white men, Hispanic men have more advanced stage tumors, higher prostate specific antigen (PSA) levels, and higher grade tumors at the time of diagnosis. In a retrospective review, Hispanic men and white men with prostate cancer were compared for clinical and pathologic features, outcomes after radical prostatectomy, and the impact of Hispanic race on outcome.

Methods.—All patients included in the review had consecutively undergone radical retropubic prostatectomy for clinically localized prostate cancer between July 1995 and November 2002. Two of the investigators performed all procedures. After exclusion of 11 patients who received preoperative therapy, 451 men (315 white and 136 Hispanic) were eligible for review. Treatment failure was defined as a PSA of 0.2 or greater more than 8 weeks after surgery or receiving any adjuvant therapy. Variables known to affect outcome and race of the patient were evaluated for their ability to predict treatment failure.

Results.—Compared with white patients, the Hispanic men were older and had a higher percentage of abnormal rectal examinations, Gleason 7 tumors, and preoperative PSA levels greater than 10. With a mean follow-up of 36 months for white and 32 months for Hispanic men, treatment failure rates were similar in the 2 groups (17.8% and 18.7%, respectively). Variables strongly associated with treatment failure were higher pre-PSA, postoperative Gleason scores, pathologic stages, positive surgical margins, and positive lymph nodes. There was no association between race and positive surgical margins, and mean age of the treatment failure group was similar to that of the treatment success group.

Conclusion.—After controlling for other known predictive factors, Hispanic race had no significant effect on outcome after radical prostatectomy. Hispanic men did have higher pre-PSAs and Gleason grade tumor at diagnosis compared with white men, a finding that may suggest socioeconomic factors that delayed diagnosis or intrinsic biologic differences. But the decision to pursue curative therapies in Hispanic men should be based on the same preoperative clinical factors used for all patients.

▶ In this retrospective case series, 136 Hispanic men and 315 white men underwent radical prostatectomy for localized prostate cancer over a 7-year period exclusive of men with neoadjuvant therapy or radiation therapy. Hispanic ethnicity was based on self-report. In their time to failure analyses, the authors were unable to find a difference in time to recurrence. Although this study was limited by short follow-up and small numbers, it does represent 1 of the few studies that examine Hispanic men. Not unlike studies of predominantly white men, preoperative PSA, Gleason score, pathologic stage, and surgical margins were each independently associated with treatment failure.

The causes of the racial disparities in prostate cancer have haunted clinicians and scientists since the first report of a racial difference in prostate cancer survival between white and black men. Despite several decades of research, no single risk factor, hormone, or gene has yet been identified that explains the basis for these racial differences. Studies of race and health in the United States have been dominated by a biologic paradigm that views racial disparities largely as being genetically determined. This model is based on the wealth of data that support racial differences in molecular data and the prevalence of certain diseases (eg, terminal CAG repeats encoding the androgen receptor are shorter for black men with prostate cancer). However, in recent decades, the construct of race as a contributing factor has been refined as it appeared that genetic predispositions alone did not explain the range of variation in disease prevalence and mortality. In fact, there is a growing body of literature to suggest that race is a sociologic intermediary to health and that behavioral (biosocial) risk factors such as tobacco and alcohol use contribute significantly to disease development. As such, race, in and of itself, may not be a risk factor but rather a marker that we can use to better understand what factors influence prostate cancer treatment. Diet, health behaviors, access to health care, and health literacy are just a few examples of plausible nonbiologic factors. The authors of this article concluded that future work should focus on health services and attitudes. The fact that no racial difference was identified in this study does not obviate the importance of examining health disparities. As we continue to use population sciences to study prostate cancer, placing a greater emphasis on racial disparities in the delivery of health care and decision making is not only appropriate but necessary.

J. T. Wei, MD, MSc

Impact of Unilateral Interposition Sural Nerve Grafting on Recovery of Urinary Function After Radical Prostatectomy

Singh H, Karakiewicz P, Shariat SF, et al (Baylor College of Medicine, Houston; Mem Sloan-Kettering Cancer Ctr, New York; Univ of Texas, Dallas)

Urology 63:1122-1127, 2004 15–28

Objectives.—To test the hypothesis that unilateral sural nerve graft (SNG) interposition may improve the rate of urinary function (UF) recovery after radical retropubic prostatectomy (RRP) in patients undergoing unilateral nerve resection (UNR).

Methods.—We studied 111 consecutive patients who underwent RRP with purposeful UNR performed by a single surgeon. Of the 111 patients, 53 underwent unilateral SNG interposition. All patients were invited to complete a questionnaire that included the validated University of California, Los Angeles, Prostate Cancer Index. The time to UF recovery above the median value of the group and urinary control status were evaluated.

Results.—The median follow-up was 26 and 12 months for the UNR and UNR+SNG patients, respectively. At 12 months after RRP, 94.7% of patients with UNR+SNG reported having complete urinary control or leakage of only a few drops of urine compared with 58.3% of patients with UNR alone ($P = 0.012$). In multivariate Cox regression models, UNR+SNG was associated with a 9.95 times greater rate of reaching a UF score above the median versus UNR alone ($P < 0.001$). In multivariate logistic regression analyses, SNG status increased the odds of having complete urinary control or leakage of only a few drops of urine by 14.99 and 29.19 at 6 and 12 months after RRP, respectively (both $P < 0.05$).

Conclusions.—In patients undergoing UNR surgery, SNG interposition is associated with a greater rate of UF recovery and a higher likelihood of urinary control after RRP. These findings need to be validated in larger, multicenter, prospective, randomized studies.

► Sural nerve grafts have been touted as a method of improving sexual function following resection of neurovascular bundle. As an added benefit, several groups including this one have reported improve continence rates in patients who have undergone sural nerve graft. I think these results are intriguing. However, I am concerned that patient selection may have been the predominant reason for the patients receiving sural nerve grafts did better. In addition, the apical dissection needs to be precise in order to identify the location of the nerve for anastomosis. This improved apical dissection may be the primary reason for the improved continence rates.

A. S. Kibel, MD

Radiation Therapy

6-Month Androgen Suppression Plus Radiation Therapy vs Radiation Therapy Alone for Patients With Clinically Localized Prostate Cancer: A Randomized Controlled Trial

D'Amico AV, Manola J, Loffredo M, et al (Brigham and Women's Hosp, Boston; Dana Farber Cancer Inst, Boston)

JAMA 292:821-827, 2004 15–29

Introduction.—There is a survival benefit among patients with high-grade clinically localized prostate cancer who undergo 70 Gy radiation therapy combined with 3 years of androgen suppression therapy (AST). Long-term treatment with AST is associated with several adverse events. The survival benefit of 3-dimensional conformational radiation therapy (3D-CRT) alone versus in combination with 6 months of AST was prospectively evaluated in 206 patients with clinically localized prostate cancer.

Methods.—Patients were randomly assigned to receive 70 Gy 3D-CRT alone or in combination with 6 months of AST. All patients had a prostate-specific antigen (PSA) level of at least 10 ng/mL, a Gleason score of at least 7, or radiographic evidence of extraprostate disease. The primary outcome measures were time to PSA failure (PSA >1.0 ng/mL and increasing > 0.2 ng/mL on 2 consecutive visits) and overall survival.

Results.—After a median follow-up of 4.52 years, patients assigned to the 3D-CRT plus AST group had significantly higher survival rates (P = .04), lower prostate cancer–specific mortality rates (P = .02), and higher survival rates free of salvage AST (P = .002) compared with patients in the 3D-CRT group. Kaplan-Meier estimates of 5-year survival rates were 88% (95% confidence interval [CI], 80%-95%) in the combination therapy group versus 78% (95% CI, 68%-88%) in the 3D-CRT group. The rates of survival free of salvage AST at 5 years were 82% (95% CI, 73%-90%) in the combination therapy group and 57% (95% CI, 46%-69%) in the 3D-CRT group. The unadjusted and adjusted hazard ratios for survival without salvage AST were 2.30 (95% CI, 1.36-3.89; P = .002) and 217 (95% CI, 1.28-3.69; P = .004) for patients in the 3D-CRT group compared with the combination therapy group.

Conclusion.—The addition of 6 months of AST to 70 Gy 3D-CRT provides an overall survival benefit in patients with clinically localized prostate cancer.

▶ Studies have already demonstrated that AST in combination with radiation therapy improves overall survival rate in patients with aggressive localized prostate cancer. A concern of prior studies is that AST was delivered for up to 3 years in duration. Since AST clearly has adverse side effects, several groups, including this group from Harvard, have instituted trials of shorter-duration AST. All patients received approximately 70 Gy delivered by a 3D-CRT technique and were selected randomly to 6 months of luteinizing hormone-releasing hormone agonist with flutamide versus no treatment. The average follow-up was almost 5 years. The Kaplan-Meier curves demonstrated a clear overall survival advantage, favoring patients who received combination therapy.

In 2004, external beam therapy needs to be given in combination with androgen deprivation for patients with high-risk disease. The question that remains to be answered is

1. How long a period of androgen deprivation is required?
2. How high a dose of radiation therapy is required?
3. Should pelvic radiation also be included in all patients with high-risk disease?

I believe in the coming years, as additional trials are published, a consensus will be achieved. We will have to await the publication of these trials.

A. S. Kibel, MD

▶ This study shows that with about 5 years of follow-up, 6 months of AST in conjunction with 70 ray of 3D-CRT confers an overall survival benefit for patients with clinically localized prostate cancer. These data, in conjunction with those provided by Bolla et al,[1] show that there seems to be an emerging consensus that neoadjuvant AST is beneficial for a broad spectrum of men also receiving CRT.

G. L. Andriole, Jr, MD

Reference

1. Bolla M, Collette L, Blank L, et al: Long-term results with immediate androgen suppression and external irradiation in patients with locally advanced prostate cancer (an EORTC study): A phase III randomised trial. *Lancet* 360:103-106, 2002.

Salvage Radiotherapy for Recurrent Prostate Cancer After Radical Prostatectomy

Stephenson AJ, Shariat SF, Zelefsky MJ, et al (Baylor College of Medicine, Houston)

JAMA 291:1325-1332, 2004 15–30

Context.—Salvage radiotherapy may potentially cure patients with disease recurrence after radical prostatectomy, but previous evidence has suggested that it is ineffective in patients at the highest risk of metastatic disease progression.

Objective.—To delineate patients who may benefit from salvage radiotherapy for prostate cancer recurrence by identifying variables associated with a durable response.

Design, Setting, and Patients.—Retrospective review of a cohort of 501 patients at 5 US academic tertiary referral centers who received salvage radiotherapy between June 1987 and November 2002 for detectable and increasing prostate-specific antigen (PSA) levels after radical prostatectomy.

Main Outcome Measure.—Disease progression after salvage radiotherapy, defined as a serum PSA value ≥0.1 ng/mL above the postradiotherapy PSA nadir confirmed by a second PSA measurement that was higher than the first by any amount, by a continued increase in PSA level after treatment, or by the initiation of androgen deprivation therapy after treatment.

Results.—Over a median follow-up of 45 months, 250 patients (50%) experienced disease progression after treatment, 49 (10%) developed distant metastases, 20 (4%) died from prostate cancer, and 21 (4%) died from other or unknown causes. The 4-year progression-free probability (PFP) was 45% (95% confidence interval [CI], 40%-50%). By multivariable analysis, predictors of progression were Gleason score of 8 to 10 (hazard ratio [HR], 2.6; 95% CI, 1.7-4.1; *P*<.001), preradiotherapy PSA level greater than 2.0 ng/mL (HR, 2.3; 95% CI, 1.7-3.2; *P*<.001), negative surgical margins (HR, 1.9; 95% CI, 1.4-2.5; *P*<.001), PSA doubling time (PSADT) of 10 months or less (HR, 1.7; 95% CI, 1.2-2.2; *P*=.001), and seminal vesicle invasion (HR, 1.4; 95% CI, 1.1-1.9; *P*=.02). Patients with no adverse features had a 4-year PFP of 77% (95% CI, 64%-91%). When treatment was given for early recurrence (PSA level ≤2.0 ng/mL), patients with Gleason scores of 4 to 7 and a rapid PSADT had a 4-year PFP of 64% (95% CI, 51%-76%) and of 22% (95% CI, 6%-38%) when the surgical margins were positive and negative, respectively. Patients with Gleason scores of 8 to 10, positive margins, and receiving early salvage radiotherapy had a 4-year PFP of 81% (95% CI,

57%-100%) when the PSADT was longer than 10 months and of 37% (95% CI, 16%-58%) when the PSADT was 10 months or less.

Conclusions.—Gleason score, preradiotherapy PSA level, surgical margins, PSADT, and seminal vesicle invasion are prognostic variables for a durable response to salvage radiotherapy. Selected patients with high-grade disease and/or a rapid PSADT who were previously thought to be destined to develop progressive metastatic disease may achieve a durable response to salvage radiotherapy.

▶ PSA failure after radical prostatectomy is a clinical conundrum. The patient has been treated aggressively for his disease with the promise of cure and feels healthy, yet we know that disease has recurred. The treatment alternatives are limited, and all have significant side effects. This multi-institutional retrospective analysis attempts to shed light on who will benefit from salvage radiotherapy. On multivariate analysis, patients appeared to do poorly if they had a Gleason score of 8 to 10 on the prostatectomy specimen, preradiotherapy PSAs greater than 2, negative surgical margins, PSADTs of less than 10 months, and seminal vesicle invasion.

The authors point out that some high-risk patients were cured with adjuvant radiation therapy. For example, while only 29% of patients with Gleason score of 8 to 10 had a 4-year progression-free survival, if one looked at the subset of patients that had PSAs of less than 2 at the time of radiation therapy, positive surgical margin, and PSADTs of greater than 10 months, fully 81% of these patients showed no evidence of disease at 4 years. They conclude that salvage radiotherapy is a potentially curative option in patients with aggressive prostate cancer.

With good patient selection, a reasonably high percentage of patients can have excellent PSA responses. Of particular importance is that if salvage radiotherapy is going to be delivered, it needs to be given early while the preradiotherapy PSA is low. With that said, there are still several concerns. First, PSA failure is a surrogate end point. What we really care about is metastasis-free and overall survival. Second, many of the pathologic variables that predict success for radiation therapy in this paper, such as prolonged PSADT and low Gleason score, have been shown to predict a long metastasis-free and overall survival in patients who received no adjuvant therapy.[1] For this reason, the patients who are most successfully treated may be the ones who require no treatment at all. Soon to be published randomized trials from Southwest Oncology Group and European Organization for the Research and Treatment of Cancer will hopefully shed some light on this subject.

A. S. Kibel, MD

Reference

1. Pound CR, Partin AW, Eisenberger MA, et al: Natural history of progression after PSA elevation following radical prostatectomy. *JAMA* 281:1591-1597, 1999.

▶ This large multi-institutional study attempts to identify predictors of PSA progression after salvage radiation therapy. Relatively low Gleason scores

(≤7) and relatively low preradiotherapy PSA levels (<2) as well as PSADT of less than 10 months are predictors of response. It would be good for practitioners to consult this report when considering use of salvage radiation therapy for men after radical prostatectomy.

G. L. Andriole, Jr, MD

Systemic Chemotherapy

Docetaxel and Estramustine Compared With Mitoxantrone and Prednisone for Advanced Refractory Prostate Cancer

Petrylak DP, Tangen CM, Hussain MHA, et al (Columbia Univ, New York; Southwest Oncology Group Statistical Ctr, Seattle; Univ of Michigan, Ann Arbor)

N Engl J Med 351:1513-1520, 2004 15–31

Background.—In men with progressive androgen-independent prostate cancer, mitoxantrone-based chemotherapy palliates pain but does not extend survival. Docetaxel plus estramustine with mitoxantrone plus prednisone was compared in this patient population.

Methods.—Seven hundred seventy men were assigned randomly to 1 of 2 treatments given in 21-day cycles. Three hundred thirty-eight received 280 mg of estramustine 3 times a day on days 1 through 5, 60 mg of docetaxel per square meter of body-surface area on day 2, and 60 mg of dexamethasone in 3 divided doses before docetaxel (group 1). Three hundred thirty-six patients received 12 mg of mitoxantrone per square meter on day 1 plus 5 mg of prednisone twice a day (group 2).

Findings.—Intention-to-treat analysis demonstrated an overall survival of 17.5 months in group 1 compared with 15.6 months in group 2. The corresponding hazard ratio for death was 0.80. The median time to progression in groups 1 and 2 were 6.3 and 3.2 months, respectively. Decreases in prostate-specific antigen (PSA) of at least 50% were documented in 50% of group 1 and 27% of group 2. Objective tumor responses were observed in 17% and 11%, respectively, of patients with bidimensionally measurable disease. Grade 3 or 4 neutropenic fevers, nausea and vomiting, and cardiovascular events were more common in group 1 than in group 2. Pain relief in the 2 groups was comparable.

Conclusions.—First-line treatment with estramustine and docetaxel, compared with mitoxantrone and prednisone, moderately increases survival in men with metastatic androgen-independent prostate cancer. However, this benefit must be weighed against the increased rate of adverse events.

Docetaxel Plus Prednisone or Mitoxantrone Plus Prednisone for Advanced Prostate Cancer

Tannock IF, for the TAX 327 Investigators (Univ of Toronto; et al)

N Engl J Med 351:1502-1512, 2004 15–32

Background.—The treatment of metastatic prostate cancer remains palliative, although androgen ablation typically improves symptoms and reduces serum prostate-specific antigen (PSA) levels in these patients. For those who become refractory to hormone treatment, chemotherapy is an option. Some evidence suggests mitoxantrone plus low-dose prednisone relieves pain and improves quality of life (QOL) more frequently than prednisone alone, but the combination has no effect on survival. This Phase III study compared the effects of docetaxel plus prednisone on PSA levels, pain control, QOL, and survival with those of mitoxantrone plus prednisone in patients with metastatic, hormone-refractory prostate cancer.

Methods.—The subjects were 1006 men with metastatic, hormone-refractory prostate cancer (median age, 68 years) recruited from 24 countries from March 2000 through June 2002. All patients were treated with prednisone, 5 mg twice a day, and were randomized into 3 groups. Group 1 received mitoxantrone, 12 mg/m^2, every 3 weeks. Group 2 received docetaxel, 75 mg/m^2, every 3 weeks. Group 3 received docetaxel, 30 mg/m^2 per week for 5 of every 6 weeks. Up to 10 treatment cycles were planned for groups 1 and 3, and up to 5 cycles were planned for group 1. Serum PSA levels were measured every 3 weeks. Each day patients recorded their level of pain according to the Present Pain Intensity scale from the McGill-Melzack questionnaire. The QOL was assessed with the Functional Assessment of Cancer Therapy-Prostate (FACT-P) questionnaire at baseline, every 3 weeks during therapy, and every month after the end of therapy. The primary endpoint was overall survival.

Results.—The mean follow-up was 20.7 to 20.8 months in the 3 groups. The risk of death did not differ significantly in group 1 (mitoxantrone) and group 3 (weekly docetaxel)(hazard ratio for death 0.91 vs group 1). However, the risk of death was significantly lower in group 2 (docetaxel every 3 weeks) than in group 1 (hazard ratio for death 0.76). Median survival was 18.9 months in group 2, 17.4 months in group 3, and 16.5 months in group 1. The proportions of patients with ≥50% reduction in serum PSA level were significantly higher in groups 2 and 3 than in group 1 (45% and 48% vs 32%, respectively). Patients in groups 2 and 3 were also significantly more likely than those in group 1 to meet the pain reduction criterion (35% and 31% vs 22%, respectively). Additionally, patients in groups 2 and 3 were significantly more likely to have improvements in their QOL (22% and 23% vs 13%, respectively). However, patients in groups 2 and 3 were also more likely to have ≥1 serious adverse event (26% and 29% vs 20%, respectively); most adverse events associated with docetaxel were more bothersome than life threatening.

Conclusion.—Compared with mitoxantrone plus low-dose prednisone, docetaxel plus low-dose prednisone in both regimens examined achieved significantly better PSA levels, pain control, and QOL in men with hormone-refractory prostate cancer. Importantly, the regimen of docetaxel every 3 weeks plus prednisone (group 2) led to superior survival compared with mitoxantrone plus prednisone. These findings suggest docetaxel in combination with prednisone may greatly contribute to our armamentarium for treating this devastating disease.

► Until now, no therapy has provided survival advantage for patients with hormone-refractory prostate cancer. These 2 studies (Abstracts 15–31 and 15–32) demonstrate that docetaxel, either combined with prednisone or with estramustine, provides approximately a 2-month survival advantage. In my opinion, these are landmark articles. While the survival advantage is modest at 2 months, we now have a foundation of effective therapy to build on. In the coming years, docetaxel will be used in combination with other cytotoxic and cytostatic agents in hormone-refractory prostate cancer. In addition, chemotherapy will be used earlier in the disease process, such as for PSA failures or for high-risk localized disease. There are some small differences between the 2 articles. First and foremost, the pain and QOL scores in Tannock et al (Abstract 15–32) were better in the docetaxel/prednisone arm than in the mitoxantrone/prednisone arm. This is particularly striking when one recognizes that mitoxantrone was approved by the Food and Drug Administration on the basis of its ability to decrease pain and improve QOL. What does this mean for the practicing urologist? Simply put, we need to refer our hormone-refractory patients to the medical oncologist earlier.

A. S. Kibel, MD

Humoral Immune Response to α-Methylacyl-CoA Racemase and Prostate Cancer

Sreekumar A, Laxman B, Rhodes DR, et al (Univ of Michigan, Ann Arbor; Harvard Med School, Boston)

J Natl Cancer Inst 96:834-943, 2004 15–33

Background.—Prostate cancer is the second-leading cause of cancer in men in the United States. Prostate-specific antigen (PSA) screening has resulted in earlier detection of prostate cancer, but the effects of PSA screening on cancer-specific mortality rate is unknown, and the specificity of this screening method is poor. As the use of serum PSA testing has increased, so has the number of prostate needle biopsies. A recent study has suggested lowering the threshold of PSA for recommending prostate biopsy from 4.1 ng/mL to 2.6 ng/mL to correct for verification bias and improve the clinical value of the PSA test; however, lowering the threshold will result in an additional increase in the number of prostate biopsies performed. Thus, additional serum and tissue biomarkers are needed to supplement PSA. The expression of α-methylacyl-CoA racemase (AMACR), which is involved in the conversion of R-stereoisomers of branched-chain fatty acids to S-stereoisomers, has been shown to be specifically increased in prostate cancer epithelia. However, no attempts have been successful to detect AMACR in circulation. Whether an immune response to AMACR could be used as a serum biomarker for prostate cancer was determined.

Methods.—Serum from 46 patients with biopsy-proved prostate cancer and 28 control subjects was screened for a humoral immune response to selected tumor antigens, including AMACR, using protein microarrays. The humoral immune response to AMACR was then validated using high-throughput immunoblot analysis in 151 patients and 259 control subjects and enzyme-linked immunosorbent assay (ELISA) in 54 patients and 55 control subjects. Receiver operating characteristic curves were used to determine the sensitivity and specificity of the immune response to AMACR for the detection of prostate cancer.

Results.—Immunoreactivity against AMACR was statistically significantly higher in sera from patients with prostate cancer than in control subjects by all 3 techniques. High-throughput immunoblot analysis showed that, in subjects with intermediate PSA levels of 4 to 10 ng/mL, the immune response against AMACR was more sensitive and specific than was PSA in distinguishing sera from prostate cancer patients versus control subjects (sensitivity and specificity of 77.8% and 80.6%, respectively vs 45.6% and 50%, respectively).

Conclusions.—Assays for detection of a humoral response against AMACR may provide an effective supplement to PSA screening in the identification of patients with clinically significant prostate cancer, particularly patients with intermediate PSA levels.

▶ We all know that PSA is an imperfect screening tool for detecting prostate cancer, and a significant effort is going into discovering a better test. This group from the University of Michigan attempted to identify better markers by using a protein microarray to determine relative levels of 12 tumor antigens, 1 of which was AMACR. They found that AMACR was preferentially elevated in patients with cancer over benign disease. None of the other markers tested were preferentially elevated, including CEA, HSC-70, HSP-47, HSP-60, and interestingly PSA.

Unfortunately, the group found that levels of AMACR were so low that it was difficult to detect actual protein levels, and therefore, they had to resort to detecting autoantibodies against AMACR. This demonstrated, in a validation cohort, a specificity of 80.6%% and a sensitivity of 77.8%%. The authors believed that the test would be most useful in combination with PSA screening and envisioned patients with an elevated PSA undergoing AMACR testing.

The major shortcoming of this test is that AMACR levels can be elevated in other cancers besides prostate. I find this of particular concern since a patient with an elevated AMACR level could be biopsied, found to have prostate cancer (which was incidental), and a more serious malignancy could be missed. A second issue is that since their test depends on antibodies, freezing may alter its sensitivity. As AMACR levels is validated in other patient populations, it may be important to pay close attention to how the samples are stored. With that said, I think this is an exciting new test for prostate carcinoma, and I expect we will be hearing much more about it in the near future.

A. S. Kibel, MD

Advanced Disease—Imaging and Treatment

Intermediate End Point for Prostate Cancer-Specific Mortality Following Salvage Hormonal Therapy for Prostate-Specific Antigen Failure

D'Amico AV, Moul JW, Carroll PR, et al (Brigham and Women's Hosp, Boston; Uniformed Services Univ, Bethesda, Md; Univ of California, San Francisco; et al)

J Natl Cancer Inst 96:509-515, 2004 15–34

Background.—Increasing prostate-specific antigen (PSA) levels are generally used for identification of patients with prostate cancer, but also define disease recurrence after initial therapy with radical prostatectomy or external beam radiation therapy. In many cases, increasing PSA levels will also trigger the start of secondary therapy. The most widely practiced secondary therapy is some form of salvage hormonal therapy, which nearly always reduces the serum PSA level. However, whether the PSA response to salvage hormonal therapy can act as an intermediate endpoint for prostate cancer-specific mortality (PCSM) is unclear. Whether PSA response, which was defined as the absolute value of the ratio of the rate of PSA change after salvage hormonal therapy to the rate of PSA changes before salvage therapy, is associated with the time to PCSM after salvage hormonal therapy was determined.

Methods.—The study cohort included a single-institution database of 199 patients who received salvage hormonal therapy for PSA failure after surgery or radiation therapy. The validation cohort, totaling 1255 patients, was formed from 2 pooled multi-institution databases containing baseline, treatment, and follow-up data on similar patients. The ability of PSA response and its constituents (ie, presalvage hormonal therapy PSA slope and postsalvage hormonal therapy PSA slope) to predict the time to PCSM after salvage hormonal therapy was assessed using Cox regression analysis.

Results.—A statistically significant association of PSA response with time to PCSM after salvage hormonal therapy was noted in both the study and validation cohorts. However, the constituents of PSA response were not significantly associated with time to PCSM after salvage hormonal therapy. Patients with a PSA response of 1 or less had a statistically significantly shorter time to PCSM than patients with a PSA response of more than 1 in both the study and validation cohorts.

Conclusions.—The PSA response to salvage hormonal therapy can be used as an intermediate endpoint for PCSM in patients with an increasing PSA level after surgery or radiation therapy.

► D'Amico and colleagues examined the PSA kinetics of patients who had PSA-only failure after radical prostatectomy or curative radiation therapy, and were then treated with hormone ablation. The long and the short of this article is that changes in PSA levels before and after hormone ablation can predict survival. A rapidly rising PSA before hormone ablation and a PSA value that does not fall with hormone ablation are poor prognostic signs. By combining these 2 variables, the authors could identify patients who are going to progress much more rapidly to death.

How should this study influence your practice? Identification of patients at high risk for progressing to metastatic disease and subsequent death should allow early referral to medical oncologists for systemic treatment. Now that docetaxel-based chemotherapy has proven to be effective, I think it behooves all of us to refer these high-risk patients more rapidly.

A. S. Kibel, MD

Bicalutamide 150 mg in Addition to Standard Care in Patients With Localized or Locally Advanced Prostate Cancer: Results From the Second Analysis of the Early Prostate Cancer Program at Median Followup of 5.4 Years

Wirth MP, See WA, McLeod DG, et al (Technical Univ, Dresden, Germany; Med College of Wisconsin, Milwaukee; Walter Reed Army Med Ctr, Washington, DC; et al)

J Urol 172:1865-1870, 2004 15–35

Purpose.—We evaluated the efficacy and tolerability of 150 mg bicalutamide daily given in addition to standard care, in patients with localized or locally advanced prostate cancer.

Materials and Methods.—The bicalutamide Early Prostate Cancer program consists of 3 randomized, double blind, placebo controlled trials prospectively designed for combined analysis. A total of 8,113 men with T1b-T4, M0, any N (N0 in 1 trial) prostate cancer were randomized to bicalutamide 150 mg/day (4,052) or placebo (4,061) in addition to standard care (radical prostatectomy, radiotherapy or watchful waiting). Primary end points were objective progression-free survival (PFS) and overall survival.

Results.—At median 5.4 years of followup (21.6% progression events) bicalutamide significantly improved PFS in the overall population. This result was driven by positive results in trials 24 and 25, with the North American trial (trial 23) showing no difference. Patients with locally advanced disease gained most benefit from bicalutamide in terms of PFS, irrespective of underlying therapy. Overall survival was similar in the bicalutamide and placebo groups, across the program and in each trial. Among watchful waiting patients survival appeared to be improved with bicalutamide in those with locally advanced disease, whereas survival appeared to be reduced with bicalutamide in those with localized disease. The most common adverse events with bicalutamide were gynecomastia and breast pain. Other adverse events occurred with a similarly low incidence in the 2 treatment groups.

Conclusions.—This analysis confirms that bicalutamide provides benefit in patients with locally advanced disease. The current data suggest that early or adjuvant hormonal therapy for patients at low risk of disease progression, such as those with localized disease, is not appropriate.

▶ This is a rather impressive effort to study over 8000 patients to determine if early high-dose (150 mg) bicalutamide alters prostate cancer outcome. While progression-free survival did favor the bicalutamide arm in the trial as a whole, there was no advantage to bicalutamide treatment in the North American arm of the trial, and patients with clinically localized disease actually appeared to do worse when treated with bicalutamide.

I believe this trial will eventually boil down to that age-old urologic question: Which is better—early or delayed hormone ablation? Patients with a reasonable likelihood of having occult metastatic disease are probably going to benefit from earlier ablation. I think the most interesting facet of the trial is that patients with minimal likelihood of having occult metastatic disease may actually do worse. Even a drug as safe as bicalutamide can have significant side effects and increase mortality.

I do not believe that the results of this trial should impact routine clinical practice at the current time. However, I think we need to continue to follow it closely.

A. S. Kibel, MD

Preoperative PSA Velocity and the Risk of Death From Prostate Cancer After Radical Prostatectomy

D'Amico AV, Chen M-H, Roehl KA, et al (Brigham and Women's Hosp, Boston; Harvard Med School, Boston; Univ of Connecticut, Storrs; et al)

N Engl J Med 351:125-135, 2004 15–36

Background.—Watchful waiting is an option for the management of localized prostate cancer when the patient and physician agree that the potential adverse effects of treatment exceed the expected benefit. Methods for identifying men who are unlikely to be cured of prostate cancer despite treatment with radical prostatectomy could facilitate the decision-making process regarding the treatment of these patients. It was determined whether men at risk for death from prostate cancer after radical prostatectomy can be identified by the rate of rise in prostate-specific antigen (PSA) levels (PSA velocity).

Methods.—A total of 1095 men with localized prostate cancer were studied to determine whether several factors—the PSA velocity, the PSA level at diagnosis, the Gleason score, and the clinical tumor stage—could predict the time of death from prostate cancer and death from any cause after radical prostatectomy.

Results.—In comparison with an annual PSA velocity of 2.0 ng/mL or less, an annual PSA velocity of more than 2.0 ng/mL was associated with a significantly shorter time to death from prostate cancer and death from any cause. An increasing PSA level at diagnosis, a Gleason score of 8, 9, or 10, and a clinical tumor stage of T2 were also predictive of the time to death from prostate cancer. The estimates of the risk of death from prostate cancer and death from any cause 7 years after radical prostatectomy in men with an annual PSA velocity of more than 2.0 ng/mL were also influenced by the PSA level, tumor stage, and Gleason score at diagnosis.

Conclusions.—Men with increases in their PSA level of more than 2.0 ng/mL in the year before a diagnosis of prostate cancer may have a relatively high risk of death from prostate cancer despite being treated with radical prostatectomy.

▶ The latest buzz word in prostate cancer is PSA kinetics. The concept is fairly simple: Patients with a rapidly rising PSA at the time of diagnosis are more likely to have prostate cancer and at the time of failure are more likely to die of prostate cancer. This has been true for patients failing primary local treatment, failing hormone ablation, and now even patients who have not yet been treated for their prostate cancer. This rather nice study from Dr D'Amico and colleagues demonstrated that patients with an annual PSA velocity of 2.0 ng/mL or greater were associated with a significantly shorter time to death from prostate cancer and death from any cause.

One of the things that I found most striking about this article is the relatively high number of patients that had this high PSA velocity. Out of the 1095 patients studied, 262, or around 25%, had this rather rapid PSA rise. Twenty-four of these 262 patients, or just under 10%, died of prostate cancer. In comparison, of the roughly 800 patients with PSA velocities less than 2.0 ng/mL per year, only 3 died of prostate cancer.

What this study does not answer is, "What would the outcome have been if the patients were not operated on?" Clearly, an aggressive surgical approach cured many of the patients. I therefore don't think this study should be used to identify patients for whom we have "no effective therapy" but instead to identify patients who may need multimodality therapy, possibly within the confines of a clinical trial.

A. S. Kibel, MD

Is the Efficacy of Hormonal Therapy Affected by Lymph Node Status? Data From the Bicalutamide (Casodex) Early Prostate Cancer Program

Iversen P, for the Casodex Early Prostate Cancer Trialists' Group (Rigshospitalet, Copenhagen; Technical Univ of Dresden, Germany; Med College of Wisconsin, Milwaukee; et al)

Urology 63:928-933, 2004 15–37

Background.—The value of adding bicalutamide (150 mg daily) to the standard care of patients with localized or locally advanced prostate cancer is being investigated in the ongoing bicalutamide Early Prostate Cancer program. The first combined analysis of this program at a 3-year median follow-up indicated that bicalutamide plus standard care (radical prostatectomy, radiotherapy, or watchful waiting) significantly reduces the risk of objective progression and prostate-specific antigen (PSA) doubling in patients with

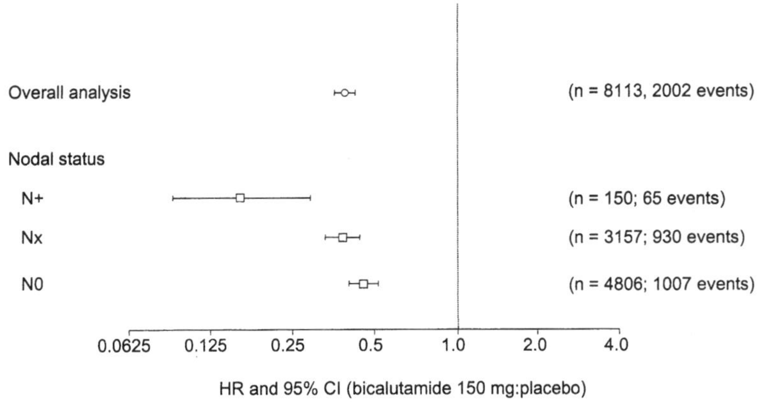

FIGURE 3.—Hazard ratios (*HRs*) and 95% confidence intervals (*CIs*) for time to prostate-specific antigen doubling for overall population and by nodal status at 3 years' median follow-up. (Reprinted from Iversen P, for the Casodex Early Prostate Cancer Trialists' Group: Is the efficacy of hormonal therapy affected by lymph node status? Data from the bicalutamide (Casodex) early prostate cancer program. *Urology* 63:928-933, 2004. Copyright 2004, with permission from Elsevier Science.)

localized/locally advanced prostate cancer. An exploratory subgroup analysis was reported that assessed the extent to which the overall benefit identified in the Early Prostate Cancer program is dependent on lymph node status at randomization.

Methods.—The study group was composed of 8113 men with localized/locally advanced disease receiving bicalutamide, 150 mg or placebo once daily, plus standard care. The time to event data (objective progression, PSA doubling) was analyzed by lymph node status at randomization.

Results.—When compared with standard care alone, bicalutamide significantly reduced the risk of objective progression, regardless of lymph node status. The most significant reduction occurred in patients with N+ compared with those with N0 and Nx disease. The greatest decline in risk of PSA doubling with bicalutamide was observed in N+ disease, with significantly reduced risks seen in patients with N0 and Nx disease (Fig 3).

Conclusion.—Bicalutamide was shown to significantly reduce the risk of objective disease progression and PSA doubling in patients with locally advanced prostate cancer, irrespective of lymph node status, when the bicalutamide is given in addition to standard care. There is a significant benefit of bicalutamide for patients with N+ disease, which suggests a benefit of early endocrine therapy for patients with N+ disease.

► This is another interim report from the Early Prostate Cancer trial that randomized men to immediate bicalutamide therapy, 150 mg once daily, or to standard of care. In this report, the authors say that patients with node-positive disease seem to have the greatest reduction in the hazard rate for time to PSA doubling (see Fig 3). The authors are correct in pointing out that the end point of time to PSA doubling is not established to correlate with survival. Nonetheless, this study provides additional data to the question of whether early hormonal therapy improves survival of men with node-positive prostate cancer. Further follow-up of this cohort will be necessary.

G. L. Andriole, Jr, MD

The Diagnosis and Treatment of Osteoporosis in Men On Androgen Deprivation Therapy for Advanced Carcinoma of the Prostate

Bae DC, Stein BS (Rhode Island Hosp; Brown Med School, Providence, RI)

J Urol 172:2137-2144, 2004 15–38

Purpose.—Androgen deprivation therapy (ADT) for advanced prostate cancer increases the risk of osteoporosis. Thus, the practicing urologist should be aware of the appropriate assessment and management. In this article we review the tests designed to diagnose osteoporosis as well as treatment options. We also review methods to monitor the response to therapy and make recommendations for management.

Material and Methods.—We performed a MEDLINE (1966 to 2004) search for the terms male, osteoporosis, bone mineral density, prostate cancer, androgen deprivation therapy, bisphosphonates, estrogen and the combinations thereof. We then constructed a management algorithm based on the best evidence available.

Results.—Dual energy x-ray absorptiometry of the hip is the gold standard test for osteoporosis. Biochemical markers of bone turnover are not suitable for diagnosis but they have been shown to be useful for monitoring the response to treatment. Smoking cessation, weight bearing exercise, and vitamin D and calcium have been shown to help improve bone mineral density (BMD). Bisphosphonates have been demonstrated to increase BMD and decrease fracture risk in men with osteoporosis. Estrogens have also recently been shown to decrease bone turnover and increase BMD in men on ADT.

Conclusions.—Hip dual energy x-ray absorptiometry should be performed in all men who are anticipated to be on long-term ADT. In addition, all men on ADT should receive vitamin D and calcium supplementation, and perform regular weight bearing exercise. The value of smoking cessation cannot be overstated. In men who have osteopenia or osteoporosis bisphosphonate therapy should be initiated. Estrogen therapy has shown promise but specific recommendations cannot be made at this time.

Hip Fractures in Men With Prostate Cancer Treated With Orchiectomy

Dickman PW, Adolfsson J, Åström K, et al (Karolinska Institutet, Stockholm)

J Urol 172:2208-2212, 2004 15–39

Purpose.—Androgen deprivation therapy increases the risk of osteoporosis related fractures. This issue is of increasing importance in men with prostate cancer as increasingly more undergo androgen deprivation therapy and therapy is administered sooner following diagnosis. Data directly addressing the long-term fracture risk in men diagnosed with prostate cancer are limited.

Materials and Methods.—Using population based registries in Sweden we studied the incidence of hip fractures in 17,731 men diagnosed with prostate cancer from 1964 to 1996 who were treated with bilateral orchiectomy within 6 months of diagnosis. The fracture incidence was compared to the incidence in 43,230 men diagnosed with prostate cancer but not treated with orchiectomy and in 362,354 of similar age who were randomly selected from the general population.

Results.—Men treated with orchiectomy were at increased risk for hip fracture. The estimated relative risk comparing men who underwent orchiectomy to population controls was 2.11 (95% CI 1.94 to 2.29) for femoral neck fractures and 2.16 (95% CI 1.97 to 2.36) for intertrochanter fractures. An increased risk of hip fracture was observed as early as 6 months after orchiectomy and the relative risk remained fairly constant up to 15 years following orchiectomy.

Conclusions.—Hip fracture risk increases almost immediately following orchiectomy and the excess risk persists for at least 15 years. This side effect should be considered when assessing the merits of androgen deprivation therapy, particularly in symptom-free men diagnosed with localized prostate cancer. Measures to prevent osteoporosis should be considered in men undergoing androgen deprivation therapy.

Risk of Fracture After Androgen Deprivation for Prostate Cancer

Shahinian VB, Kuo Y-F, Freeman JL, et al (Univ of Texas, Galveston)

N Engl J Med 352:154-164, 2005 15–40

Background.—The use of androgen-deprivation therapy for prostate cancer has increased substantially over the past 15 years. This treatment is associated with a loss of bone-mineral density, but the risk of fracture after androgen-deprivation therapy has not been well studied.

Methods.—We studied the records of 50,613 men who were listed in the linked database of the Surveillance, Epidemiology, and End Results program and Medicare as having received a diagnosis of prostate cancer in the period from 1992 through 1997. The primary outcomes were the occurrence of any fracture and the occurrence of a fracture resulting in hospitalization. Cox proportional-hazards analyses were adjusted for characteristics of the patients and the cancer, other cancer treatment received, and the occurrence of a fracture or the diagnosis of osteoporosis during the 12 months preceding the diagnosis of cancer.

Results.—Of men surviving at least five years after diagnosis, 19.4 percent of those who received androgen-deprivation therapy had a fracture, as compared with 12.6 percent of those not receiving androgen-deprivation therapy ($P<0.001$). In the Cox proportional-hazards analyses, adjusted for characteristics of the patient and the tumor, there was a statistically significant relation between the number of doses of gonadotropin-releasing hormone received during the 12 months after diagnosis and the subsequent risk of fracture.

Conclusions.—Androgen-deprivation therapy for prostate cancer increases the risk of fracture.

► There is a growing body of evidence that long-term hormone ablation causes significant morbidity, including osteoporosis and fracture. Since the average urologist sees only a few patients with these complications, it is often difficult to appreciate the magnitude of the risk. I would argue that Dickman et al (Abstract 15–39) and Shahinian et al (Abstract 15–40) provide fairly concrete evidence that androgen deprivation causes substantial harm to the patient. Dickman et al examined over 17,000 men diagnosed with prostate cancer in the 1960s through 1990s who were subsequently treated with bilateral orchiectomy. They compared this cohort of men to over 40,000 men diagnosed with prostate cancer but not treated with orchiectomy, and over 300,000 men without prostate cancer randomly selected from the general population. The end point they were looking at was admission to hospital for hip fracture. I would point out this is a very hard endpoint with clear clinical relevance. The authors found that the risk of femoral neck and intertrochanteric fractures was more than double that of control populations.

Many will question this studies relevance in the PSA era, however the results of Shahinian et al, a PSA era study, are remarkably similar. This study only included men diagnosed since 1992 and used the SEER database. They found that the risk of fracture increased from 12.6% to 19.5%. Importantly, there was no increased risk in individuals who received short-term hormone ablation (1 and 4 doses of a GnRH agonist). However, as you increase the number of doses received, the risk increased proportionately. The group with the highest risk were those who underwent orchiectomy. In a nutshell, long-term androgen ablation, causes significant morbidity. This does not mean that patients should not be treated, simply that we should not pull the trigger too soon.

What can urologists do to prevent fractures? This nice review article by Bae and Stein (Abstract 15–38) outlines different tests and treatments for osteoporosis secondary to androgen deprivation. Briefly, I believe that the standard of care in the United States requires patients receiving androgen deprivation to be encouraged to take Vitamin D and calcium. I believe that regular monitoring of bone marrow density is required, and patients who become osteoporotic should be made aware of at least the potential benefits of bisphosphonate therapy.

A. S. Kibel, MD

The Influence of Androgen Deprivation Therapy on Dihydrotestosterone Levels in Prostatic Tissue of Patients With Prostate Cancer

Nishiyama T, Hashimoto Y, Takahashi K (Niigata Univ, Japan; Nippon Kayaku Co Ltd, Tokyo)

Clin Cancer Res 10:7121-7126, 2004 15–41

Background.—First-line hormonal therapy has been used to impair the production or activity in androgens since it was first discovered that disseminated prostate cancer reacts favorable to castration or the administration of estrogenic hormones. However, the influence of androgen deprivation therapy on levels of dihydrotestosterone in prostatic tissue has not been clearly elucidated. Changes in these levels in the prostatic tissue during androgen deprivation therapy in the same patients have not been reported. Dihydrotestosterone levels in prostatic tissue before and after androgen deprivation therapy were analyzed.

Methods.—Prostatic biopsy was performed in 103 patients suspected of having prostate cancer. Of these patients, 69 were given a diagnosis of prostate cancer, while the remaining 34 patients received a negative diagnosis. Serum samples were collected before biopsy or prostatectomy. Dihydrotestosterone levels in prostatic tissue and serum were analyzed by liquid chromatography/electrospray ionization–mass spectrometry after polar derivatization. Of the 30 patients with prostate cancer, dihydrotestosterone levels in prostatic tissue were determined by performing rebiopsy or with prostate tissues excised after 6 months of androgen deprivation therapy with castration and flutamide.

Results.—The dihydrotestosterone levels in prostate tissue after androgen deprivation therapy remained at about 25% of the pretherapy measurement. Dihydrotestosterone levels in serum decreased to about 7.5% after androgen deprivation therapy. The level of dihydrotestosterone in prostatic tissue before androgen deprivation therapy was not correlated with the serum level of testosterone. Serum levels of adrenal androgens were reduced to approximately 60% after androgen deprivation therapy.

Conclusion.—The origin of dihydrotestosterone in prostatic tissue after androgen deprivation therapy involves intracrine production within the prostate, converting adrenal androgens to dihydrotestosterone. New therapies may be required, such as treatment with a combination of 5α-reductase inhibitors and antiandrogens, as well as castration.

▶ This interesting article shows that, among castrated patients, approximately 25% of the dihydrotestosterone concentration remains within the prostate tissue. It is unclear whether this dihydrotestosterone derives from metabolism of adrenal androgens. Persistence of dihydrotestosterone concentration is supportive of previous observations that there is usually a modest but measurable response to secondary and tertiary hormone manipulations for patients with recurrent prostate cancer after primary hormonal therapy.

This particularly lends credence to the possibility of using 5α-reductase inhibitors, such as dutasteride, to maximally inhibit formation of dihydrotestosterone within the prostate. Dutasteride may be preferable to finasteride as it inhibits both isoforms of 5α-reductase, whereas finasteride only inhibits the type II isoform. Recent studies have shown the presence of the type I isoform within prostate cancers.

G. L. Andriole, Jr, MD

16 Scrotum

Spermatic Cord Anesthesia Block for Scrotal Procedures in Outpatient Clinic Setting

Issa MM, Hsiao K, Bassel YS, et al (Emory Univ, Atlanta, Ga)

J Urol 172:2358-2361, 2004 16–1

Purpose.—We evaluated the safety and effectiveness of spermatic cord anesthetic block (SCAB) as the only method of anesthesia for bilateral simple orchiectomy in an outpatient clinic setting.

Materials and Methods.—The study included 141 consecutive bilateral simple orchiectomy (BSO) procedures performed at Atlanta Veterans Affairs Medical Center during a 33-month period. All procedures were performed in an outpatient clinic setting using SCAB as the only method of anesthesia. The anesthetic solution consisted of an equal mixture of 1% lidocaine with epinephrine at 1:100,000 and 0.25% bupivacaine. A 10-point visual analog pain scale was used to assess pain/discomfort at baseline, during SCAB instillation and during BSO. Postoperatively overall patient impression/satisfaction with SCAB as a method of anesthesia was determined.

Results.—Nine of the 141 available cases (6.4%) were excluded from study. The remaining 132 cases were included in data analysis. Mean patient age was 75.4 years (range 44 to 86). A total of 76 patients (57.6%) were receiving luteinizing hormone releasing hormone agonist therapy at the time of the procedure. The mean time needed to perform SCAB and BSO was 3.9 (range 2 to 6) and 33.0 minutes (range 12 to 70), respectively. The average volume of anesthetic solution was 20.1 ml per case (range 10 to 32). The mean pain score was 0.36 (range 0 to 8), 1.96 (range 0 to 8) and 0.33 (range 0 to 5) at baseline, and during SCAB and BSO, respectively. Of the patients 102 (77.3%) underwent a painless procedure (pain score = 0), 29 (21.9%) experienced transient pain that was mild in nature (pain score 4 or less) and only 1 (0.7%) had a pain score of 5. Pain scores were similar in patients who were and were not receiving luteinizing hormone releasing hormone agonists at baseline ($P = 0.36$), during SCAB instillation ($P = 0.89$) and during BSO ($P = 0.36$). The overall impression/satisfaction with SCAB as a method of anesthesia was rated as highly satisfactory by 91.7% of patients and satisfactory by 8.3%. There were no intraoperative adverse events related to SCAB.

Conclusions.—SCAB is a simple, safe and highly effective method of anesthesia for scrotal procedures. It allows such procedures to be performed in an outpatient clinic setting, offering convenience and the potential for cost savings.

► While the use of local anesthetics during office procedures is not an alien concept to urologists, this small but well-done case series illustrates how effective it can be. Using validated pain scales, the authors report that the median pain experienced by patients during a simple orchiectomy was 0 (essentially no pain). A similar technique has been used for years by urologists who perform vasectomy. The use of local anesthetics in the office also extends beyond just scrotal surgery. Issa and colleagues have previously reported use of nerve block during prostate biopsies.

Several caveats should be considered. First, make certain that the patient is not allergic to the local anesthetic agent. Second, aspirate before injection to avoid intravascular delivery of the anesthetic, and calculate the maximum dose that can safely be delivered. Last, this technique may not be suitable for all patients. For those patients who exhibit a high degree of anxiety, sedation in addition to the local anesthetic or use of a general anesthetic may still be appropriate.

J. T. Wei, MD, MSc

17 Infertility

Regeneration of Male Germline Stem Cells by Spermatogonial Dedifferentiation In Vivo

Brawley C, Matunis E (Johns Hopkins Univ, Baltimore, Md)

Science 304:1331-1334, 2004 17–1

Background.—The ability of engrafted stem cells to regenerate tissue has been well-studied, but the molecular mechanisms controlling regeneration are not well understood. The ligand Unpaired (Upd) is produced in the *Drosophila* testis after germline stem cells (GSCs) attach to a cluster of quiescent somatic cells, called the hub. The Janus kinase–signal transducer and Jak-STAT pathway within GSCs is locally activated by Upd for maintenance of stem cell fate. GSC divisions are stereotypically oriented, a situation that ensures that one daughter remains at the hub while the other differentiates. Studies have shown that GSCs null for the *Drosophila* STAT homolog *stat92E* differentiate, and so it was hypothesized that a temperature-sensitive allele of *stat92E* (*stat92E*^{F}) would allow the reversible control of GSC differentiation.

Methods.—*stat92E*^{F}/*stat92E*^{F06346} fruit flies die during embryogenesis at 29°C but are viable and fertile at 18°C, so the effects of removing *stat92E* on adult GSCs were studied using confocal microscopy for analysis of testes from *stat92E*^{F}/*stat92E*^{F06346} flies raised at 18°C and then shifted to 29°C.

Results.—It was suspected that spermatogonia reverted to stem cell fate because all or part of the testes from *stat92E*^{F}/*stat92E*^{F06346} flies shifted to 29°C for 2 and 4 days contained spermatogonia. In addition, males that were shifted to 29°C for 6 days and which lacked spermatogonia but contained spermatocytes never regained lost GSCs when returned to 18°C. Thus, it was determined that spermatogonia, not spermatocytes, revert to GSCs. An interesting finding is that somatic stem cells always returned in testes undergoing repopulation but were absent in 14% of day 2 testes. Spermatogonia that produce GSCs were found in clusters of 8 or 16 interconnected cells, which indicated that these multicellular cysts must break apart to produce GSCs when signaling is restored.

Conclusions.—Conditional manipulation of Jak-STAT signaling showed that spermatogonia that have initiated differentiation and are undergoing limited mitotic divisions can repopulate the niche and revert to stem cell identity. In the appropriate microenvironment, transit-amplifying cells de-differentiate and become functional stem cells during tissue regeneration.

► Spermatogenesis is a multi-step process by which type A spermatogonial stem cells divide and differentiate to produce mature spermatozoa. Based on the stem-cell renewal model, the type A spermatogonial stem cells proliferate to produce 2 types of spermatogonial cells; specifically, those that retain their stem cell potential and produce more spermatogonial stem cells, A_0; and, those cells that are committed down the path of differentiation (type A_1,A_2,A_3,A_4, intermediate, and type B spermatogonia). The type A_4 spermatogonial cell is thought to be able to maintain the renewal of more differentiation-committed type A_1 spermatogonia, as well as differentiate into intermediate spermatogonia. The type A_0 spermatogonial stem cells are thought to divide slowly and are kept in reserve to repopulate the testis following injury, or to maintain normal numbers of type A_1 spermatogonia.

Although the present study involves Drosophila spermatogonial cells, the concept that spermatogonial cells that have already committed down the path of differentiation may in fact be able to de-differentiate to maintain the testis stem cell population, is intriguing and deserves further investigation.

C. K. Naughton, MD

Prediction of Successful Outcome of Microdissection Testicular Sperm Extraction in Men With Idiopathic Nonobstructive Azoospermia

Tsujimura A, Matsumiya K, Miyagawa Y, et al (Osaka Univ, Suita, Japan; Osaka Central Hosp, Japan; Osaka Police Hosp, Japan)

J Urol 172:1944-1947, 2004 17–2

Purpose.—Microsurgical techniques in testicular sperm extraction can improve sperm retrieval in patients with nonobstructive azoospermia (NOA). However, spermatozoa retrieval rates have still been reported to be around 50% for patients with NOA. Thus, a reliable prediction method for successful outcome is needed to avoid unnecessary surgery. In this retrospective study we determined the diagnostic and predictive values of noninvasive parameters used in the treatment of patients with NOA.

Materials and Methods.—We analyzed 9 preoperative factors including patient age, testicular volume and endocrinological data of 100 patients with NOA using multivariate logistic modeling. Testicular spermatozoa were retrieved successfully in 41 of the 100 patients (41%).

Results.—We found that the concentrations of follicle-stimulating hormone (FSH), total testosterone (TT) and inhibin B were considered the most influential preoperative factors. We developed a formula to calculate the probability of successful outcome, $P = [1 + \exp(5.201 - 0.048 \times FSH - 0.449 \times TT - 0.021 \times \text{inhibin B})]^{-1}$. Association of predicted probabilities and observed responses was 0.77. A predicted probability of more than 15.7% was found to be the best cutoff. Sensitivity was 71.0% and specificity was 71.4% as determined by receiver operating characteristic analysis.

Conclusions.—We concluded that our formula should be useful for doctors considering microdissection testicular sperm extraction for patients with NOA because our equation uses noninvasive parameters without a preoperative testicular biopsy, which is a relatively invasive examination.

An Artificial Neural Network for Predicting the Presence of Spermatozoa in the Testes of Men With Nonobstructive Azoospermia

Samli MM, Dogan I (Afyon Kocatepe Univ, Turkey)

J Urol 171:2354-2357, 2004 17–3

Purpose.—We developed an artificial neural network (ANN) for predicting spermatozoa prior to testicular biopsy in men with nonobstructive azoospermia. The performance of this ANN was compared to that of the standard logistic regression (LR) model.

Materials and Methods.—Data were retrospectively collected from the physical examination and laboratory records of 303 patients who presented with infertility due to nonobstructive azoospermia. Input factors were patient age, duration of infertility, serum follicle-stimulating hormone, luteinizing hormone, total testosterone and prolactin, and left and right testicular volume. The ANN and LR models were constructed based on data on cases in which spermatozoa were and were not detected on testicular sperm extraction. The ANN was trained and validated with the data in the training (200 cases) and validation (30 cases) sets, and the model was then used to predict findings in the test set (73 cases). The LR model was constructed using the same data on the 230 training and validation cases. The same 73 patients served as the test set.

Results.—The sensitivity of the ANN model was significantly higher than that of the LR model (68% vs 28%, $p < 0.0001$). The neural network correctly predicted the outcome in 59 of the 73 test set patients (80.8%), whereas LR correctly predicted the outcome in 48 (65.7%, $p = 0.07$).

Conclusions.—This ANN model, which is based on age, duration of infertility, serum hormone levels and testicular volumes, has clinically acceptable sensitivity. It may be of value for predicting spermatozoa in men with nonobstructive azoospermia.

▶ Presently, the only option to establish a biologic pregnancy for men who present with NOA is assisted reproduction with testis sperm extraction. However, successful retrieval of spermatozoa suitable for in vitro fertilization combined with intracytoplasmic sperm injection varies between 24% and 79% based on testicular histology.[1]

The ability to predict successful spermatozoa retrieval rates from testis sperm extraction procedures would be a valuable tool in counseling couples considering assisted reproductive techniques. Tsujimura et al (Abstract 17–2) found preoperative hormone levels to be the most influential predictive factors and proposed a formula to predict the probability of successful outcome. However, some of these parameters have not been predictive in other studies.

Another approach suggested by Samli and Dogan (Abstract 17–3) is the use of an ANN. Unfortunately, the significant variables identified by this group as predictors of successful spermatozoa retrieval were different.

The differences in these 2 and other studies may simply reflect clinical differences among men with NOA. It is important to remember that predictors of successful spermatozoa retrieval for men with maturation arrest may not necessarily be identical for men with Sertoli cell only and/or hypospermatogenesis. Indeed, a combination of several clinical factors may be important in predicting successful spermatozoa retrieval; however, a better-defined patient population may be necessary before predictive models are generated.

C. K. Naughton, MD

Reference

1. Su LM, Palermo GD, Goldstein M, et al: Testicular sperm extraction with intracytoplasmic sperm injection for nonobstructive azoospermia: Testicular histology can predict success of sperm retrieval. *J Urol* 161:112-116, 1999.

Impaired Leydig Cell Function in Infertile Men: A Study of 357 Idiopathic Infertile Men and 318 Proven Fertile Controls

Andersson A-M, Jørgensen N, Frydelund-Larsen L, et al (Copenhagen Univ)

J Clin Endocrinol Metab 89:3161-3167, 2004 17–4

Introduction.—To investigate whether an impaired Leydig cell function is present in severely oligospermic men, serum testosterone (T), LH, estradiol (E_2), and SHBG levels in 357 idiopathic infertile men were compared with levels in 318 proven fertile men. In addition, the T/LH ratio, E_2/T ratio, and calculated free T index (cFT) were compared between the two groups. A shift toward lower serum T levels, cFT, and T/LH ratio and higher serum LH, E_2, and E_2/T levels was observed in the group of infertile men. On average, the infertile men had 18, 26, and 34% lower serum T, cFT, and T/LH levels, respectively, and 19, 18, and 33% higher serum LH, E_2, and E_2/T levels, respectively, than the fertile men. Twelve percent of the infertile men had a serum T level that fell below the 2.5 percentile of the fertile levels, and 15% of the infertile men had a LH level that was above the 97.5 percentile of the fertile levels. Thus, the group of infertile men showed significant signs of impaired Leydig cell function in parallel to their impaired spermatogenesis. The association of decreased spermatogenesis and impaired Leydig cell function might reflect a disturbed paracrine communication between the seminiferous epithelium and the Leydig cells, triggered by distorted function of the seminiferous epithelium. On the other hand, the parallel impairment of spermatogenesis and Leydig cells may reflect a congenital dysfunction of both compartments caused by a testicular dysgenesis during fetal/infant development.

▶ Germ cell dysfunction is extensively studied in models of aberrant spermatogenesis. This relatively large human study highlights the important role of non–germ cells, such as Leydig cells, in the testis for spermatogenesis. This study is simply based on blood hormone levels. As such, the authors address the importance of timing of blood sampling but admit that blood was drawn between a 5.5-hour period. To ensure that the time of day the blood was drawn did not affect hormone level results, a comparison of blood draw times between fertile and infertile men is needed. The observed differences in the hormone profile between fertile and infertile men should stimulate future studies of testicular non–germ cell function and its impact on spermatogenesis.

C. K. Naughton, MD

Association of Meiotic Arrest With Lack of *BOULE* Protein Expression in Infertile Men

Luetjens CM, Xu EY, Pera RAR, et al (Westphalian Wilhelms-Univ, Muenster, Germany; Univ of California, San Francisco)

J Clin Endocrinol Metab 89:1926-1933, 2004 17–5

Introduction.—Spermatogenesis is a complex developmental process of mitotic and meiotic cell divisions that ultimately results in production of haploid spermatozoa. Recent studies in flies demonstrate that the *BOULE* gene encodes a key factor of meiosis in male germ cells, regulating the expression of *twine*, a *cdc25* phosphatase, which promotes progression through meiosis. In this study, we investigated whether a common mechanism underlies the block of germ cell maturation observed in idiopathic and nonidiopathic azoospermic patients with meiotic arrest. We examined, by immunohistochemistry, *BOULE* and *CDC25A* phosphatase protein, the human homolog of twine, expression in 47 men with meiotic arrest, mixed atrophy, or normal spermatogenesis. The presence of genetic alterations within the *BOULE* gene was investigated by single-stranded conformation polymorphism. *BOULE* protein expression in men with complete spermatogenesis can be restricted to stages from leptotene up to stages of late spermatocytes, whereas *CDC25A* expression ranges from leptotene spermatocytes to elongating spermatids. Although spermatocytes were present in all testicular biopsies with meiotic arrest (28 testes), *BOULE* protein expression was completely lacking. In addition, in nearly all biopsies in which *BOULE* was absent, *CDC25A* was concomitantly lacking. However, no mutations or polymorphisms in the BOULE gene were identified, which could explain the lack of *BOULE* or *CDC25A* expression. These results indicate that a major group of infertile men with meiotic arrest lack *BOULE* protein and its putative target, *CDC25A* expression. The spermatogenic failure seems to arise from factor(s) upstream of *BOULE*, which are possibly involved in regulating transcription and/or translation of *BOULE*. Thus, the spermatogenic damage leading to meiotic arrest is independent of the etiology and indicates that *BOULE* is a possible fundamental mediator of meiotic transition in the human.

▶ This study characterized *BOULE* and downstream *CDC25A* protein expression in 18 men with complete meiotic arrest (maturation arrest), 16 men with "mixed atrophy," and 17 men with complete spermatogenesis (vasectomized patients). The authors suggest that *BOULE* is a possible mediator of germ cell meiotic transition in human beings, as all testicular biopsies with complete spermatogenesis demonstrated *BOULE* protein expression in spermatocytes, while no *BOULE* protein expression was observed in spermatocytes of testis biopsy histology of maturation arrest.

Although all testis tissues from vasectomized patients demonstrated *CDC25A* protein expression, 4 of 28 testicular units from 18 patients with complete maturation arrest demonstrated *CDC25A* protein expression despite lack of *BOULE* expression. Another concern is the difference in staining of right versus left testicles from the same patient with the identical histology. The number of samples are most likely too small to determine if this observation is real or technical. Furthermore, the heterogeneity of the patient population makes interpretation of results even more difficult. The authors recognize and acknowledge the diverse patient population in this group, but then suggest that the lack of *BOULE* expression independent of the etiology of the spermatogenetic damage makes *BOULE* more convincingly involved in meiotic arrest. Alternatively, it may suggest that lack of *BOULE* expression is a result of, and not necessarily a cause of, maturation arrest. The problems with this study are even more evident when carefully studying the 22 testicular units of the 16 men with "mixed atrophy." This group showed "moderate" *BOULE* spermatocyte staining in the majority of the seminiferous tubules. However, the status of germ cell maturation in tubules with staining versus those without staining was not reported. The staining results of these biopsies are potentially the most convincing, as seminiferous tubules with complete spermatogenesis are typically juxtaposed to seminiferous tubules with maturation arrest and Sertoli cell only pattern. Therefore, *BOULE* staining of spermatocytes in tubules with complete spermatogenesis and lack of staining of spermatocytes in tubules with maturation arrest would provide more convincing evidence that *BOULE* is a mediator of germ cell meiotic transition. The testicular sections that contain tubules of different histologies on the same slide are of most interest, as they serve as their own controls. Fortunately, the group of vasectomized patients demonstrates consistent *BOULE* and *CDC25A* staining in a defined patient population with complete spermatogenesis.

This study demonstrates the difficulty in interpreting results without a defined group of patients with identical clinical histories. It highlights the importance of strictly defining clinical criteria in patient study selection to contribute to the understanding of molecular mechanisms of these clinical entities.

C. K. Naughton, MD

Are Volunteers Delivering Semen Samples in Fertility Studies a Biased Population?

Eustache F, Auger J, Cabrol D, et al (Université Paris V; Hôpital Cochin, Paris)

Hum Reprod 19:2831-2837, 2004 17–6

Background.—It is not known to what extent the results of epidemiological studies on male fertility and semen quality based on voluntary participation in the general population are relevant.

Methods.—In a study on the reproductive health of male partners of pregnant women, information was obtained from a group of men agreeing to collect a semen sample and to complete a questionnaire (group A), a group only completing the questionnaire (group B) and from men refusing to participate altogether (group C).

Results.—The participation rate (group A) was 15.8% for 1409 men approached. Ages and socio-professional status were similar in the three groups. Time to pregnancy (TTP) was not significantly different in groups A and B, although there appeared to be an insignificantly higher proportion of couples taking longer than 12 months to conceive in group A than in group B. A history of urogenital disease appeared to be more frequent in groups A and B than in the general population. However, comparable semen characteristics were found for men with or without a history of urogenital disease. Pregnancy outcomes were similar in the three groups.

Conclusions.—The present study does not suggest major selection bias, although the social and reproductive histories of these men may prompt them to participate. Such factors need to be accounted for in similar studies.

Selection Bias in Semen Studies Due to Self-Selection of Volunteers

Muller A, De La Rochebrochard E, Labbé-Declèves C, et al (INSERM, Le Kremlin-Bicêtre, France; Université Paris 5; CECOS Midi-Pyrénées; et al)

Hum Reprod 19:2838-2844, 2004 17–7

Background.—Reports of a secular decrease in semen quality remain controversial, particularly due to the possibility of selection bias. We aimed to describe the potential bias due to self-selection of volunteers in semen studies involving fecund men.

Methods.—Using data from the French multicentre study REPRHOM, we compared the characteristics of the partners of pregnant women for three levels of participation: completion of a refusal questionnaire (n = 698), agreement to complete the study questionnaires only (n = 676) and agreement to complete the study questionnaires and give a semen sample (n = 331, 13% of the subjects approached).

Results.—Poorly educated men refused more often to participate than highly educated men. Semen providers were more likely to have experienced unfavourable pregnancy outcomes (odds ratio 1.68, 95% confidence interval 1.14-2.49) compared with participants completing the questionnaires only. Time to pregnancy was similar for all participants.

Conclusions.—This study demonstrates the existence of selection bias in semen studies associated with fertility and socio-demographic characteristics of men. The results of semen analysis for this population sample cannot be extrapolated to the whole population from which the volunteers originate. More information is required on who participates, and participation rates should be reported in semen studies to make it possible to interpret the results correctly.

► Clinical studies involving semen parameters often collect control data from fertile male donor volunteers. These 2 articles (Abstracts 17-6 and 17–7) address possible selection bias in this population attributable to self-selection of volunteers.

Although one study noted presence of selection bias while the other study did not, both found that men with higher educational levels were more likely to agree to participation than less-educated men. In one study, the volunteers tended to be those who were concerned about their fertility because of previous urogenital history.

These studies highlight potential selection bias of semen samples from men who agree to participate. Each donor population should be characterized separately, and identified factors should be taken into consideration before interpreting results.

C. K. Naughton, MD

Adolescents With Open-Identity Sperm Donors: Reports From 12-17 Year Olds

Scheib JE, Riordan M, Rubin S (Univ of California, Davis; Sperm Bank of California, Berkeley; World, Oakland; et al)

Hum Reprod 20:239-252, 2004 17–8

Background.—Donor insemination programs can include 'open-identity' sperm donors, who are willing to release their identities to adult offspring. We report findings from adolescent offspring who have open-identity donors.

Methods.—Using mail-back questionnaires, youths from 29 households (41.4% headed by lesbian couples, 37.9% by single women, 20.7% by heterosexual couples) reported their experience growing up knowing how they were conceived and their interest in the donor's identity.

Results.—Most youths (75.9%) reported always knowing, and were somewhat to very comfortable with their conception origins. All but one felt knowing had a neutral to positive impact on their relationship with their birth mother and, separately, co-parent. The youths' top question about the donor was, 'What's he like?' and >80% felt at least moderately likely to request his identity and pursue contact. Finally, of those who might contact the donor, 82.8% would do so to learn more about him, with many believing it would help them learn more about themselves. No youth reported wanting money and few (6.9%) wanted a father/child relationship. We also discuss differences found among youths from different household types.

Conclusions.—The majority of the youths felt comfortable with their origins and planned to obtain their donor's identity, although not necessarily at age 18.

▶ The increasing number of donor insemination programs worldwide offering "open-identity" sperm donors has sparked interest in learning how adolescent offspring perceive and respond to available information. No formal recommendations exist as to when and how children born from open-identity donors should be counseled. This descriptive report from adolescents born from open-identity sperm donors is the first step in defining guidelines for parents using this resource.

C. K. Naughton, MD

A Sertoli Cell-Selective Knockout of the Androgen Receptor Causes Spermatogenic Arrest in Meiosis

De Gendt K, Swinnen JV, Kaunders PTK, et al (Flanders Interuniversity Inst for Biotechnology, Belgium; Catholic Univ of Leuven, Belgium; Centre for Reproductive Biology, Edinburgh, Scotland; et al)

Proc Natl Acad Sci U S A 101:1327-1332, 2004 17–9

Introduction.—Androgens control spermatogenesis, but germ cells themselves do not express a functional androgen receptor (AR). Androgen regulation is thought to be mediated by Sertoli and peritubular myoid cells, but their relative roles and the mechanisms involved remain largely unknown. Using *Cre/loxP* technology, we have generated mice with a ubiquitous knockout of the AR as well as mice with a selective AR knockout in Sertoli cells (SC) only. Mice with a floxed exon 2 of the AR gene were crossed with mice expressing Cre recombinase ubiquitously or selectively in SC (under control of the anti-Mullerian hormone gene promoter). AR knockout males displayed a complete androgen insensitivity phenotype. Testes were located abdominally, and germ cell development was severely disrupted. In contrast, SC AR knockout males showed normal testis descent and development of the male urogenital tract. Expression of the homeobox gene *Pem*, which is androgen-regulated in SC, was severely decreased. Testis weight was reduced to 28% of that in WT littermates. Stereological analysis indicated that the number of SC was unchanged, whereas numbers of spermatocytes, round spermatids, and elongated spermatids were reduced to 64%, 3%, and 0% respectively of WT. These changes were associated with increased germ cell apoptosis and grossly reduced expression of genes specific for late spermatocyte or spermatid development. It is concluded that cell-autonomous action of the AR in SC is an absolute requirement for androgen maintenance of complete spermatogenesis, and that spermatocyte/spermatid development/survival critically depends on androgens.

► Androgenic regulation of spermatogenesis is thought to be mediated through Sertoli cells, as germ cells themselves do not express a functional AR. These investigators were able to selectively knock out the AR expression of Sertoli cells, driven by an anti-Müllerian hormone gene promoter, and show that SC-selective knockout (SCARKO) mice testes display a spermatogenic arrest at the late spermatocyte/spermatid developmental stage.

Mice with ubiquitous knockout of the AR (ARKO) are phenotypically different from SCARKO, as ARKO mice display complete androgen insensitivity. Testes of ARKO mice are much smaller than normal males and are located in the abdominal or inguinal region. Wolffian duct structures, specifically the vas deferens, epididymis, and seminal vesicles, and urogenital sinus (prostate) are absent. In contrast, SCARKO mice show normal external sexual development and normal Wolffian duct development without evidence of cryptorchidism. Further, serum levels of total testosterone, luteinizing hormone, and follicle stimulating hormone were indistinguishable from wild-type animals. However, histologic analyses of SCARKO testes demonstrate spermatogenic arrest at the primary spermatocyte to secondary spermatocyte stage. Secondary spermatocytes and round spermatids were observed, but in significantly reduced numbers. No elongated spermatids were detected in mutant testes.

The generation of SCARKO mice has answered some interesting questions regarding selective inactivation of the AR in mouse SCs. First, it does not prevent testicular descent and allows normal development of Wolffian duct structures. Second, direct actions of androgens on SC, mediated by AR, are critical for subsequent maturation of spermatocytes.

The "normal" number of SCs in SCARKO mice in this report was based on measurements of nuclear volume per testis, or simply morphology. It would be more convincing to base the unchanged SC number with available SC markers. Even more convincing would have been to perform double immunohistochemical studies to demonstrate normal number of SCs and absence of AR in mutant testes compared with WT. Further, the mechanism of how the lack of AR expression regulates spermatogenesis was not sufficient. The authors note an increase in apoptotic germ cells in SCARKO testes; however, the cell type undergoing apoptosis is not clear. Is it a decrease in the spermatogonial cell population, so that these cells never have a chance to mature into spermatocytes, or is it cell death of the spermatocytes, which results in absence of spermatids? What does the loss of AR expression do to intratesticular testosterone levels? Could aberrant intratesticular testosterone levels be involved in the mechanism of observed abnormal spermatogenesis?

Although the answers to these questions are not clear from this report, the phenotype may carry insight into a potential mechanism for the human condition of maturation arrest.

C. K. Naughton, MD

Infertility With Defective Spermatogenesis and Hypotestosteronemia in Male Mice Lacking the Androgen Receptor in Sertoli Cells

Chang C, Chen Y-T, Yeh S-D, et al (Univ of Rochester, NY; Chang Gun Mem Hosp, Kaohsiung, Taiwan; Taipei Med Univ, Taiwan; et al)

Proc Natl Acad Sci U S A 101:6876-6881, 2004 17–10

Introduction.—Androgens and the androgen receptor (AR) play important roles in male fertility, although the detailed mechanisms, particularly how androgen/AR influences spermatogenesis in particular cell types, remain unclear. Using a Cre-Lox conditional knockout strategy, we generated a tissue-specific knockout mouse with the AR gene deleted only in Sertoli cells (S-AR$^{-/y}$). Phenotype analyses show the S-AR$^{-/y}$ mice were indistinguishable from WT AR mice (B6 AR$^{+/y}$) with the exception of testes, which were significantly atrophied. S-AR$^{-/y}$ mice were infertile, with spermatogenic arrest predominately at the diplotene premeiotic stage and almost no sperm detected in the epididymides. S-AR$^{-/y}$ mice also have lower serum testosterone concentrations and higher serum leuteinizing hormone concentrations than B6 AR$^{+/y}$ mice. Further mechanistic studies demonstrated that S-AR$^{-/y}$ mice have defects in the expression of anti-Müllerian hormone, androgen-binding protein, cyclin A1, and sperm-1, which play important roles in the control of spermatogenesis and/or steroidogenesis. Together, our Sertoli cell-specific AR knockout mice provide in vivo evidence of the need for functional AR in Sertoli cells to maintain normal spermatogenesis and testosterone production, and ensure normal male fertility.

► Another group generated a tissue-specific knockout mouse with the AR deleted only in Sertoli cells by the Cre-Lox conditional knockout strategy. Similar to the SCARKO mouse discussed in Abstract 17–9, the knockout mice were indistinguishable from wild-type mice except for significantly atrophied testes. Histology revealed spermatogenic arrest predominantly at the premeiotic stage. These mice were also found to have defects in the expression of anti-Müllerian hormone (AMH), androgen-binding protein, cyclin A1, and sperm-1. The increased expression of AMH suggests that the loss of AR in Sertoli cells causes increased AMH that affects Leydig cell production and secretion of testosterone.

This study, in combination with the study in Abstract 17–9, provides in vivo evidence that AR expression of Sertoli cells is important for meiosis of spermatocytes. What is unclear from this report is when the Cre-Lox system was activated, that is, at what age the animals were mated to produce the mutant mice. I assume matings were performed when the mice were mature, usually at 6 to 8 weeks. We know that when AR expression is lost from birth, the phenotype also shows maturation arrest (SCARKO mice). It would be interesting to mate these conditional animals at different times during the first wave of spermatogenesis to determine the spermatogenetic effect if AR is lost after the first wave is completed. Does it affect subsequent waves of spermatogenesis the same way?

C. K. Naughton, MD

Deletion of the Parkin Coregulated Gene Causes Male Sterility in the *quaking*^{viable} Mouse Mutant

Lorenzetti D, Bishop CE, Justice MJ (Baylor College of Medicine, Houston)
Proc Natl Acad Sci U S A 101:8402-8407, 2004 17–11

Introduction.—Quaking^{viable} (*qk*^{v}) is a recessive neurological mouse mutation with severe dysmyelination of the CNS and spermiogenesis failure. The molecular lesion in the *qk*^{v} mutant is a deletion of approximately 1 Mb on mouse chromosome 17 that alters the expression of the qk gene in oligodendrocytes. Complementation analysis between the *qk*^{v} mutation and *qk* mutant alleles generated through chemical mutagenesis showed that the male sterility is a distinctive feature of the *qk*^{v} allele. This observation suggested that the sperm differentiation defect in *qk*^{v} is due to the deletion of a gene(s) distinct from *qk*. Here, we demonstrate that the deletion of *Pacrg* is the cause of male sterility in the *qk*^{v} mutant. *Pacrg* is the mouse homologue of the human *PARKIN*-coregulated gene (*PACRG*), which encodes for a protein whose biochemical function remains unclear. We show that *Pacrg* is highly expressed in the testes in both mice and humans. In addition, the expression pattern of *Pacrg* during spermiogenesis suggests that it plays a role in sperm differentiation. In support of this hypothesis, we show that transgenic expression of *Pacrg* in testes restores spermiogenesis and fertility in *qk*^{v} males. This finding provides the first in vivo evidence, to our knowledge, for the function of Pacrg in a model organism. Immunolocalization experiments on isolated spermatozoa show that the Pacrg protein is present in mature sperm. Remarkably, the mammalian Pacrg protein shares significant sequence similarities with gene products from flagellated protozoans, suggesting that Pacrg may be necessary for proper flagellar formation in many organisms.

► One of 2 genes mapped to the *qk*^{v} deletion of approximately 1 Mb on mouse chromosome 17, which alters expression of the *qk* gene in oligodendrocytes, termed *PARKIN*-coregulated gene (*PACRG*), was found to be the cause of male infertility in *qk*^{v} mice.

Pacrg protein was localized to the postacrosomal region of the sperm head and to the flagellum midpiece. Based on protein expression, one would suspect abnormalities in sperm motility. Indeed, authors report only rare abnormal sperm in the epididymis of nontransgenic *qk*^{v}/*qk*^{v} males compared with numerous motile spermatozoa of *qk*^{v}/*qk*^{v} transgenic animals produced by breeding rescue experiments. Unfortunately, these important differences were data not shown in the report. Instead, the authors include testicular histology, attempting to demonstrate presence of long-tailed spermatozoa in the lumen of testes of rescued animals versus nontransgenic *qk*^{v}/*qk*^{v} males. Differences in testicular histology would suggest aberrant spermatogenesis, which should be accompanied by quantitative testicular histology analyses (ie, the percentage of seminiferous tubules restored with rescue breeding). The structural presence of long-tailed spermatozoa in the epididymis of nontransgenic animals, however, suggests that the abnormal motility observed in these animals is not caused by aberrant spermiogenesis.

This study reports restoration of sperm motility with rescue breeding experiments of nontransgenic qk^v/qk^v animals. *Pacrg* may be involved in cases of male infertility caused by sperm motility dysfunction.

C. K. Naughton, MD

Transgenic Zebrafish Produced by Retroviral Infection of *in Vitro*-Cultured Sperm

Kurita K, Burgess SM, Sakai N (Fukui Prefectural Univ, Obama, Japan; NIH, Bethesda, Md)

Psychiatr Serv 101:1263-1267, 2004 17–12

Introduction.—Transgenic modification of sperm before fertilization has distinct advantages over conventional transgenic methods. The primary advantage is that the mosaicism inherent in those other techniques is avoided. A culture system using primary cultures of zebrafish male germ cells, in which the differentiation from spermatogonia to functional sperm can occur *in vitro*, provides the opportunity for genetic modification of sperm *in vitro*. Here, we report the production of transgenic zebrafish from cultured sperm. The sperm were differentiated from premeiotic germ cells infected with a pseudotyped retrovirus *in vitro*. The collected sperm were used to perform successful *in vitro* fertilizations, and transgenic embryos were identified. The transgenic fish transmitted the proviral integration to the next generation in a Mendelian fashion. We report the generation of a transgenic animal by cultured sperm and open the door to many exciting possibilities for the rapid generation of transgenic lines in model organisms such as zebrafish or other animal systems that are otherwise intractable to transgenesis.

▶ The ability to genetically manipulate testicular germ cells has tremendous clinical potential in the treatment of genetic disease. However, genetic manipulation of male germ cells is challenging because of the small population of testicular stem cells, difficulties in maintaining a male stem cell line, and low intrinsic infectivity of germ cells. Indeed, in this study, despite use of high-titer retrovirus, total efficiency of transgenic fish production from 12-day cultured sperm was only 5%. The observed efficiency further demonstrates the intrinsically low infection rate of these particular cells. This study highlights the challenge of overcoming these recognized limitations before gene therapy may be applied clinically.

C. K. Naughton, MD

18 Sexual Function

What Is the Relationship Between Male Sexual Function and Lower Urinary Tract Symptoms (LUTS)?

Sak SC, Hussain Z, Johnston C, et al (St James Univ, Leeds, England; Univ of Leeds, England)

Eur Urol 46:482-487, 2004 18–1

Introduction.—There is considerable current interest in the relationship between LUTS and sexual function in men, and in particular whether there is a causative relationship between them. This observational study, performed in a single centre, seeks to explore this area further.

Methods.—1420 patients attending a prostate assessment clinic were assessed by International Prostate Symptoms Score (IPSS), BPH impact index (BPH-II), Urinary flow rate (Q_{max}), post-void residual volume (PVR) and the O'Leary sexual questionnaire (which assesses erectile, ejaculatory and sexual drive). The results were analyzed using univariate and multivariate techniques.

Results.—Following exclusion of those with incomplete data, those who were not sexually active, those with PSA >20 ng/ml and those who refused to fill in the questionnaire, there were 696 evaluable patients. Using univariate techniques, age, IPSS, Quality of life (QOL), BPH-II, Q_{max} and PVR all correlated with differing domains of sexual function including erectile and ejaculatory function. Multiple regression analysis demonstrated that age was overwhelmingly the most important predictor of sexual function, but that BPH-II and QOL were also predictive for some domains, while the IPSS score was not.

Conclusion.—This study confirms that a significant proportion of men with LUTS have sexual dysfunction. The relationship is complex and differs according to the type of sexual dysfunction.

▶ There is an ever-growing body of evidence from the epidemiologic literature relating LUTS and their severity to male sexual dysfunction. These investigators from the United Kingdom assessed 1420 patients attending a prostate assessment clinic and gave them the IPSS and BPH-Impact Index as well as a sexual questionnaire. The O'Leary sexual questionnaire was utilized rather than the more standardized International Index of Erectile Function questionnaire. The authors demonstrated a significant correlation between LUTS and the various domains of the O'Leary sexual questionnaire, namely interest, erection, ejaculation problem, and overall satisfaction domain. These relationships, however, are complex and differ according to the type of the sexual dysfunction. Nonetheless, this rather large cross-sectional assessment adds to a growing body of knowledge regarding the relationship between male sexual dysfunction and LUTS and suggests the need for a more translational and basic research regarding the pathophysiologic mechanism underlying it.

C. G. Roehrborn, MD

AUA Guideline on the Pharmacologic Management of Premature Ejaculation

Montague DK, Jarow J, Broderick GA, et al (American Urological Association, Inc)

J Urol 172:290-294, 2004 18–2

Background.—Most epidemiologic studies have suggested that premature ejaculation (PE) may be the most common sexual disorder in men. Data from the National Health and Social Life Survey have suggested a prevalence of 21% in men aged 18 to 59 years in the United States. Other studies (using varying definitions of PE) have reported prevalences ranging from fewer than 5% to greater than 30%. As yet there is no universally accepted definition of PE, and the exact cause of this disorder is unknown. Recommendations on the use of medications currently available in the United States for treatment of PE were presented.

Methods.—A search of the MEDLINE database was conducted by the Erectile Dysfunction Guideline Update Panel of the American Urological Association for relevant articles in the English language. However, the lack of standardization in studying PE, lack of agreement in quantitating the amount of stimulation the patients experienced, and a lack of consistency and accuracy in measuring the time to ejaculation and other outcomes precluded the use of a meta-analysis. The guidelines developed by the panel were based solely on consensus or consensus combined with a review of the available evidence.

Results.—Several recommendations were developed. First, the diagnosis of PE is made on the basis of sexual history alone, and a detailed sexual history should be obtained from all patients with ejaculatory symptoms Second, patients with concomitant PE and erectile dysfunction should be treated for the erectile dysfunction first. Third, the risks and benefits of all treatment options should be discussed with the patients before any interventions. The primary goal of treatment in PE is patient and partner satisfaction. Substantial evidence shows that patients can benefit from the use of several oral or topical medications, including serotonin reuptake inhibitors and topical anesthetics. The optimal treatment choice should be based on the judgment of the physician and patient preference.

Conclusions.—PE has traditionally been treated with psychotherapy or behavioral therapy. This report is the first to address the pharmacologic treatment of PE.

▶ Even though PE may be the most common male sexual disorder, its etiology is poorly understood. Since urologists rarely prescribe behavioral approaches, these guidelines deal solely with pharmacologic management. None of the discussed treatments is approved by the Food and Drug Administration for this indication, but both oral antidepressants and topical anesthetics do delay ejaculation with minimal side effects.

D. E. Coplen, MD

Erectile Dysfunction After a Long-distance Cycling Event: Associations With Bicycle Characteristics

Dettori JR, Koepsell TD, Cummings P, et al (Univ of Washington, Seattle)

J Urol 172:637-641, 2004 18–3

Purpose.—We conducted a prospective cohort study to examine the relationship between bicycle characteristics and the occurrence of erectile dysfunction.

Materials and Methods.—Subjects consisted of 463 cyclists completing a cycling event of at least 320 km who were free of erectile dysfunction before their event.

Results.—The cumulative incidence of erectile dysfunction after the ride was 4.2% (95% confidence interval [CI] 2.4%-6.8%) and 1.8% (95% CI 0.7%-3.8%) 1 week and 1 month after the event, respectively. Bicycle characteristics associated with an increased risk of erectile dysfunction included a mountain bicycle compared with a road bicycle (risk ratio [RR] 4.1, 95% CI 1.6-12.5), and the relative height of the handlebars parallel with or higher than the saddle compared with the relative handlebar height lower than the saddle (RR 3.0, 95% CI 1.1-9.3). Perineal numbness during the ride was experienced by 31% of the cyclists and was associated with erectile dysfunction (RR 4.4, 95% CI 1.6-12.7). Saddle cutouts were associated with an increased risk of erectile dysfunction among those who experienced numbness (RR 6.0, 95% CI 1.3-27.1), but the association was reversed among those who did not report numbness (RR 0.3, 95% CI 0.0-2.5).

Conclusions.—If the associations described are causal, then cyclists on a long-distance ride may be able to decrease the risk of erectile dysfunction by riding a road bicycle instead of a mountain bicycle, keeping handlebar height lower than saddle height and using a saddle without a cutout if perineal numbness is experienced.

Bicycle Riding and its Relationship to the Development of Erectile Dysfunction

Taylor JA III, Kao T-C, Albertsen PC, et al (Univ of Connecticut Health Ctr, Farmington; Uniformed Services Univ of the Health Sciences, Bethesda, Md; Columbia Univ, New York)

J Urol 172:1028-1031, 2004 18–4

Purpose.—Researchers have suggested that cycling is a hazard to the sexual health of men. Insufficient data have left cyclists skeptical of this claim. We explore risk factors within cycling that may put riders at risk for the development of erectile dysfunction (ED).

Materials and Methods.—We performed an Internet based survey of cyclists to examine factors associated with cycling that might contribute to ED as defined by the International Index of Erectile Function. A total of 688 cyclists were included in the analysis ranging in age from 18 to 77 years.

Results.—ED prevalence was 17% (115 of 688). Although results from univariate analysis revealed a correlation between ED and several tested variables, none proved to be statistically significant after controlling for age.

Conclusions.—The overall prevalence of ED in the cycling community does not appear to be greater than that of historical controls. Previously suggested alterations in riding habits may not change the prevalence of ED among cyclists.

▶ A relationship between ED and bicycle riding has been hypothesized. There may be a relationship between saddle design, perineal pressure, and ED,[1] although there has never been a clinical trial showing the efficacy of new "anatomically correct" saddles. Taylor et al (Abstract 18–4) performed an internet-based survey of recreational cyclists. They were unable to demonstrate a significant correlation between pudendal pressure and ED. The study is potentially limited by small sample size and response bias. This may have resulted in insufficient power to detect subtle relationships between some of the risk factors and ED. Dettori et al (Abstract 18–3) report a cumulative incidence of 4.2% and 1.8% of ED 1 week and 1 month after 200-mile bike rides. Mountain bikes and high handlebars seem to be the largest risk factor for ED. A saddle cutout was not protective. Perineal numbness during riding seemed to be the most significant association with the development of ED. Bicycling is an excellent form of exercise and attention to bicycle fit and posture should help to eliminate the small risk of developing ED.

D. E. Coplen, MD

Reference

1. Lowe BD, Schrader SM, Breitenstein MJ: Effect of bicycle saddle designs on the pressure to the perineum of the bicyclist. *Med Sci Sports Exerc* 36:1055-1062, 2004.

Evaluation of the Safety of Sildenafil for Male Erectile Dysfunction: Experience Gained in General Practice Use in England in 1999

Boshier A, Wilton LV, Shakir SAW (Drug Safety Research Unit, Southampton, England)

BJU Int 93:796-801, 2004 18–5

Objective.—To examine the safety of sildenafil, the first of the phosphodiesterase type 5 inhibitors licensed for the treatment of male erectile dysfunction (ED), as used in general medical practice in England, quantifying the incidence of a range of events in patients treated with sildenafil, and identifying any previously unrecognized adverse drug reactions.

Methods.—In a postmarketing observational cohort study using prescription-event monitoring (PEM), exposure data were derived from dispensed prescription details for patients who started treatment between April and August 1999. Outcome data were derived from 'green form' questionnaires (GFs) returned by general practitioners (GPs).

Results.—In all, 24,835 (54.7%) of GFs posted to GPs were returned, of which 22,473 contained useful data for 22,471 male and two female patients. The major primary indications/clinical context of prescribing were impotence (16,583, 73.8%) and diabetes mellitus (183, 0.8%); 145 events were reported as adverse drug reactions to sildenafil. GPs recorded 3951 reasons for stopping sildenafil, and ischemic heart disease (IHD) in 135 patients was the commonest clinical reason reported. The clinical condition reported most frequently in the first month of observation was diabetes mellitus and/or hyperglycemia (in 99 events). A standardized mortality ratio (SMR) for deaths caused by IHD in the first 8893 of 22,473 patients was 31.41 (95% confidence interval, 18.29-50.29), using the comparator population of males in England in 1998.

Conclusion.—This study identified the safety profile of sildenafil as used in the community, showing no unexpected events. The SMR analysis of deaths from IHD provided no evidence to suggest a higher incidence of deaths in the study cohort than in the male population in England.

▶ The evaluation of long-term safety of medications is very important. Sildenafil was first approved for use in the United Kingdom in 1988. A major concern with the medication is the potential for cardiac events related either to concomitant use of nitrates or increases in physical stress associated with sexual activity. This is a very large study (22,000 men) that suggests no higher incidence of myocardial infarction or fatal ischemic heart disease in users of sildenafil. In addition, other severe adverse events were very rare. These findings may be limited by underreporting but give some useful information regarding the safety of the product.

D. E. Coplen, MD

On-Demand Treatment of Premature Ejaculation with Clomipramine and Paroxetine: A Randomized, Double-blind Fixed-dose Study With Stopwatch Assessment

Waldinger MD, Zwinderman AH, Olivier B (Leyenburg Hosp, The Hague, The Netherlands; Utrecht Univ, The Netherlands; Univ of Amsterdam)
Eur Urol 46:510-516, 2004 18–6

Objective.—To investigate the degree of ejaculation delay induced by on-demand treatment with 20 mg paroxetine and 25 mg clomipramine and to assess the type and severity of non-sexual side-effects of treatment at the day of and the day after treatment with these drugs.

Method.—A randomized, double-blind, fixed-dose, on-demand study in 30 men with lifelong premature ejaculation was performed. During a 1-month baseline period and a 4-week drug treatment period patients assessed the intravaginal ejaculation latency time (IELT) at home with a stopwatch. Only men with an IELT < 1 min were randomly assigned to drug treatment. Patients assessed the drug coitus interval time (DCIT) and used the UKU side effect scale questionnaire at baseline, the day of and the day after intercourse.

Results.—On-demand treatment with 25 mg clomipramine, with a mean DCIT of 5.14 h, led to a 4.05 (95%CI: 3.26-5.02) fold-increase of the IELT. On-demand treatment with 20 mg paroxetine, with a mean DCIT of 5.39 h, led to a 1.41 (95%CI: 1.22-1.63) fold-increase of the IELT. Both drugs had a high incidence of non-sexual side effects at the coitus day and the next day. At the day of coitus paroxetine led to significant sleepiness and yawning compared to clomipramine. At the day after coitus clomipramine induced significant nausea compared to paroxetine.

Conclusion.—On-demand treatment with 25 mg clomipramine led to a clinical relevant ejaculation delay. In contrast, 20 mg paroxetine had no clinical relevant ejaculation delay in men with lifelong premature ejaculation with an IELT of less than 1 minute. Both drugs exert mostly mild yet annoying non-sexual side effects both at the coitus day and the next day.

▶ Because the exact etiology of premature ejaculation is unknown, treatment includes both behavioral modification and pharmacotherapy. The authors show increased ejaculatory latency with on-demand use of clomipramine. For the individual patient, this benefit must be balanced against the medication side effects during the first 48 hours after administration.

D. E. Coplen, MD

19 Urethral Reconstruction

Repeat Urethrotomy and Dilation for the Treatment of Urethral Stricture Are Neither Clinically Effective Nor Cost-Effective

Greenwell TJ, Castle C, Andrich DE, et al (Inst of Urology, London; et al)

J Urol 172:275-277, 2004 19–1

Purpose.—We developed an algorithm for the management of urethral stricture based on cost-effectiveness.

Materials and Methods.—United Kingdom medical and hospital costs associated with the current management of urethral stricture were calculated using private medical insurance schedules of reimbursement and clean intermittent self-catheterization supply costs. These costs were applied to 126 new patients treated endoscopically for urethral stricture in a general urological setting between January 1, 1991 and December 31, 1999. Treatment failure was defined as recurrent symptomatic stricture requiring further operative intervention following initial intervention. Mean followup available was 25 months (range 1 to 132).

Results.—The costs were urethrotomy/urethral dilation £2,250.00 ($3,375.00, ratio 1.00), simple 1-stage urethroplasty £5,015.00 ($7,522.50, ratio 2.23), complex 1-stage urethroplasty £5,335.00 ($8,002.50, ratio 2.37) and 2-stage urethroplasty £10,370 ($15,555.00, ratio 4.61). Of the 126 patients assessed 60 (47.6%) required more than 1 endoscopic re-treatments (mean, 3.13 each), 50 performed biweekly clean intermittent self-catheterization, and 7 underwent urethroplasty during follow-up. The total cost per patient for all 126 patients for stricture treatment during follow-up was £6,113 ($9,170). This cost was calculated by multiplying procedure cost by the number of procedures performed. A strategy of urethrotomy or urethral dilation as first-line treatment, followed by urethroplasty for recurrence yielded a total cost per patient of £5,866 ($8,799).

Conclusions.—A strategy of initial urethrotomy or urethral dilation followed by urethroplasty in patients with recurrent stricture proves to be the most cost-effective strategy. This financially based strategy concurs with evidence-based best practice for urethral stricture management.

▶ Endoscopic treatment or dilation for the management of urethral strictures is simple and safe but the treatment fails to give a durable result in nearly 50% of cases. This evidence-based analysis of urethral stricture management shows that urethroplasty is both cost-effective and associated with excellent clinical outcomes. Urethroplasty should be considered as a primary therapy in very young patients and in those with strictures greater than 1 cm in length. While urethroplasty is technically demanding, it should be offered to patients with recurrent urethral stricture disease.

D. E. Coplen, MD

Long-term Results of a Self-expanding Wallstent in the Treatment of Urethral Stricture

Hussain M, Greenwell TJ, Shah J, et al (Inst of Urology, London)
BJU Int 94:1037-1039, 2004 19–2

Objective.—To report the long-term outcome over 12 years of using the urethral Urolume™ wallstent (AMS, Minnetonka, MI, USA) for treating recurrent bulbar urethral stricture disease.

Patients and Methods.—The case-notes of 60 consecutive men with urethral Urolume wallstents placed for treating recurrent bulbar strictures were reviewed retrospectively. Information was collected on patient demographics, stricture etiology, stent-related complications and the need for further surgery to treat stent- or stricture-related complications.

Results.—The mean (range) age of the men was 58 (32-76) years. The most common cause of stricture was iatrogenic, arising after previous endoscopic surgery or after an indwelling catheter (45%). Thirty-five men had complications, with reoperation required in 27 (45%) of them. The most frequent nonsurgical complications were post-micturition dribble (32%) and recurrent urinary tract infections (27%). The most common surgical interventions required were transurethral resection of obstructing stent hyperplasia (32%), urethral dilatation or urethrotomy for stent obstruction or stricture (25%) and endoscopic litholapaxy for stent encrustation or stone (17%).

Conclusions.—The Urolume wallstent should only be used in patients who are unfit for or who refuse a bulbar urethroplasty.

▶ The authors report long-term outcomes using the wallstent in the treatment of bulbar urethral strictures. Only 45% of men were successfully treated with the prosthesis. Seventy-five percent of the failures required repeat surgical intervention, including urethral dilation, resection of hyperplastic epithelial ingrowth, and prosthesis removal. The prosthesis has poor long-term success, and bulbar urethroplasty (90% success) is the preferred treatment for suitable operative candidates.

D. E. Coplen, MD

20 Pediatric Urinary Tract Infection

Febrile Urinary Tract Infections in Infants: Renal Ultrasound Remains Necessary

Giorgi LJ Jr, Bratslavsky G, Kogan BA (Albany Med College, NY)

J Urol 173:568-570, 2005 20–1

Purpose.—Current guidelines from the American Academy of Pediatrics recommend voiding cystourethrography (VCUG) and renal ultrasound for the radiographic evaluation of infants after a febrile urinary tract infection. Some recent studies have suggested that ultrasound is not necessary in the era of prenatal ultrasound. We reviewed our experience to ascertain the influence that ultrasound has on the treatment of these infants.

Materials and Methods.—We reviewed retrospectively the charts of 282 consecutive patients (5 days to 6 months old, 98 males and 184 females) who underwent radiographic evaluation for a febrile urinary tract infection between October 1995 and August 2001. All patients were evaluated at our institution with VCUG and renal ultrasound.

Results.—Of 203 patients with normal VCUG ultrasound was abnormal in 32 (16%). Subsequent evaluation demonstrated 1 case each of significant ureteropelvic junction obstruction, ectopic ureter in a bilaterally duplicated system, renal duplication, renal duplication with calculus, ectopic ureter, renal cysts, multicystic dysplastic kidney and renal scarring. In addition, there were 3 cases of ureterovesical obstruction. No significant renal pathology was identified in the other cases. Two of these patients underwent operative intervention. Treatment or parental counseling was altered in 7 others, for a total of 9 of the 203 patients (4.4%).

Conclusions.—In our population renal ultrasound adds information to the radiographic evaluation of infants after a febrile urinary tract infection. This information alters treatment and parental counseling in a significant number of patients.

▶ It has been suggested that because prenatal US is obtained in nearly all pregnancies, US is not required in the evaluation of infants with febrile urinary infections. The authors identified renal abnormalities in 32 infants with normal cystograms. Patient management was altered in 9 infants. While this represented only 5% of the population, it is reflective of variations in the quality and timing (gestational age) of prenatal imaging. It is reasonable to obtain renal and bladder USs in infants with febrile urinary infections.

D. E. Coplen, MD

Follow-up Urine Cultures and Fever in Children With Urinary Tract Infection

Currie ML, Mitz L, Raasch CS, et al (Med College of Wisconsin, Milwaukee)
Arch Pediatr Adolesc Med 157:1237-1240, 2003 20–2

Background.—The American Academy of Pediatrics practice parameter for urinary tract infection suggests a repeat urine culture if the expected clinical response is not achieved within the first 48 hours of therapy. The utility of repeat urine cultures and clinical significance of fever at 48 hours is unclear.

Objectives.—To determine the frequency of positive repeat urine cultures in children admitted to the hospital with urinary tract infection, and to describe the fever curves of children admitted to the hospital with urinary tract infection.

Design and Methods.—We reviewed all cases of urinary tract infection in children 18 years and younger who were admitted during a 5-year period to Children's Hospital of Wisconsin (Milwaukee). We recorded temperatures from hospital admission to discharge, age, sex, initial and follow-up culture results, antibiotics received, imaging performed, and medical history.

Results.—Urinary tract infection was identified in 364 patients, and 291 (79.9%) had follow-up urine cultures. None were positive. Follow-up cultures produced $21,388.50 in patient charges. Fever lasted beyond 48 hours in 32% of patients. Older children were more likely to have fever beyond 48 hours.

Conclusions.—Follow-up urine cultures were of no utility in children hospitalized for urinary tract infection, including those with fever lasting beyond 48 hours or those with an underlying urologic disease. Fever beyond 48 hours is common and should not be used as a criterion for obtaining a repeat urine culture. These conclusions are valid for children with vesicoureteral reflux. Such an approach would result in significant cost savings.

▶ Fevers often persist for 48 to 72 hours after initiation of antibiotic therapy. In this retrospective review, fever lasted longer in older children and in those with vesicoureteral reflux. Persistent fever beyond 48 hours does not indicate a failure of therapy. Even though the American Academy of Pediatrics UTI guidelines[1] recommends a repeat urine culture, if bacterial sensitivities indicate an appropriate antibiotic choice, there is limited utility in obtaining a repeat culture.

D. E. Coplen, MD

Reference

1. American Academy of Pediatrics, Committee on Quality Improvement. Subcommittee on Urinary Tract Infection. Practice parameter: the diagnosis, treatment and evaluation of the initial urinary tract infections in febrile infants and young children. *Pediatrics* 103:843-852, 1999.

Correlation of Renal Ultrasonographic Findings With Inflammatory Volume From Dimercaptosuccinic Acid Renal Scans in Children With Acute Pyelonephritis

Wang Y-T, Chiu N-T, Chen M-J, et al (Chi-Mei Found Hosp, Liouying, Taiwan; Natl Cheng Kung Univ, Tainan, Taiwan; Chung Hwa Inst of Technology, Tainan, Taiwan)

J Urol 173:190-194, 2005 20–3

Purpose.—We correlated abnormal findings on renal ultrasonography (US) and inflammatory volume (Volume) on ^{99m}technetium dimercaptosuccinic acid renal single photon emission computerized tomography (DMSA) in children with acute pyelonephritis (APN) with renal scars.

Materials and Methods.—A total of 31 males and 14 females (9 days to 9.8 years old) who fulfilled diagnostic criteria for APN and who underwent initial DMSA between January 1995 and July 2002 and followup DMSA at least 6 months later were enrolled in the study. APN was diagnosed by initial DMSA, and placement in the scar or scar-free group was determined by followup DMSA. Photopenic areas on initial DMSA were calculated as Volume, and were compared to US findings.

Results.—Ultrasound demonstrated 35 abnormal kidneys (38.9%) among these children with APN. Significant differences in age, Volume (11.19 ± 2.52 ml vs 3.02 ± 0.75 ml, $P < 0.005$), C-reactive protein (CRP) and photopenic lesion on initial DMSA were found between children with abnormal and normal US. Of 65 children with initial APN foci 33 (50.8%) recovered, and the others had development of scars. The sensitivity of US for detecting APN (identified by DMSA scan) was 49.2%, and the specificity was 88% (OR 7.1, 95% CI 2.18 to 24.41). The sensitivity of US for predicting renal scarring was 59.4%, and the specificity was 60.6% (OR 2.3, 95% CI 0.82 to 7.65). Patients with abnormal US findings and high serum CRP (greater than 70 mg/l) had a large Volume (10.96 ± 3.05 ml) and a 76.2% chance of being in the scar group.

Conclusions.—US findings are significantly correlated to Volume in APN. Along with a high level of CRP, US is helpful in predicting development of renal scarring.

▶ The authors evaluate the ability of US to detect renal inflammation and renal scarring in children with clinical pyelonephritis. When compared with DMSA, US detected nearly 50% of APN and nearly 60% of renal scars. The question is whether DMSA is too sensitive or whether US misses clinically significant renal inflammation and scarring that lead to hypertension and renal compromise.

CRP elevation (>70) correctly identified 81% of children that eventually developed renal scars with a false positive of 25%. DMSA remains the gold standard but perhaps could be obtained in late follow-up of children with US and serologic abnormalities suggestive of significant renal risk.

D. E. Coplen, MD

Adverse Reactions of Nitrofurantoin, Trimethoprim and Sulfamethoxazole in Children

Karpman E, Kurzrock EA (Univ of California, Sacramento)
J Urol 172:448-453, 2004 20–4

Purpose.—Many children with urological disease require long-term treatment with antibiotics. In many cases the choice of medical instead of surgical management hinges on the implied safety of certain drugs. Recently some groups have advocated subureteral injection procedures to avoid long-term antibiotics for low grade reflux. We present a concise and relevant review on the use and adverse reactions of nitrofurantoin, trimethoprim and sulfamethoxazole in children.

Materials and Methods.—We reviewed the literature regarding the safety and toxicity of these drugs. Information regarding absorption, excretion and dosing was also gathered to explain better the mechanisms of toxicity.

Results.—Adverse reactions in children reported in the literature related to nitrofurantoin are gastrointestinal disturbance (4.4/100 person-years at risk), cutaneous reactions (2% to 3%), pulmonary toxicity (9 patients), hepatoxicity (12 patients and 3 deaths), hematological toxicity (12 patients), neurotoxicity and an increased rate of sister chromatid exchanges. Adverse reactions in children related to trimethoprim/sulfamethoxazole are almost exclusively due to the sulfamethoxazole component, including cutaneous reactions (1.4 to 7.4 events per 100 person-years at risk), hematological toxicity (0% to 72% of patients) and hepatotoxicity (5 patients). The majority of adverse reactions were found in children on full dose therapy and not prophylaxis.

Conclusions.—The use of nitrofurantoin, trimethoprim and sulfamethoxazole is safe in children for long-term prophylactic therapy. The antibiotic safety issue should not be misconstrued as an argument for surgical therapy, whether minimally invasive or not. Adverse reactions exist to these medicines but they are less common than seen in adults, presumably because of the lower dose used for therapy, and the lack of significant comorbidities and drug interactions in children. Serious side effects are extremely rare and most are reversible by discontinuing therapy. The extremely low potential for significant adverse reactions should be discussed with parents.

▶ Low-dose antimicrobial prevention is commonly used in the medical management of vesicoureteral reflux and recurrent urinary tract infections. This is an excellent review that discusses the safety of these medications when used at very low doses in the pediatric population. Serious complications are exceedingly rare and are usually self-limiting. This is very useful information that should be shared with parents.

D. E. Coplen, MD

The Physical and Antimicrobial Effects of Microwave Heating and Alcohol Immersion on Catheters That Are Reused for Clean Intermittent Catheterisation

Bogaert GA, Goeman L, de Ridder D, et al (UZ Gasthuisberg, Leuven, Belgium; KU, Leuven, Belgium)

Eur Urol 46:641-646, 2004 20–5

Introduction.—Due to worldwide different health insurance policies, patients are often forced to reuse the catheters when performing Clean Intermittent Catheterisation (CIC). We have compared the physical qualities and the antimicrobial effects of two methods of reusing catheters: microwave heating and storage of the catheters in a 70% alcohol solution. The studies were performed during different lengths of time.

Materials and Methods.—Three types of catheters (a standard polyvinylchloride catheter, a special polyvinylchloride catheter with flexible Ergothan® tip and a prelubrified catheter), normally intended for single use, were submitted to the effect of a microwave oven (Multitech 215 High Grade and Whirlpool M220 750 W and 1000 W with rotating plate) or preservation in a 70% alcohol solution. To study the effects of microwave heating, a recipient of water was placed in the oven to spread the microwaves and to absorb the heat. The catheters were placed in a resealable plastic bag (Ziploc®). To study the effects of preservation in a 70% alcohol solution, the catheters were immersed in the solution for different lengths of time. Thereafter the physical qualities of the catheters were evaluated by using the technique of Differential Scanning Calorimetry (DSC). The antimicrobial effect of the method was evaluated after grafting the catheters with pathogenic *E. coli, P. aeruginosa* or *S. aureus* strains.

Results.—Microwave heating up to 12 minutes at 750 W caused only minimal changes in the physical qualities of all the catheters. However, there was only an antimicrobial effect of the microwave heating on *E. coli* and not on *P. aeruginosa* or *S. aureus*. If the catheter remained longer than 45 minutes in a 70% alcohol solution, the physical qualities of the catheter changed either minimal in the special polyvinylchloride catheter with flexible Ergothan® top but changed significantly in the prelubrified catheter). However, already after 5 minutes of immersion in the 70% alcohol solution there was a complete antimicrobial effect on *E. coli, P. aeruginosa* and *S. aureus* in all catheters.

Conclusions.—It should be recommended to patients on CIC to use a sterile packed and not previously used catheter. In this study we have shown that immersing the catheters in a 70% alcohol solution during 5 minutes can effectively disinfect the catheter without jeopardising the physical qualities. Thereafter, the catheters could be placed in a resealable (e.g. Ziploc®) bag without being rinsed under water, in order that the few drops of alcohol cause alcohol vapours within the closed plastic bag and maintain the antimicrobial effect.

▶ Intermittent bladder catheterization is usually associated with asymptomatic bacteruria. Catheters can be safely reused without any attempt at sterilization. Rarely, clinically significant infections develop, and bladder management needs to be modified. Increased catheterization frequency and attention to hand washing or hygiene measures may suffice. Rarely, sterile catheterization is required. The authors show that a short immersion in 70% alcohol effectively disinfects a polyvinyl catheter without changing its physical properties. Since the cost of a new catheter 5 to 6 times per day may be prohibitive, alcohol disinfection should be tried in patients with recurrent symptomatic bacteruria.

D. E. Coplen, MD

21 Vesicoureteral Reflux

Timing of Follow-up Voiding Cystourethrogram in Children With Primary Vesicoureteral Reflux: Development and Application of a Clinical Algorithm

Thompson M, Simon SD, Sharma V, et al (Univ of Missouri, Kansas City)

Pediatrics 115:426-434, 2005 21–1

Background and Objectives.—Of children diagnosed with urinary tract infection, 30% to 40% have primary vesicoureteral reflux (VUR). For the majority of these children, treatment involves long-term prophylactic antibiotics (ABX) and a periodic voiding cystourethrogram (VCUG) until resolution of VUR as detected by VCUG. Radiation exposure and considerable discomfort have been associated with VCUG. To date, no clear guidelines exist regarding the timing of follow-up VCUGs. The objective of this study was to develop a clinically applicable algorithm for the optimal timing of repeat VCUGs and validate this algorithm in a retrospective cohort of children with VUR.

Methods.—Based on previously published data regarding the probability of resolution of VUR over time, a decision-tree model (DTM) was developed. The DTM compared the differential impact of 3 timing schedules of VCUGs (yearly, every 2 years, and every 3 years) on the average numbers of VCUGs performed, years of ABX exposure, and overall costs. Based on the DTM, an algorithm optimizing the timing of VCUG was developed. The algorithm then was validated in a retrospective cohort of patients at an urban pediatric referral center. Data were extracted from the medical records regarding number of VCUGs, time of ABX prophylaxis, and complications associated with either. VUR in patients in the cohort was grouped into mild VUR (grades I and II and unilateral grade III for those ≤ 2 years old), and moderate/severe VUR (other grade III and grade IV). Kaplan-Meier survival curves were created from the cohort data. From the survival curves, the median times to resolution of VUR were determined for the cohort, and these times were compared with the median times to VUR resolution of the data used for the DTM. The numbers of VCUGs performed, time of ABX exposure, and costs in the cohort were compared with those that would have occurred if the algorithm had been applied to both mild and moderate/severe VUR groups.

Results.—Using an algorithm that results in a recommendation of VCUGs every 2 years in mild VUR would reduce the average number of VCUGs by

42% and costs by 33%, with an increase in ABX exposure of 16%, compared with a schedule of yearly VCUGs. For moderate/severe VUR, a VCUG performed every 3 years would reduce the average number of VCUGs by 63% and costs by 51%, with an increase in ABX exposure of 10%. Applying this algorithm to the retrospective cohort consisting of 76 patients (between 1 month and 10 years old) with primary VUR would have reduced overall VCUGs by 19% and costs by 6%, with an increase in ABX exposure of 26%. The patterns of VUR resolution, age distribution, and prevalence of severity of VUR were comparable between previously published results and the retrospective cohort.

Conclusions.—Delaying the schedule of VCUG from yearly to every 2 years in children with mild VUR and every 3 years in children with moderate/severe VUR yields substantial reductions in the average numbers of VCUGs and costs, with a modest subsequent increase in ABX exposure.

▶ The majority of children with VUR are placed on prophylactic antibiotics while the reflux resolves. The most appropriate timing of the follow-up imaging is not known. Parents would like to stop the antibiotics but would also like to avoid repeating the VCUG. An algorithm was developed and then validated. The proposed interval of 2 to 3 years may decrease radiation exposure and overall costs but may be too long a period of uncertainty for most parents. However, given the slow resolution rate of higher grades of reflux, a decreased frequency of imaging in children without breakthrough infections is warranted.

D. E. Coplen, MD

The Modified Sting Procedure to Correct Vesicoureteral Reflux: Improved Results With Submucosal Implantation Within the Intramural Ureter

Kirsch AJ, Perez-Brayfield M, Smith EA, et al (Emory Univ, Atlanta, Ga)

J Urol 171:2413-2416, 2004 21–2

Purpose.—With the advent of tissue bulking agents, in particular dextranomer/hyaluronic acid copolymer (Dx/HA), for endoscopic implantation for vesicoureteral reflux (VUR), there has been a major shift in the surgical paradigm throughout Europe, and more recently, in the United States. We describe a modification of the technique used for implantation that has significantly improved our results.

Materials and Methods.—Between October 2001 and October 2003, 285 children 7 months to 15 years old (mean age 4.6 years) underwent endoscopic implantation of Dx/HA for VUR at our institutions. A modified STING (subureteral transurethral injection) procedure (implantation submucosally within the intramural ureter) was introduced during the last year of the study. The average volume of injected material was measured for each ureter. Renal sonography was performed to determine if hydronephrosis was present. At 3 months fluoroscopic voiding cystourethrograms were used to evaluate for the presence of VUR. A subset of 122 patients treated with STING (52) were compared to those treated with modified STING (70).

Results.—A total of 459 ureters in 231 girls and 54 boys were treated (174 bilateral cases). Mean maximum grade per patient was 2.5/5. Mean injected volume was 0.9 cc ureter. There were 181 patients with at least 3 months of followup. After 1 treatment 76% (137 of 181) of cases were cured (grade 0 reflux), while 54% (24 of 44) of the failures were improved. The overall cure rate was 94% for grade I, 85% for grade II, 78% for grade III and 71% for grade IV reflux. The patients treated with STING had a mean age of 4.8 years, mean maximum reflux grade was 2.5 and success rate was 71% (37 of 52; 86% grade I, 89% grade II, 70% grade III and 63% grade IV reflux). The patients treated with a modified STING had a mean age of 5.5 years, mean maximum grade was 2.8 and a success rate was 89% (62 of 70; 100% grade I, 92% grade II, 91% grade III and 90% grade IV reflux). Ureteral success rates were significantly ($P < .01$) greater for the modified STING (92%) vs the standard STING (79%). There were no cases of hydronephrosis at 3 months postoperatively.

Conclusions.—The majority of patients undergoing minimally invasive therapy for VUR with Dx/HA are cured after 1 treatment. The modified STING is our preferred method of implant injection for the correction of VUR and in our hands produces a resolution rate of 89% (92% of ureters). The technique optimizes ureteral coaptation, is easy to perform and is not associated with any significant short-term complications. Persistence of VUR in a minority of patients continues to be the only significant adverse effect of endoscopic implantation.

► The role of STING in the surgical correction of VUR has significantly increased with the availability of Dx/HA. Reflux resolution has always been lower with this minimally invasive approach, but the authors describe a modification of technique that resulted in 90% resolution after a single injection in a small number of children with grades III and IV reflux. The authors hypothesize that the intraureteric injection leads to more reproducible placement of the implant, thus, leading to optimal ureteral coaptation. This modification did not lead to ureteral obstruction in any cases. The role of the STING in reflux management will become better defined over the next several years. As the success of the procedure improves, it may be considered a first-line treatment (over prophylaxis) in some patients.

D. E. Coplen, MD

22 Voiding Dysfunction

Measurement of Bladder Compliance Can Be Standardized by a Dimensionless Number: Clinical Perspective

Wahl EF, Lerman SE, Lahdes-Vasama TT, et al (Univ of California, Los Angeles; Tampere Univ, Finland)

BJU Int 94:898-900, 2004 22–1

Objective.—To devise a new, practical and more accurate method for measuring bladder compliance, and to show that traditional estimates of compliance are impractical.

Materials and Methods.—Childhood bladder capacity varies greatly with age while detrusor pressure in a normal bladder does not. Consequently, traditional bladder compliance ($\Delta V/\Delta P$) increases with age, i.e. maturation. Therefore we devised a standard method that includes normal values of pressures and volumes to calculate and report bladder compliance in children, and that also applies to adults. A dimensionless number ($N_{Wahl}{}^{-1}$) was computed for standardizing bladder compliance, comparing the normalized capacity to normalized pressure by the ratio $(\Delta V/V_{cap,NL})/(\Delta P/P_{cap,NL})$, where ΔP is the pressure at bladder capacity, ΔV, the volume at bladder capacity, $V_{cap,NL}$, the volume at mean expected bladder capacity and $P_{cap,NL}$, the pressure at mean expected bladder capacity. $V_{cap,NL}$ is obtained from nomograms of published data.

Results.—The bladder compliance of patients undergoing urodynamic testing was calculated using $N_{Wahl}{}^{-1}$ and the traditional equation $\Delta V/\Delta P$. $N_{Wahl}{}^{-1}$ provided a more accurate diagnosis and therefore was of more practical use.

Conclusions.—Bladder compliance depends on patient age, sex and size; the new estimate used to standardize bladder compliance is based on these factors and is a dimensionless number. This may help when comparing patients and assessing outcomes.

▶ Bladders enlarge with aging, but ideal bladder pressures do not increase. Consequently, traditional measures of compliance ($\Delta P/\Delta V$) give a decreasing value with aging. The authors have developed a standardized compliance measurement that more correctly assesses bladder compliance because it is the same for all normal cases. It will allow comparison of patients and clinical outcomes.

D. E. Coplen, MD

Pelvic Floor Spasms in Children: An Unknown Condition Responding Well to Pelvic Floor Therapy

Hoebeke P, Van Laecke E, Renson C, et al (Ghent Univ Hosp, Gent, Belgium)
Eur Urol 46:651-654, 2004 22–2

Objective.—During a study period of 4 years, 21 children are seen for night time pelvic pain. These children typical wake up in the middle of the night with severe lower abdominal or perineal pain. During day some of them suffer urge syndrome. During urodynamic investigation extremely high pelvic floor activity as recorded by high urethral pressure was observed in these children. We therefore started pelvic floor relaxation biofeedback in these children.

Methods.—All children diagnosed with pelvic floor spasms underwent biofeedback pelvic floor relaxation therapy in order to learn them to counteract pelvic pain due to these spasms. In those girls in whom detrusor hyperactivity was seen on urodynamics concomitant anticholinergic treatment was given (oxybutynin).

Results.—Between January 1998 and January 2002 symptomatic pelvic floor spasms were diagnosed in 21 children (19 girls/2 boys). Pelvic floor relaxation biofeedback was successful for treatment of this condition in 17 of 21 children. The mean duration of therapy was 3 months (12 weekly sessions) and on long term follow-up relapse was seen in 3 of 17 successfully treated children. 10 of 17 successfully treated children received anticholinergics.

Conclusion.—Pelvic floor spasms in children (which can be secondary to detrusor overactivity) respond well to pelvic floor relaxation therapy.

▶ Abnormalities of pelvic muscle control are the common thread in dysfunctional bowel and bladder elimination. Failure or inability to relax these muscles leads to incomplete bladder emptying, bladder instability, infections, and incontinence. Children infrequently present with severe postvoid genital discomfort or random complaints of lower abdominal pain. This discomfort can be either referred bladder spasm pain or pelvic muscle spasm. The former will usually respond to behavioral modification and anticholinergics. Successful treatment of the latter is more difficult and, historically, has required sitz baths, urethral dilation, diazepam, botulinum toxin, and so forth. The authors report improvement with biofeedback in a group of these children diagnosed with pelvic muscle spasms on the basis of high urethral pressures (UPP) on urodynamics. The UPP is subjective, and, in a child, the mere presence of a catheter may increase the tone. That being said, most of the children had a normal uroflow and did not have staccato voiding, as is typically seen in children with pelvic muscle spasms. Regardless, the authors used an anal plug to teach pelvic relaxation and successfully treated 17 of 21 patients. Biofeedback may have utility in this unique group of children.

D. E. Coplen, MD

Impact of Urodynamics in Treatment of Primary Nocturnal Enuresis Persisting Into Adulthood

Yucel S, Kutlu O, Kukul E, et al (Akdeniz Univ, Antalya, Turkey)

Urology 64:1020-1025, 2004 22–3

Objectives.—To investigate the urodynamic profiles of adults with primary nocturnal enuresis (PNE) and the association of the urodynamic profile findings with the efficacy of desmopressin and/or tolterodine pharmacotherapy. At least 2% of adults are enuretic during the night. The diagnostic and treatment approach for PNE is empirically the same in children and adults.

Methods.—A total of 20 nocturnal enuretic patients (12 women and 8 men) with a mean age of 27.1 years (range 20 to 42) were studied. They had wet their bed at least twice per week for the past 6 months. Urodynamic studies, including filling and voiding cystometry, pressure-flow study, and pelvic floor electromyography with superficial electrodes, were performed on all patients. Two of them had daytime symptoms, and two had prior failed desmopressin therapy. All patients began taking oral desmopressin 0.4 mg for 1 month. Their continence was assessed, and tolterodine 4 mg was added for those in whom desmopressin alone failed. The patients responsive to desmopressin alone or desmopressin plus tolterodine were weaned from medication at 6 and 12 months to reassess continence. The mean follow-up period was 11.6 ± 3.3 months (range, 4 to 14).

Results.—Urodynamic studies of 20 PNE adult patients revealed detrusor instability in 10 (50%), hypocompliance in 8 (40%), nonneurogenic detrusor-sphincter dyssynergy in 1 (5%), and no abnormality in 10 (50%). Of the 20 patients, 19 (95%) had no voiding bladder problems. Of the 10 patients responsive to desmopressin alone, 6 (60%) had a normal urodynamic profile; the remaining 4 (40%) had detrusor instability and/or hypocompliance. Of the 5 patients who received desmopressin and tolterodine, 3 achieved continence. The overall continence rate was 86% (13 of 15), and 12 (92%) of the 15 patients required maintenance therapy. In 2 patients (13.3%), desmopressin and tolterodine therapy failed. The efficacy of desmopressin alone and of desmopressin plus tolterodine were not related to the urodynamic profile findings ($P > 0.05$). The urodynamic profile was also not related to the relapse rate after any form of pharmacotherapy ($P > 0.05$).

Conclusions.—PNE persisting into adulthood may be associated with abnormal urodynamic findings. Patients may benefit from urodynamic studies, because if the findings are abnormal, they might have the best chance of successful treatment.

► PNE in adulthood is rare but is also unlikely to spontaneously resolve. In adults with PNE, a sleep disorder or urinary tract abnormality is much more likely than in children who are typically anatomically and neurologically normal. The authors identified urodynamic abnormalities in 50% of the patients even though none of them had any daytime voiding symptoms. The patients were treated with desmopressin or a combination of desmopressin and tolterodine. The response to treatment was not related to the urodynamic findings, so it is unclear that these results could be used to direct therapy. Urodynamics could probably be reserved for those adults that do not respond to empiric therapy.

D. E. Coplen, MD

23 Neurogenic Bladder

Efficacy and Safety of Oxybutynin in Children With Detrusor Hyperreflexia Secondary to Neurogenic Bladder Dysfunction

Franco I, Horowitz M, Grady R, et al (Cornell Univ, New York; Univ of Washington, Seattle; Texas Scottish Rite Hosp for Children, Dallas; et al)

J Urol 173:221-225, 2005 23–1

Purpose.—We evaluated the efficacy and safety of oxybutynin in children with detrusor hyperreflexia due to neurological conditions.

Materials and Methods.—*Study 1*—A prospective, open label trial of 3 formulations of oxybutynin (tablets, syrup and extended release tablets) was conducted for 24 weeks in children 6 to 15 years old with detrusor hyperreflexia who used oxybutynin and clean intermittent catheterization. The effect of treatment on average urine volume per catheterization and on secondary urodynamic outcomes was evaluated. *Study 2*—The efficacy and safety of oxybutynin syrup were evaluated urodynamically in an open label study of children 1 to 5 years old with detrusor hyperreflexia who used oxybutynin and clean intermittent catheterization.

Results.—*Study 1*—Mean urine volume per catheterization (±SEM) increased by 25.5 ± 5.9 ml (P < 0.001). Maximal cystometric capacity increased by 75.4 ± 9.8 ml (P < 0.001). Mean detrusor and intravesical pressures were significantly decreased by −9.2 ± 2.3 ($P \leq 0.001$) and −7.5 ± 2.5 cm H_2O (P < 0.004), respectively, at week 24. Of 61 children with uninhibited detrusor contractions 15 cm H_2O or greater at baseline 34 did not have them at week 24 (P < 0.001). Improvements in bladder function were consistent across all oxybutynin formulations. *Study 2*—Mean maximal cystometric capacity increased significantly by 71.5 ± 21.99 ml (P = 0.005). At study end only 12.5% of patients had uninhibited detrusor contractions 15 cm H_2O or greater compared with 68.8% at baseline (P = 0.004). Oxybutynin was well tolerated in both studies. There were no serious treatment related adverse events.

Conclusions.—All 3 formulations of oxybutynin are safe and effective in children with neurogenic bladder dysfunction.

▶ This was a large prospective trial evaluating 3 different forms of oral oxybutynin in children with neurogenic bladder and urinary incontinence. All 3 forms were well tolerated. All forms appeared to have equal efficacy, and even though there was no attempt to compare side-effect profiles, there did not seem to be a significant difference between the 3 forms.

D. E. Coplen, MD

Transitional Cell Carcinoma of the Bladder Following Augmentation Cystoplasty for the Neuropathic Bladder

Soergel TM, Cain MP, Misseri R, et al (Indiana Univ, Indianapolis)
J Urol 172:1649-1652, 2004 23–2

Purpose.—Cancer following augmentation cystoplasty is a recognized risk factor. The procedure has only gained popularity in pediatric urology within the last 25 years, limiting the population being studied by statistical power and the lack of long-term followup. The majority of reported cases of post-augmentation malignancy have occurred in adults with multiple risk factors. Currently the most common indication for augmentation cystoplasty in children and adolescents is neuropathic bladder. We review 3 cases of transitional cell carcinoma (TCC) following augmentation cystoplasty in this unique population with no additional risk factors for bladder cancer.

Materials and Methods.—We reviewed our clinical database of children and adolescents who underwent bladder augmentation since 1978 to evaluate the incidence of cancer. This study represents a captured population within a single institutional practice. There were 483 cases entered into the database, and particular attention was paid to 260 augmentations with at least 10 years of followup. We reviewed medical history, clinical outcomes, cancer risk factors, augmentation type and pathology of the 3 patients who presented with TCC after augmentation cystoplasty.

Results.—Three patients presented with grade 2 to 3 TCC following bladder augmentation, all of whom underwent exploratory laparotomy and eventually died of metastatic disease. No patient had a history of smoking exposure greater than 10 packs per year or other known risk factors for bladder cancer. Two patients had an ileocecal augmentation and 1 had a cecal augmentation for neuropathic bladder. Patient age at augmentation was 8, 20 and 24 years, and age at diagnosis of TCC was 29, 37 and 44 years, respectively. Mean time from augmentation to TCC was 19 years. Assuming a 10-year lag period before the risk of cancer, in at least 1.2% of bladder augmentation cases in our database, cancer has developed.

Conclusions.—This study supports the hypothesis that bladder augmentation appears to be an independent risk factor for TCC, with a lag time of less than 20 years. We recommend endoscopic surveillance of all patients with a history of bladder augmentation beginning 10 years after initial surgery.

► This study clearly shows that bladder augmentation is an independent risk factor for the development of TCC in children with a neuropathic bladder. The majority of previously reported cancer in augmented bladders occurred in those with tuberculous cystitis. The inciting factors in this series are unknown but likely include inflammation and disordered cell-cell signaling between the transitional and colonic epithelium. Because the lag time for development of tumors is unknown, the appropriate screening during follow-up of these patients is unknown. The potential malignancy risk should be discussed with parents and patients before augmentation. Hopefully, bladder augmentation with autologous tissue will reduce the incidence of malignancy.

The reader is directed to a recent review article that further discusses secondary malignancies in urinary diversion.[1]

D. E. Coplen, MD

Reference

1. Austen M and Kalble T: Secondary malignancies in different forms of urinary diversion using isolated gut. *J Urol* 172:831-838, 2004.

24 Antenatal Hydronephrosis

Prenatal Mild Pyelectasis: Evaluating the Thresholds of Renal Pelvic Diameter Associated With Normal Postnatal Renal Function

Odibo AO, Raab E, Elovitz M, et al (Univ of Pennsylvania, Philadelphia)

J Ultrasound Med 23:513-517, 2004 24–1

Objective.—To determine the threshold of the renal pelvic anteroposterior (AP) diameter that predicts normal postnatal renal outcome in the follow-up of cases with mild pyelectasis.

Methods.—A retrospective review of our sonography database was conducted over a 3-year period for cases of mild pyelectasis diagnosed between 18 and 30 weeks. Cases were evaluated for the association between different thresholds of renal pelvic anteroposterior diameter and normal postnatal function after 32 weeks' gestation and also for the initial renalpelvic anteroposterior diameter at 18 to 30 weeks.

Results.—In the 3-year period, 7416 women were evaluated, and 150 cases with a diagnosis of pyelectasis (2%) were identified. Among the 115 women meeting our inclusion criteria, complete outcomes were available for 66. Persistent postnatal renal anomalies were seen in 20 cases (30%). On the basis of receiver operating characteristic curves, the renal threshold that best predicted normal postnatal outcome was an anteroposterior diameter of less than 7.0 mm after 32 weeks, yielding sensitivity and specificity of 87% and 85%, respectively (odds ratio, 0.31; 95% confidence interval, 0.11-0.86; $P <$ .02).

Conclusions.—In the follow-up of fetuses with a diagnosis of mild pyelectasis between 18 and 30 weeks, a renal pelvic anteroposterior diameter of less than 7.0 mm after 32 weeks is highly predictive of normal postnatal renal function. Therefore, only those with an anteroposterior diameter of greater than 6 mm after 32 weeks deserve follow-up.

▶ The authors generate receiver operating characteristics (ROC) curves based upon a small number of infants with antenatally detected hydronephrosis (isolated renal pelvic dilation). The false positive rate with a cutoff of 7 mm was 15%. This means that there is a low likelihood of obstruction if renal pelvic dilation is less than 7 mm after 32 weeks' gestation. While the follow-up is short, and the number of patients is small, these data are similar to those reported in other small series, and I think the ROC curve gives a good visual image as to the sensitivity and specificity of renal pelvic dimensions. It should be noted that even though the title claims an evaluation of renal function, the authors are only evaluating US anatomy and not function.

D. E. Coplen, MD

Long-term Clinical Outcome of Infants With Mild and Moderate Fetal Pyelectasis: Validation of Neonatal Ultrasound as a Screening Tool to Detect Significant Nephrouropathies

Ismaili K, for the Brussels Free Univ Perinatal Nephrology Study Group (Hôpital Universitaire des Enfants—Reine Fabiola, Brussels, Belgium; et al)

J Pediatr 144:759-765, 2004 24–2

Objective.—To assess the long-term outcome of infants with mild and moderate fetal pyelectasis and to determine the predictive value of neonatal ultrasound imaging in identifying significant nephrouropathies.

Study Design.—This prospective study included 213 infants with antenatal mild to moderate pyelectasis who were followed for up to 2 years. Postnatal renal ultrasound examinations were performed at day 5 and months 1, 3, 6, 12 and 24 after birth. Voiding cystourethrography was performed in all infants.

Results.—Normal or nonsignificant findings were diagnosed in 130 of 213 (61%) infants. Significant nephrouropathies were diagnosed in 83 of 213 (39%) infants. The sensitivity, specificity, positive predictive value, and negative predictive value of two successive neonatal renal ultrasound examinations performed at day 5 and 1 month to predict significant nephrouropathies were 96%, 76%, 72%, and 97%, respectively. In 102 of 213 (48%) infants with normal neonatal renal ultrasound scans, we later found only three of 102 (3%) cases with significant nephrouropathies.

Conclusions.—We found in a population of infants with mild to moderate fetal pyelectasis a 39% incidence of significant nephrouropathies. Ultrasound is an excellent screening tool with high sensitivity and negative predictive value that allows avoidance of unjustified medical follow-up in patients with two normal neonatal ultrasound scans.

▶ This is a 2-year evaluation of infants with antenatally detected pyelectasis. All infants were evaluated with US and radiologic imaging. The authors state that significant abnormalities were identified in nearly 40% of infants with isolated pyelectasis. However, they fail to define the significance. Only 2 of 27 with a "UPJ obstruction" required surgery. Reflux resolved in 16 of 23 within 1 year, and no reimplantations were required in the remainder. Isolated pyelectasis measuring less than 10 mm in anteroposterior diameter is usually a benign condition.

D. E. Coplen, MD

Antenatal Renal Pelvis Dilatation Emphasizing Vesicoureteric Reflux: Two-Year Follow-up of Minor Postnatal Dilatation

Kapadia H, Lidefelt K-J, Erasmie U, et al (Sachs' Children's Hosp, Stockholm; South Stockholm Gen Hosp)

Acta Paediatr 93:336-339, 2004 24–3

Aim.—To describe the occurrence of foetal renal pelvis dilatation in an unselected population of pregnancies and to describe the clinical course in a subgroup of infants with minor renal pelvis dilatation (RPD).

Methods.—During 1996-1999 the foetuses of 17,850 consecutive pregnant women were scanned with ultrasonography (USG) in the 16th-19th gestational week and later in the pregnancy when indicated. RPD was defined as anterior-posterior pelvic diameter ≥ 5 mm. After birth, all infants were examined with USG twice. If any postnatal USG showed RPD ≥10 mm, extended radiological investigation was performed. Infants with pelvis dilatation < 10 mm and no calyceal or ureteric dilatation were not investigated further and antibiotic prophylaxis was discontinued. The children were followed up at 2 y of age.

Results.—109 foetuses (0.6%) with RPD were identified. Postnatally, 94/109 were available for follow-up: 43 had postnatal dilatation ≥ 10 mm and were investigated and treated according to clinical routine, while 51 had dilatation < 10 mm and were followed up after they had reached at least 2 y of age. No case of pyelonephritis was recorded. USG in 48/51 children was normal.

Conclusion.—The data indicate that infants with minor RPD do not constitute a risk group for renal morbidity and thus, do not need antibiotic prophylaxis and extensive radiological examination.

▶ This study evaluates postnatal outcomes in prospectively identified minimal renal pelvic dilation (<10 mm) without caliectasis or ureteral dilation. These children were not placed on prophylaxis and a voiding cystourethrogram was not obtained in any of the infants. All of the children had follow-up imaging at 2 years and no hydronephrosis or scarring was identified. On the basis of this study, it is clear that the routine antibiotics and radiologic imaging in children with minimal renal pelvic dilation should be questioned and further studied.

D. E. Coplen, MD

Diagnosis and Outcome of Fetal Lower Urinary Tract Obstruction in the Northern Region of England

Anumba DO, Scott JE, Plant ND, et al (Univ of Newcastle upon Tyne, England; Univ of Sheffield, England)

Prenat Diagn 25:7-13, 2005 24–4

Objective.—We reviewed the prenatal and postnatal management of fetal lower urinary tract obstruction (LUTO) in a large geographically defined population.

Methods.—The records of 113 cases of LUTO seen over a 14-year period were examined. The predictive accuracy of prenatal findings for chronic renal failure (CRF) and a comparison of prenatal-suspected and non-suspected cases were made.

Results.—The incidence of LUTO was 2.2 in 10,000 births. During the study period, prenatal detection improved from 33% to 62%. Sensitivity of prenatal ultrasound detection of renal dysplasia and fetal urinary sodium, calcium, and beta2-microglobulin for CRF or renal dysplasia on autopsy were 59, 33, 66, and 63% respectively. Compared to undetected cases, those detected prenatally had higher mortality and a higher rate of CRF at 24 months (17% vs 57%, $P < 0.01$).

Conclusion.—Our observations confirm the poor prognosis associated with fetal LUTO. The value of serial fetal urine biochemistry, other prenatal predictors of postnatal renal function, and the benefits of vesicoamniotic shunting require larger series and longer follow-up.

▶ This is a population-based study evaluating the incidence and outcomes of LUTO. The ascertainment level in this region is 95%, and the incidence of LUTO was 2.2 per 10,000 births. Nearly one half of these were prenatally detected. Prenatal diagnosis was associated with a poorer outcome.

Prenatal diagnosis is not perfect, and this series highlights its limitations. Obstructive uropathy was not confirmed in 26 of 82 cases of prenatally suspected LUTO. These observations should help during prenatal counseling, but definitive information regarding the value of biochemistry and prenatal intervention cannot be ascertained from this series.

D. E. Coplen, MD

Outcome Analysis of Prenatally Detected Ureteroceles Associated With Multicystic Dysplasia

Coplen DE, Austin PF (Washington Univ, St Louis)

J Urol 172:1637-1639, 2004 24–5

Purpose.—We assessed the outcome of a nonoperative approach in infants with prenatally detected ureteroceles associated with multicystic dysplasia.

Materials and Methods.—A retrospective analysis of all infants with ureteroceles referred for evaluation of prenatally hydronephrosis was conducted. Ultrasound, cystogram and scintigraphy findings were tabulated. Clinical outcomes including infections and the need for surgical intervention were assessed.

Results.—We identified 5 female and 3 male infants with prenatally detected ureteroceles and associated multicystic dysplasia. There were 4 cases with renal duplication and 4 with single systems. All infants were treated expectantly. One infant had a single urinary tract infection. The multicystic dysplastic moiety involuted by age 18 months in all children. The ureterocele collapsed in 3 children and remained stable in the remainder. None of the children required surgical intervention with a median and mean follow-up of 36 months (range, 14 to 54).

Conclusions.—We identified a subset of prenatally diagnosed ureteroceles that had a benign clinical course and did not require surgical intervention with available followup. Careful evaluation and interpretation of postnatal studies will allow identification and observational management of this unique subset of ureteroceles associated with multicystic dysplasia and absence of hydroureteronephrosis.

► Historically, ureteroceles present with urinary tract infections and usually require some form of surgical intervention. The authors describe a subset of antenatally detected ureteroceles that have a benign postnatal course. The anatomical features predictive of this benign course include multicystic dysplasia in the affected moiety, absence of a dilated ureter or hydronephrosis, absent of low-grade vesicoureteral reflux and a ureterocele that does not obstruct the bladder outlet. The multicystic dysplastic ureterocele moiety involutes, so it is unlikely that infections will be a future concern. Renal scintigraphy revealed absent function in these infants. In my experience, there is also a subset of antenatally detected ureteroceles that function and have normal drainage. These can also be observed and rarely develop infections or require surgical intervention. While postnatally detected ureteroceles usually require surgical intervention, careful evaluation of antenatally detected ureteroceles allows conservative management in some infants.

D. E. Coplen, MD

25 Neurogenic Reconstruction

Lessons Learned From Stomal Complications in Children With Cutaneous Catheterizable Continent Stomas

Barqawi A, de Valdenebro M, Furness PD III, et al (Univ of Colorado, Denver; Children's Hosp, Denver)

BJU Int 94:1344-1347, 2004 25–1

Objective.—To evaluate the impact of various factors that might ultimately influence the stoma complication rate associated with the construction of a continent catheterizable urinary (CCU) and Malone antegrade colonic enema (MACE) stoma in children.

Patients and Methods.—Retrospectively, we reviewed our experience in patients who had a CCU and/or MACE stoma reconstructed at our institution from 1992 to 2003. Diagnosis, type of stoma constructed (CCU vs MACE), single vs dual stomas, stomal site, conduit material (appendix, split appendix, Monti-Yang or ureter), sex, age, patient mobility and body mass index, race and concomitant surgery (e.g. bladder augmentation with or without bladder neck reconstruction) were evaluated for stoma-related complications. In all, 109 patients (64 males and 45 female), with a mean (SD, range) age of 8.6 (5.7, 2-37) years, had 151 stomas constructed during the period of analysis, comprising 56 CCU only, 11 MACE only and 42 (84 stomas) both simultaneously.

Results.—The mean (range) follow-up was 48 (6-144) months. The primary diagnoses were neurogenic bladder in 60 (55%), bladder exstrophy/epispadias in 17 (16%) and posterior urethral valves in 11 (9%) patients. The umbilicus was the primary site for the CCU stoma in 88 of 98 (90%) cases, while the right lower quadrant was the primary site for MACE in 46 of 53 (87%). After surgery complete stomal continence was provided in 95 of 98 (97%) CCU stoma, whereas the MACE was successful in 52 of 53 (99%). The stoma-related complications included stenosis in 27, leakage in eight, false passage in four, atrophy in two, keloid in one, and breakdown of the stoma in two. Individually, only greater age and a primary diagnosis of neurogenic bladder were independent risk factors associated with an increased rate of stomal complications and higher incidence of revision ($P < 0.05$).

Conclusion.—Stomal complications are extremely common whether CCU or MACE stomas are constructed individually or together. Nevertheless, despite the need for revision, the high stoma continence rate supports their use. Greater age at surgery and a primary diagnosis of neurogenic bladder were associated with a significant increase in the stoma-related complications and the need for revision.

► Continent catheterizable channels are routinely created in complex pediatric reconstructions but complications frequently occur. Stomal stenosis occurs in nearly 20% of the patients. The continent colonic stoma (MACE) also has a higher rate of stenosis that may be related to relative ischemia of the end blood supply at the tip of the in-situ appendix. The complications do not appear to be related to the stoma site but are clearly related to patient body mass index and patient age. Exacting surgical technique is imperative in the construction of continent stomas.

D. E. Coplen, MD

In Situ Malone Antegrade Continence Enema in 127 Patients: A 6-Year Experience

Herndon CDA, Rink RC, Cain MP, et al (Riley Hosp for Children, Indianapolis, Ind)

J Urol 172:1689-1691, 2004 25–2

Purpose.—The initial description of the Malone antegrade continence enema (MACE) relied on a reversed, tunneled, and reimplanted appendix. In 1999, we reported our in-situ technique that uses windows developed in the appendiceal mesentery for imbrication. We present our long-term results.

Materials and Methods.—From 1997 to 2003, 168 patients were identified who had undergone a MACE procedure. An in situ technique was performed in 76 females and 51 males. Average patient age at the time of surgery was 9.6 years (range 2.9 to 28.4). Diagnoses included myelomeningocele in 116 cases, lipomeningocele in 6, spinal cord injury in 2, posterior urethral valves in 1, sacral agenesis in 1 and functional constipation in 1.

Results.—Cecal plication/imbrication was performed in 100 patients, appendix intussusception and imbrication in 24, and creation of tenia flaps in 3. The abdominal stoma was umbilical in 50 cases, right lower quadrant in 74 and periumbilical in 3. Concomitant genitourinary reconstruction was performed in 87% of patients. Mean follow-up was 26.9 months (range, 0.7 to 68.1). Fecal continence was reported by 91% of the patients. Thirteen stomal revisions (stenosis 10, prolapse 2 and leakage 1) were required in 11 patients. Major complications included a cecal volvulus requiring a right hemicolectomy in 1 patient, small bowel obstruction in 2, and shunt infection and/or malfunction in 2. Four patients have elected to no longer use the MACE for nontechnical reasons.

Conclusions.—The in situ MACE procedure has reliable long-term results for treating fecal incontinence associated with neuropathic bowel.

▶ Successful management of constipation and fecal incontinence in children with neurologic bowel dysfunction is a time-consuming venture. Dietary modification, stool softeners, and timed elimination are successful in some patients. Retrograde enemas can be successful but a lax external sphincter often precludes retention of the fluid.

The Malone (MACE) is a continent colonic stoma that is used for antegrade administration of an enema or colonic washout. Most children evacuate the enema within 30 minutes of once-daily administration and do not soil between administrations. In many circumstances, the quality-of-life improvement with fecal continence exceeds that achieved with continent urinary reconstruction.

Stomal complications are common and related to ischemia of the distal end of the appendix. Retubularized ileum (Monti) or a cecal flap can also be used and may decrease this complication. Electrolyte abnormalities are rare, using tap water because of the short retention time. The MACE is an excellent adjunct to urinary reconstruction in children with neurogenic bladder and bowel.

D. E. Coplen, MD

Paediatric Urology: Experience With Non-cycled Artificial Urinary Sphincters

Herndon CDA, Rink RC, Shaw MBK, et al (Indiana Univ, Indianapolis)

BJU Int 93:1049-1062, 2004 25–3

Objective.—To report our experience in children and adolescents with a non-cycled artificial urinary sphincter (AUS). While some children with the AUS can void, others require clean intermittent catheterization (CIC) through the sphincter or an alternative site for catheterization; in some of the latter, we have either not cycled (pumped) an activated AUS or the AUS has failed, and there is concern about ischaemia in some adults with a non-cycled AUS.

Patients and Methods.—In all, 143 patients who had an AUS placed between 1980 and 2002 were reviewed retrospectively; 15 (10 boys and five girls) no longer cycled (pumped) their AUS. The mean age at AUS insertion was 11 years and the mean (range) follow-up after insertion was 10.4 (1.64-22.2) years. The diagnoses included myelomeningocele in 11, sacral agenesis in three and cloaca in one. Nine patients have an activated functioning AUS and in six the AUS does not function; in the first nine the sphincter has not routinely been cycled (pumped) for a mean (range) of 1.6 (0.6-2.9) years. In the other six with a nonfunctioning AUS the mean (range) observation period is 6.4 (1.5-10) years since the system has not functioned.

Results.—All patients were completely continent, including the six with a nonfunctioning AUS. After inserting the AUS, two patients voided in combination with CIC (one each urethral and abdominal stoma) and 13 emptied by CIC (nine abdominal stoma, four urethral). There was a mechanical complication in eight patients; three had the AUS repaired and are dry, and five are dry with no repair. In one patient the AUS was never activated. To date there has been no erosion of the cuff in any of the 15 patients with a non-cycled AUS.

Conclusion.—The AUS remains an extremely reliable procedure to achieve continence in children and young adults. It is versatile and can be combined with other procedures that provide an alternative means for catheterization. While some have noted the need to routinely cycle the AUS to prevent erosion, this has not been our experience in these 15 patients.

▶ Achieving urinary continence in children with abnormal bladder outlets (anatomical [exstrophy] or neuropathic [spinal dysraphism]) may be one of the most demanding surgical challenges for pediatric urologists. Bulking agents, bladder neck reconstructions, bladder neck suspensions and slings, and AUSs have utility in some patients, although none is the ideal approach in all patients.

The AUS provides a continence rate of 90%. Since it is a mechanical device, the majority will require some type of revision with extended follow-up. Cuff-erosion is a potentially devastating complication related to tissue ischemia. In theory, intermittent deflation of the cuff decreases the risk of erosion. The authors report excellent outcomes in a small series of patients managed with a continuously inflated cuff or a broken cuff (6 patients) that was left in situ. Most of the patients catheterized through an abdominal stoma. Continence in the presence of an empty cuff implies that fibrosis or the bulk of the device alone has some long-term efficacy.

D. E. Coplen, MD

26 Urinary Reconstruction

Long-term Outcome Analysis of Starr Plication for Primary Obstructive Megaureters

Fretz PC, Austin JC, Cooper CS, et al (Univ of Iowa, Iowa City)

J Urol 172:703-705, 2004 26–1

Purpose.—The Starr technique of tapering megaureters was first reported in 1979. Although this method of ureteral plication is well known, to our knowledge there are no clinical studies regarding outcomes. We report the first long-term outcome results with the Starr technique for primary obstructive megaureters.

Materials and Methods.—Three girls and 10 boys with a total of 16 primary obstructive megaureters (3 bilateral) underwent reimplantation with Starr plication between 1988 and 2000. Baseline and followup renal function (average followup 6.2 years) was determined with renal scan and/or 24-hour urinary creatinine clearance. Average age at operation was 5.6 years (range 2 months to 13 years). All ureters were plicated using the Starr technique with interrupted polydioxanone sutures performed by a single surgeon. Reimplantation methods were the Hendren technique in 7 and Politano-Leadbetter in 9.

Results.—No ureter demonstrated obstruction postoperatively. One ureter refluxed, which resolved with subureteral collagen injection. Seven patients had mean preoperative and postoperative creatinine clearance ± SD 72.9 ± 14.8 and 102.1 ± 10.9 cc/min, respectively ($P < 0.05$). Six patients underwent preoperative and postoperative renal scans. Average preoperative relative renal function on renal scan in the kidney with a megaureter was 53.0% ± 6.7% (range 37% to 84%). Long-term followup (average 4.1 years) renal scan revealed a relative function of 53.3% ± 9.2% (range 37% to 100%).

Conclusions.—Our data demonstrate that Starr plication is a safe procedure that provides long-term stabilization of renal function in the management of primary obstructive megaureter.

▶ Reimplantation of the megaureter is technically more challenging than a normal caliber ureter. Historically, recurrent obstruction or new vesicoureteral reflux occurred in 20% to 30% of megaureter reimplants. Excisional ureteral tapering or ureteral plication is required to achieve the appropriate reimplantation tunnel length (5:1) that prevents postoperative reflux. The authors report excellent results using the Starr imbrication technique. The bulk of the ureter did not present a technical problem. In younger children (smaller bladder), excision of the ureter may be beneficial and with care should not result in ureteral ischemia.

D. E. Coplen, MD

Primary Lower Urinary Tract Reconstruction for Nonfunctioning Renal Moieties Associated With Obstructing Ureteroceles

Gran CD, Kropp BP, Cheng EY, et al (Univ of Oklahoma, Oklahoma City; Northwestern Univ, Chicago; Med College of Ohio, Toledo)

J Urol 173:198-201, 2005 26–2

Purpose.—Upper pole heminephrectomy is the conventional treatment for severely compromised nonfunctioning renal units associated with ureteroceles due to the potential morbidity of leaving a nonfunctioning renal moiety in place. This approach often fails to address the pathological anatomical defect present at the bladder level, and during long-term followup the majority of patients require subsequent lower tract surgery due to persistent ureterocele, new or persistent vesicoureteral reflux, or recurrent infections. We determined the success of primary lower urinary tract reconstruction for nonfunctioning renal moieties and the morbidity associated with leaving nonfunctioning renal units in situ.

Materials and Methods.—We present the collective experience of 2 institutions using definitive lower urinary tract reconstruction without upper tract ablative surgery in 16 patients with duplex collecting systems and an associated nonfunctioning renal moiety due to obstructing ureteroceles.

Results.—At a mean followup of 62 months upper tract dilatation was decreased or completely resolved in all patients, no loss of renal function was present and 15 of 16 patients (94%) had no evidence of persistent reflux. Postoperative complications in the form of a urinary tract infection occurred in 2 of 16 patients (13%). No patient was febrile. No patient had development of hypertension, proteinuria or tumor during followup.

Conclusions.—We believe that primary, single stage, lower urinary tract reconstruction in children with severely compromised or nonfunctioning renal moieties damaged by ureteroceles is superior to upper urinary tract ablative surgery, successfully correcting the obstructive or refluxing pathology with minimal morbidity and risk during long-term followup.

► Ureterocele management is complex and a single surgical approach is not appropriate for all patients. In addition, a variety of surgical approaches may achieve an excellent surgical outcome (absence of infections and normal continence) in a given patient. The authors show that a tapered reimplant of a dilated nonfunctioning ureter can be safely performed in conjunction with the bladder neck reconstruction that is usually required in the presence of a ureterocele. This avoids the potential complications associated with nephron-sparing surgery. Cosmetic advantages of a Pfannenstiel incision versus a flank incision have been decreased with laparoscopy. While most children with ureteroceles eventually require a bladder level surgery, those without reflux may be best served with an upper-tract ablative approach that avoids the complexity of the bladder level surgery.

D. E. Coplen, MD

Symptomatic Refluxing Distal Ureteral Stumps After Nephroureterectomy and Heminephroureterectomy: What Should We Do?

Casale P, Grady RW, Lee RS, et al (Univ of Pennsylvania, Philadelphia; Univ of Washington, Seattle)

J Urol 173:204-206, 2005 26–3

Purpose.—We hypothesize that residual ureteral stumps following nephroureterectomy (NU) or heminephroureterectomy (HNU) are associated with an increased risk of urinary tract infection (UTI) that is decreased by distal ureterectomy.

Materials and Methods.—We performed a retrospective review of 71 patients who underwent NU or HNU for reflux into a nonfunctioning system between 1990 and 2003. The indications for all renal surgery included recurrent UTIs in 44 patients, hypertension in 8 and a combination of these conditions in 19. Voiding cystourethrogram and urine cultures were performed in all patients with recurrent symptomatic UTIs.

Results.—Followup in all 71 patients averaged 52 months. A total of 11 patients who underwent laparoscopic NU or HNU to the hiatus of the bladder were excluded because they did not have a ureteral remnant. The remaining 60 patients all underwent an open procedure. Of these patients 32 (53%) had refluxing distal ureteral remnants. Six of these 32 patients with refluxing stumps (19%), all girls, became symptomatic during followup. Symptomatic UTIs recurred in these 6 patients an average of 12 times per year (range 8 to 21), which significantly decreased after distal ureterectomy.

Conclusions.—If surgery is indicated in patients with reflux into a poorly functioning system, we recommend NU or HNU to the level of the bladder hiatus. If a symptomatic ureteral remnant is present, then distal ureterectomy decreases the rate of symptomatic UTIs in these patients. Laparoscopic distal ureterectomy is a viable surgical technique for this patient population.

► A refluxing ureteral stump may act as a bladder diverticulum, and the stasis may predispose to recurrent UTIs. In this series, a minority (19%) of children with refluxing stumps developed recurrent urinary infections. The authors describe their technique of laparoscopic removal of the retained distal ureteral stump. It is difficult to recommend routine removal of the distal ureter in all patients, but if the initial nephrectomy is performed laparoscopically, then removal of the distal ureter seems reasonable at that time. If the procedure is open, then a second incision is usually required to adequately remove the majority of the distal ureter.

D. E. Coplen, MD

27 Hypospadias

Tubularized Incised Plate Urethroplasty: 5 Years' Experience

Eliçevik M, Tireli G, Sander S (Clinic of Pediatric Surgery, Istanbul, Turkey)
Eur Urol 46:655-659, 2004 27–1

Objective.—To evaluate the results of tubularized incised plate (TIP) urethroplasty in a series of primary hypospadias repairs.

Patients and Method.—The medical records of 360 children (mean age, 4.3 years; range, 2-14 years) with primary hypospadias undergoing TIP urethroplasty repair and treatment of complications were reviewed. A good result is a direct urinary stream through a slit and vertically oriented meatus and mild angled urinary stream through a slightly regressed meatus is a satisfactory result.

Results.—The sum of good (74%) and satisfactory results (3%) was the overall success rate (77%), which was increased to 95% after a second surgical procedure for the treatment of complications. In 30 patients with single fistula (8%), fistula healed spontaneously in 2 patients and 20 patients had successful fistula closure. Redo TIP urethroplasty (n = 30) was performed for dehiscence (n = 15, 3%), neourethral stricture (n = 3, 1%) and multiple fistula with meatal stenosis (n = 12, 3%). The complication rate after redo TIP urethroplasty is 30%. Twenty-four (7%) patients underwent meatoplasty for meatal stenosis.

Conclusion.—TIP urethroplasty can be used to repair primary hypospadias. After a learning curve and attention to surgical details, cosmetic and functional outcome become excellent. Redo TIP urethroplasty can be performed in the treatment of complications.

Tubularized Incised Plate Hypospadias Reoperation

Nguyen MT, Snodgrass WT (Univ of Texas, Dallas)
J Urol 171:2404-2406, 2004 27–2

Purpose.—We report our updated experience with tubularized incised plate hypospadias reoperations in a series of patients of whom the majority had undergone prior urethral plate incision.

Materials and Methods.—Records of 31 consecutive patients undergoing tubularized incised plate reoperation were reviewed. The decision for this repair was based on a preserved urethral plate that appeared supple despite prior surgery.

Results.—Of the 31 patients the mean number of prior operations was 1.1, including 18 (58%) who had undergone primary repairs that involved midline plate incision. Overall, 28 (90%) patients had a successful outcome with a functional neourethra and vertical slit meatus. Complications occurred in 7 (23%) patients, consisting mostly of fistulas. Among 27 cases in which dartos was used as a barrier layer, fistulas occurred in 1 (6%) of 18 when a ventral flap was placed over the neourethra versus 3 (33%) of 9 when adjacent tissues alongside the neourethra were approximated in the midline ($P = 0.055$). The rate of complications was not affected by history of urethral plate incision. In 3 patients partial or complete glans dehiscence or a large fistula occurred, and 2 subsequently required staged buccal graft urethroplasty.

Conclusions.—Tubularized incised plate reoperation results in a functional neourethra with a vertical slit meatus when the plate has been preserved and appears supple after prior surgery. Fistulas are less likely when a flap is interposed between the neourethra and skin. Complications are low despite previous urethral plate incision if there is no apparent scarring of the plate. An alternative technique for reoperative urethroplasty should be considered if the urethral plate has been excised or is grossly scarred.

► The tubularized incised plate urethroplasty (Snodgrass repair) is commonly used in hypospadias repair. It was initially described in mid to distal shaft repairs but is now being used in proximal hypospadias and in reoperative cases. The technique is relatively straightforward, but if the urethroplasty is carried out too far onto the glans, meatal stenosis will occur (7% in the Eliçevik article (Abstract 27–1). The glanular urethra may also be compromised if the glans is small and the urethral plate is very narrow as seen in some hypospadias. A second layer of coverage is important in the prevention of fistulas. The ventral urethroplasty suture line can be covered with divergent spongiosum or preferably with a de-epithelialized dorsal dartos pedicle flap.

The reported 5-year experience is an honest appraisal at a center performing 80 of these procedures a year. A single operation was successful in three fourths of patients. This complication rate is the same or no better than with other hypospadias techniques.

Nguyen and Snodgrass (Abstract 27–2) report the largest series using the technique in reoperative cases. Even in cases with prior plate incision, a repeat incision was feasible and successful in the majority of cases. The 7% complication rate is very low for a reoperative procedure. Patient selection is clearly the key, and the authors use their vast experience with the technique to determine if the urethral plate is supple and compliant before proceeding with this approach. If the urethral plate is abnormal, either a localized vascular flap or a staged skin grafting is required for repair.

D. E. Coplen, MD

The Island Tube and Island Onlay Hypospadias Repairs Offer Excellent Long-term Outcomes: A 14-Year Followup

Patel RP, Shukla AR, Snyder HM III (Children's Hosp of Philadelphia)

J Urol 172:1717-1719, 2004 27–3

Purpose.—We have used an inner preputial flap as a transverse island tube (IT) for the 1-stage repair of proximal hypospadias when the urethral plate could not be preserved and as an island onlay flap (IO) when the urethral plate could be preserved for more than 20 years at our institution. We report long-term followup and an outcome comparison of these 2 techniques.

Materials and Methods.—We retrospectively reviewed our records for all patients who underwent proximal hypospadias repair with either the IT or IO procedure between 1981 and 1992 by 1 surgeon (HMS). We randomly contacted these former patients to undergo a long-term follow-up examination, consisting of postoperative history, physical examination and uroflowmetry with post-void residual measurement. A review of patient charts was completed for perioperative complications or the need for secondary procedures.

Results.—Patient information could be retrieved for 73 of 125 patients who underwent penoscrotal or more severe hypospadias repair with either the IT or IO procedure during the defined interval. We were able to contact 49 of these former patients following a minimum of 10 years and 30 patients agreed to return for a long-term followup examination. The IT and IO repairs were performed on 14 and 16 boys, respectively, at a mean age of 16.8 months (range, 8 to 74). At a mean follow-up of 14.2 years for both groups (range, 144 to 253 months) 2 boys in the IT group (14.2%) and none in the IO group had a fistula requiring repair. Distal stenosis requiring meatoplasty occurred in 1 and 2 patients in the IT and IO groups, respectively. There were no urethral strictures and uroflowmetry was available for 11 patients in the IT group and 14 in the IO groups with mean maximal flow rates of 17.3 and 21.8 ml per second ($P = 0.343$) and mean post-void residuals of 5.0 and 2.36 ml per second, respectively ($P = 0.249$).

Conclusions.—Unlike other forms of substitution urethroplasty, vascularized flaps based on preputial skin appear to be unique in that they do not have the long-term stricture rate seen with substitution urethroplasty using nongenital skin. The IT and IO repairs provided excellent long-term cosmetic and functional results. As the IT does have a higher incidence of postoperative complications, we have continued to extend our application of the IO to more proximal hypospadias repairs with continued success.

► The authors report excellent results with preputial IT and IO repairs of hypospadias. Complications including fistula (6%) and meatal stenosis (10%) were rare, and none of the patients developed a urethral stricture. Cosmetic results were deemed excellent. This study is limited in that it is a select group of 30 patients that agreed to return for follow-up at this institution. Because of excellent results, vascularized flap repairs remain very important in the correction of hypospadias.

D. E. Coplen, MD

Initial Experience With Staged Buccal Graft (BRACKA) Hypospadias Reoperations

Snodgrass W, Elmore J (Univ of Texas, Dallas)

J Urol 172:1720-1724, 2004 27–4

Purpose.—We report outcomes from staged buccal graft urethroplasty after failed hypospadias surgery.

Materials and Methods.—When the urethral plate had been excised or was visibly scarred after prior surgery patients underwent staged buccal graft repair. In the first operation persistent penile curvature was corrected, a proximal cutaneous urethrostomy was created, scarred tissues distally were excised and buccal graft was quilted into place for subsequent urethroplasty. At least 6 months later the now revascularized buccal strip was tubularized and covered with a dartos or tunica vaginalis flap.

Results.—A total of 25 patients underwent stage 1 repair following an average of 4.4 prior hypospadias surgeries. Complete graft take occurred in 22 (88%) cases while the remaining 3 had focal scar or graft contracture that was successfully patched before tubularization. To date 20 patients have undergone the stage 2. There were no cases of meatal stenosis, neourethral stricture or diverticulum. A fistula occurred in 1 (5%) of 18 cases in which a flap barrier layer was used. Partial glans dehiscence occurred in 4 prepubertal boys with graft obtained from the cheek, and they have undergone successful reoperative glansplasty. All patients completing surgery have a vertical slit neomeatus.

Conclusions.—Staged buccal graft reoperation reliably creates a well vascularized substitute urethral plate for tubularization with low complication rates and good cosmetic outcomes. Inner lip, which is thinner than cheek, may be a better source of graft for the glanular urethra.

▶ Reoperative hypospadias can be very challenging. While a small fistula may be easily closed in multiple layers, achieving a normal functional and cosmetic result in cases with significant glans loss, persistent curvature, or significant scarring after multiple prior surgeries can be difficult. While most hypospadias are now corrected with a single operation, a staged approach with preputial transposition in preparation for urethroplasty is used primarily in some children with very severe curvature. A vascularized pedicle is frequently used in reoperation although the surgeon must realize that the dartos blood supply may have been compromised at the first surgery. Bracka has described a 2-stage skin graft technique in both primary and reoperative cases.[1] The authors report preliminary results using a 2-stage buccal graft technique. Three patients required a second grafting procedure before the planned second stage. With a mean 5-month follow-up, 25% of patients required another surgery after the urethroplasty. Historically, single- stage buccal mucosal urethroplasty has a 40% to 50% long-term failure rate. Long-term follow-up will be required to determine whether the staged approach gives durable results.

D. E. Coplen, MD

Reference

1. Bracka A: Hypospadias repair: The two-stage alternative. *BJU Int* 76:31, 1995.

Long-term Followup of Buccal Mucosa Onlay Graft for Hypospadias Repair: Analysis of Complications

Fichtner J, Filipas D, Fisch M, et al (Johannes Gutenberg Univ, Mainz, Germany)

J Urol 172:1970-1972, 2004 27–5

Purpose.—We review the long-term results of buccal mucosa onlay grafting for urethral reconstruction in hypospadias surgery in patients with followup of at least 5 years.

Materials and Methods.—We retrospectively evaluated 132 patients who underwent buccal mucosa onlay graft for hypospadias repair, including 34 who underwent "salvage" grafting, during a 10-year period at our institution. In 49 cases with available followup longer than 5 years (average 6.2) complications were analyzed in detail.

Results.—The overall complication rate was 24% (12 of 49 patients), with all but 3 complications occurring during the first postoperative year (3 fistulas, 1 stricture, 1 meatal stenosis, 2 graft contractures, 2 scars at oral harvesting site). The remaining 3 complications manifested during postoperative years 2 and 3, and encompassed 2 anastomotic strictures at the proximal anastomosis and 1 meatal stenosis.

Conclusions.—Buccal mucosa onlay grafts for urethral reconstruction in hypospadias repair seem to provide stable long-term results, with complications occurring primarily during the first 12 months postoperatively.

► The authors report reasonably long-term outcomes using buccal mucosa in primary and salvage hypospadias repairs. Complications occurred in 24% of the patients. The complication rate was higher in the reoperative cases. Most of these occurred within the first year, although long-term follow-up is obviously required in these patients. Donor-site scarring was the significant complication in 2 patients who had large grafts from the upper and lower lips. No difference was noted in the complication rate using single or 2-stage repairs. These are complex cases, and the key is an excellent vascularized bed that facilitates graft survival and a successful surgical outcome.

D. E. Coplen, MD

Sexual Behavior and Sexual Function of Adults After Hypospadias Surgery: A Comparative Study

Bubanj TB, Perovic SV, Milicevic RM, et al (Univ Children's Hosp, Nis; Univ Children's Hosp Belgrade, Serbia)

J Urol 171:1876-1879, 2004 27–6

Purpose.—We assessed sexual behavior and sexual function in adults operated on for hypospadias.

Materials and Methods.—Long-term psychosexual adjustment was assessed with a standardized questionnaire which was mailed to 57 patients with hypospadias older than 18 years and 60 age matched normal control subjects.

Results.—A total of 37 patients with hypospadias and 39 controls participated. Self-reported strength of libido on a scale of 1 to 5 was shown to be similar in the 2 groups. Patients with hypospadias did not have problems in achieving erection, and average self-rated quality of erection ranging from 1 to 5 was the same as that of controls (mean value, 4.5). Patients with hypospadias noted curvature in a downward direction in a significantly higher proportion compared to controls (40% vs 18%, respectively). There were 13 patients with hypospadias who had ejaculation difficulties, of whom 6 had spraying and 7 had only dribbling of ejaculate. Patients with hypospadias masturbated significantly less often, were significantly less sexually active and had a smaller total number of sexual partners compared to control subjects. Control subjects were significantly more completely satisfied with their sexual life compared to patients with hypospadias (76.92% vs 51.35%, respectively).

Conclusions.—Sexual function of patients who underwent surgery for hypospadias in general is not affected. However, there is clearly a difference in certain aspects of sexual behavior between patients with hypospadias and controls. Follow-up and adequate counseling of patients who underwent surgery for hypospadias in adult life is necessary.

► This is a small case-control study evaluating sexual function and sexual behavior in adult men with a history of hypospadias repair. These men had surgical correction 15 to 20 years ago. Even though the majority had distal hypospadias and milder functional abnormalities, only half were completely satisfied with their sexual life. There is clearly room for continued improvement in surgical techniques and outcomes.

D. E. Coplen, MD

A Cost-Utility Analysis of Neonatal Circumcision

Van Howe RS (Michigan State Univ, Marquette)

Med Decis Making 24:584-601, 2004 27–7

Introduction.—A cost-utility analysis, based on published data from multiple observational studies, comparing boys circumcised at birth and those not circumcised was undertaken using the Quality of Well-being Scale, a Markov analysis, the standard reference case, and a societal perspective. Neonatal circumcision increased incremental costs by $828.42 per patient and resulted in an incremental 15.30 well-years lost per 1000 males. If neonatal circumcision was cost-free, pain-free, and had no immediate complications, it was still more costly than not circumcising. Using sensitivity analysis, it was impossible to arrange a scenario that made neonatal circumcision cost-effective. Neonatal circumcision is not good health policy, and support for it as a medical procedure cannot be justified financially or medically.

► This is an excellent cost-utility analysis based on published data. The pros and cons of circumcision are discussed in detail from clinical outcomes and financial standpoints. For example, it is well known that the uncircumcised male has a higher incidence of urinary infection but the rate would have to be 10% to 15% higher for circumcision to be cost effective. Cultural considerations do not factor into these data, so this analysis will probably have minimal impact on the performance of circumcision.

D. E. Coplen, MD

28 Genital Ambiguity

A 7-Year Experience of Genetic Males With Severe Phallic Inadequacy Assigned Female

Reiner WG, Kropp BP (Univ of Oklahoma, Oklahoma City)

J Urol 172:2395-2398, 2004 28–1

Purpose.—We examine the hypotheses underlying the clinical decision to assign female gender at birth in male neonates with severe phallic inadequacy.

Materials And Methods.—A total of 18 genetic males with severe phallic inadequacy were assessed longitudinally for physical, social, psychological and sexual identity development. Diagnoses included cloacal (11) and classic (1) exstrophy, partial androgen resistance (3), mixed gonadal dysgenesis (2) and penile agenesis (1). Neonatal sex assignment was female in 15 and male in 3 patients.

Results.—All patients demonstrated marked male typical behaviors and interests. Of the 15 female assigned patients 1 died, 1 refused to declare sexual identity or orientation, 1 converted to male before initial evaluation, 1 was reassigned male by the parents and 5 others declared male sexual identity. Thus, of 17 living patients 10 live as males and 6 as females. Of patients 17 years or older only those living as male lived independently. The 4 oldest patients living as male but only 1 patient living as female would discuss sexual orientation—all 5 declared orientation toward females, and 3 of these 4 males had girlfriends or were married. The sexually undeclared patient lived in a residential treatment center because of major behavioral difficulties since age 15. Only patients living as male had dated.

Conclusions.—This longitudinal study implies that males with severe phallic inadequacy reared male and those reared female but converting to male can have functional psychosocial developmental trajectories. Those reared female have a realistic likelihood of recognizing male sexual identity and converting to male. Those not converting to male appear to have less successful psychosocial developmental trajectories.

► The study of this small group of patients reinforces the difficulty with predicting ultimate sexual identity. Eight of 15 patients raised as females declared a male identity later in life. Current data do not support routine assignment of female sex to neonates with a Y chromosome and prenatal androgen exposure.

D. E. Coplen, MD

29 Cryptorchidism

Difference in Prevalence of Congenital Cryptorchidism in Infants Between Two Nordic Countries

Boisen KA, Kaleva M, Main KM, et al (Rigshospitalet, Copenhagen; Univ of Turku, Finland)

Lancet 363:1264-1269, 2004 29–1

Background.—Several investigators have shown striking differences in semen quality and testicular cancer rate between Denmark and Finland. Since maldescent of the testis is a shared risk factor for these conditions we undertook a joint prospective study for the prevalence of congenital cryptorchidism.

Methods.—1068 Danish (1997–2001) and 1494 Finnish boys (1997–99) were consecutively recruited prenatally. We also established prevalence data for all newborns at Turku University Central Hospital, Finland (1997–99, n=5798). Testicular position was assessed by a standardised technique. All subtypes of congenital cryptorchidism were included, but retractile testes were considered normal.

Findings.—Prevalence of cryptorchidism at birth was 9.0% (95% CI 7.3–10.8) in Denmark and 2.4% (1.7–3.3) in Finland. At 3 months of age, prevalence rates were 1.9% (1.2–3.0) and 1.0% (0.5–1.7), respectively. Significant geographic differences were still present after adjustment for confounding factors (birthweight, gestational age, being small for gestational age, maternal age, parity, mode of delivery); odds ratio (Denmark vs Finland) was 4.4 (2.9–6.7, $p<0.0001$) at birth and 2.2 (1.0–45, $p=0.039$) at three months. The rate in Denmark was significantly higher than that reported 40 years ago.

Interpretation.—Our findings of increasing and much higher prevalence of congenital cryptorchidism in Denmark than in Finland contribute evidence to the pattern of high frequency of reproductive problems such as testicular cancer and impaired semen quality in Danish men. Although genetic factors could account for the geographic difference, the increase in reproductive health problems in Denmark is more likely explained by environmental factors, including endocrine disrupters and lifestyle.

► The authors identify a high prevalence of cryptorchidism in Denmark compared with Finland. In addition, the incidence in Denmark has increased over the last 40 years. The authors have previously described a high incidence of fertility issues and testicular cancer in Danish men and hypothesize a congenital etiology. This will require further evaluation. The population differences may be genetic but could also have an environmental etiology, as has recently been hypothesized in the increasing incidence of hypospadias.

D. E. Coplen, MD

Long-term Outcome of Fowler-Stephens Orchiopexy in Boys With Prune-Belly Syndrome

Patil KK, Duffy PG, Woodhouse CRJ, et al (Univ College London Hosps)
J Urol 171:1666-1669, 2004 29–2

Purpose.—Intra-abdominal testes in boys with prune-belly syndrome have been conventionally managed by 1 or 2-stage orchiopexy with division of the gonadal vessels. We reviewed a series of adults with prune-belly syndrome to assess the morphological and functional outcome of orchiopexy in childhood with specific reference to the spontaneous onset of puberty, hormonal profiles and sexual function.

Materials and Methods.—A total of 41 boys were divided into 3 groups, depending on the type of orchiopexy performed, namely, group 1—20 with bilateral 1-stage orchiopexy, group 2—10 with unilateral 1-stage and contralateral 2-stage orchiopexy, and group 3—11 with bilateral 2-stage orchiopexy.

Results.—In group 1, 9 of 20 patients had good scrotal testes bilaterally, 6 had a good scrotal testis on 1 side and 3 had small testes on each side. Two boys required testosterone supplementation but 18 had normal hormonal and sexual function. In group 2, 6 of 10 patients had good scrotal testes bilaterally and 4 had a good scrotal testis on 1 side. All patients underwent spontaneous puberty with good sexual function. In group 3, 7 of 11 boys had good scrotal testes bilaterally, and 3 had 1 good testis with normal puberty and sexual function. These 10 patients underwent spontaneous puberty with good sexual function.

Conclusions.—The majority of boys with prune-belly syndrome had a satisfactory outcome after orchiopexy with division of the gonadal vessels with testicular function sufficient to induce puberty and maintain satisfactory sexual function in adult life.

▶ The Fowler-Stephens orchiopexy is performed in select cases of intra-abdominal cryptorchidism. The gonadal vessels are divided, and testicular viability is dependent upon collateral blood supply. This is the first report of long-term outcome after this procedure in boys with prune-belly syndrome (PBS). Only 2 of 40 boys developed bilateral testicular atrophy requiring testosterone replacement at puberty. A staged repair allows for enhanced blood supply before testicular mobilization and, theoretically, an improved surgical outcome. Assessment of fertility potential is much more difficult in this population because PBS males are azospermic. FSH (follicle stimulating hormone) is an indirect measure of spermatogenesis. Normal or minimally elevated levels were identified in three fourths of the men indicating that spermatogenic function may be present. Currently, intra-abdominal orchiopexy is performed at a much younger age and rarely requires division of the vessels to achieve adequate scrotal position. Hopefully, long-term follow-up of these patients will show success with spontaneous puberty and normal sexual function.

D. E. Coplen, MD

30 Varicocele

Paternity After Adolescent Varicocele Repair

Salzhauer EW, Sokol A, Glassberg KI (State Univ of New York, Brooklyn; Columbia Univ, New York)

Pediatrics 114:1631-1633, 2004 30–1

Objective.—Varicocelectomy has long been a therapeutic modality used in the treatment of male infertility. In the past decade, adolescent varicocelectomy has become a frequent procedure to preserve testicular growth and to help prevent future infertility. Because our clinical population includes a large portion of orthodox Jews who traditionally marry early and are forbidden to use birth control by religious law, we thought that by studying our patients, we might be able to accelerate our follow-up regarding paternity. In addition, we wanted to learn whether adolescent varicocelectomy might have any negative impact.

Methods.—Questionnaires inquiring as to the marital and paternity status, postoperative course, and complications were sent to 50 patients who had undergone a unilateral or bilateral varicocele repair during adolescence and who were at least 21 years old at the time of this review. In addition, a careful chart review was performed to examine the perioperative and postoperative parameters of each respondent.

Results.—Of the 43 responses (86% response rate), 18 of 18 patients who had attempted to father a child were successful. The remaining 25 were not married or had never attempted to father a child. In the paternity group, 10 of the fathers had undergone an Ivanissevich repair; the remaining 8 had a Palomo repair. Sixteen of the 18 had unilateral varicocelectomies, and 2 underwent bilateral repairs. Of those with a unilateral varicocele, the indication for surgery in 10 was a grade 2 to 3 varicocele associated with a > 20% volume difference when compared with the right testicle. Three had 10% to 20% volume loss, whereas the remaining three had unusually large grade 3 varicoceles without concurrent volume difference.

Conclusions.—Varicocelectomy in the adolescent population has been proposed as a therapeutic intervention to preserve both fertility and testicular growth. Although not showing a cause-and-effect relationship, it is our contention that varicocelectomy in adolescence at worst does no harm and at best preserves fertility.

▶ This a retrospective review of varicocelectomy performed before age 21. Testicular asymmetry was the indication for repair in only 11 of 43 patients.

Catch-up growth occurred in 9 of these men but this can occur even without correction. Even the complications of surgery were low, and the authors would like the reader to conclude that prophylactic varicocelectomy preserves fertility. This conclusion cannot be reached from this study design.

D. E. Coplen, MD

Is Adolescent Varicocele a Progressive Disease Process?

Diamond DA, Zurakowski D, Atala A, et al (Harvard Med School, Boston)
J Urol 172:1746-1748, 2004 30–2

Purpose.—We determined whether there was evidence of progression in either varicocele grade or testicular volume differentials over time in our adolescent varicocele population.

Materials and Methods.—A total of 41 boys, 7.3 to 19 years old, (mean age, 13.7, SD 2.5) were seen at sequential visits. At each visit, varicocele grade was determined by the attending urologist, and ultrasound calculated testicular volume differential was determined by an attending ultrasonographer. A senior staff statistician performed statistical analysis of the sequential data.

Results.—The varicocele grade data were analyzed using the nonparametric Wilcoxon test and no significant evidence of progression on sequential visits was demonstrated. Similarly, the serial volume differential data were assessed using the paired t test, and no significant evidence for progression of testicular volume differentials was demonstrated.

Conclusions.—In our study population, neither varicocele grade nor change in testicular volume differentials increased over time in a statistically significant manner. These results argue against the concept that adolescent varicocele is a progressive disease process.

▶ The authors have chosen a conservative approach to varicocele management and serially followed adolescents even in the presence of testicular asymmetry. Varicocele grade and the magnitude of the size difference rarely changed during follow-up. Semen analyses are not available in these patients, but the data argue that the adolescent varicocele may not be a progressive disease. There is no randomized study showing improved semen analysis and fertility after adolescent varicocelectomy. Observation and serial examination is a reasonable approach in this patient population.

D. E. Coplen, MD

31 Pediatric Oncology

Prepubertal Testis Tumors: Actual Prevalence Rate of Histological Types

Pohl HG, Shukla AR, Metcalf PD, et al (Children's Natl Med Ctr, Washington, DC; Children's Hosp of Philadelphia; Hosp for Sick Children, Toronto; et al)

J Urol 172:2370-2372, 2004 31–1

Purpose.—Tumor registries, urological textbooks and literature surveys all assert that yolk sac tumors are the most common primary testicular tumors in boys 12 years and younger. In contrast, several individual institutions have reported that benign tumors are more common than malignant tumors. To clarify these discordant findings, we surveyed the primary pathology records from 4 major pediatric centers.

Materials and Methods.—The pathology records of the contributing centers were culled for primary testicular masses in boys 12 years and younger. Older boys and those with either paratesticular tumors or leukemia were excluded. The prevalence of each histological subtype was calculated from the pooled cases.

Results.—A total of 98 patients met our criteria. Only 15% had yolk sac tumors. Teratomas comprised 48% of the tumors (mature 44%, immature 4%). Epidermoid cysts were found in another 14% of patients. Gonadal stromal cell tumors represented 13% of the total, divided among granulosa cell (5%), Leydig cell (4%), Sertoli cell (3%) and mixed gonadal stromal cell (1%). Other pathology, including cystic dysplasia (2), lymphoma (4), inflammatory pseudotumor (1) and gonadoblastoma (2), made up 9% of the total number of cases.

Conclusions.—We found that benign lesions represent the majority of primary testis tumors (74%), with the most common histological type being teratoma (48%). The reported high prevalence rates of prepubertal yolk sac tumors probably results from a reporting bias, since benign tumors are less likely to be submitted to tumor registries. Therefore, the primary operative approach to the majority of testis tumors in boys 12 years and younger should entail testis sparing surgery. Orchiectomy should be reserved for histologically confirmed malignancy based on increased preoperative alpha-fetoprotein and/or frozen section analysis of the tumor.

▶ This compilation of pathology records from 4 pediatric centers reveals that the majority of prepubertal testicular tumors are benign. When cystic features are present on preoperative US and the alpha fetoprotein is normal, then consideration should be given to testicular-sparing surgery. The testis can be explored through an inguinal incision and a frozen section can be obtained. Orchiectomy can be performed in yolk sac or other potentially malignant lesions and in situations where testicular sparing is not feasible.

D. E. Coplen, MD

Subject Index

A

Abdominal sacral colpopexy
  with autologous fascia lata, 67
Adolescent(s)
  (*see also* Children)
  varicocele in
    fertility and, 283
    progression in grade and volume, 284
African Americans (*see* Black American men)
Alcohol immersion
  for catheters reused for clean intermittent catheterization, 241
Alemtuzumab
  as immunosuppressive agent in kidney transplantation, 53
Alfuzosin
  once daily for acute urinary retention in benign prostatic hyperplasia, 104
α-blockers
  doxazosin with or without tolterodine in men with bladder outlet obstruction and overactive bladder, 109
  vs. finasteride for benign prostatic hyperplasia, 106
  intermittent tamsulosin therapy for lower urinary tract symptoms, 105
α-methylacyl-CoA racemase (AMACR)
  assay for humoral response as supplement to PSA screening, 201
Androgen suppression, for prostate cancer
  dihydrotestosterone levels in prostatic tissue before and after, 211
  fracture risk and, 208
  hip fracture and, 209
  immediate vs. deferred for patients not undergoing curative local treatment, 171
  osteoporosis and, diagnosis and treatment, 208
  with and without radiation therapy for clinically localized, 195
Anesthesia
  spermatic cord block for scrotal procedures, 213
Antibiotic prophylaxis
  long-term, adverse reactions of nitrofurantoin, trimethoprim, and sulfamethoxazole in children, 240
Arylamines
  as risk factor for bladder cancer in nonsmokers, 146
Azoospermia
  (*see also* Infertility, male)
  nonobstructive
    artificial neural network for predicting presence of spermatozoa in testes, 217
    prediction of successful outcome of microdissection testicular sperm extraction, 216

B

Bacillus Calmette-Guerin
  for urethral recurrence of bladder cancer following radical cystectomy and ileal bladder substitution, 157
Benign prostatic hyperplasia (BPH)
  (*see also* Lower urinary tract, symptoms)
  acute urinary retention in, alfuzosin once daily for, 104
  correlation between detrusor collagen content and urinary symptoms, 97
  dutasteride for, long-term efficacy and safety, 107
  finasteride vs. alpha-blockers for, 106
  laser vaporization of the prostate for, 117, 119
  macrophage inhibitor cytokine-1 gene down-regulation and prostatic inflammation in, 99
  microwave feedback thermotherapy vs. TURP, 113
  molecular profiling using a large scale real-time reverse transcriptase-polymerase chain reaction approach, 101
  Serenoa repens for, 103
  transurethral ethanol ablation for, 110, 112
  TUNA vs. TURP for, 5-year results, 116
  TURP for (*see* Transurethral resection of the prostate)
Bicalutamide
  for localized or locally advanced prostate cancer
    efficacy and tolerability, 204
    lymph node status and, 206
Bicycle riding
  erectile dysfunction and, 231, 232
Black American men
  longitudinal changes in lower urinary tract symptoms, 89
Bladder
  cancer (*see* Urothelial cancer)
  compliance measurement standardization, 247

contractility, noninvasive assessment in men, 95, 96
detrusor (*see* Detrusor)
intermittent catheterization, microwave heating vs. alcohol immersion for reused catheters, 241
neurogenic (*see* Neurogenic bladder)
outlet obstruction
in men
with overactive bladder symptoms, doxazosin with or without tolterodine for, 109
penile compression release maneuver as noninvasive test for diagnosis, 96
watchful waiting for mild symptoms, 90
in women
bladder neck obstruction in, diagnosis and treatment, 65
delayed treatment after sling surgery, 68
with stress incontinence, 59
overactive (*see* Overactive bladder)
reconstruction
non-cycled artificial urinary sphincter, 263
stomal complications with cutaneous catheterizable continent stomas, 261
Body mass index (*see* Obesity)
Bone anchor fixation, transvaginal complications, 79, 80
Bortezomib
for renal cell carcinoma, phase II trial, 140
Botulinum toxin
for interstitial cystitis, 62
in lower urinary tract dysfunction, 63
for refractory overactive bladder symptoms, 62
for urge incontinence, 61
BOULE protein
nonexpression, association with meiotic arrest in male infertility, 219
BPH (*see* Benign prostatic hyperplasia)
Buccal graft urethroplasty
staged, for hypospadias reoperation, 272
Buccal onlay graft
for urethral reconstruction in hypospadias repair, long-term results, 273

C

Campath-1H (*see* Alemtuzumab)
Catheters
reuse for clean intermittent catheterization, microwave heating vs. alcohol immersion for, 241
Children
(*see also* Adolescent[s]; Infants)
acute pyelonephritis, correlation of renal ultrasonography with inflammatory volume from dimercaptosuccinic acid renal scans, 239
bladder reconstruction, stomal complications with cutaneous catheterizable continent stomas, 261
detrusor hyperreflexia secondary to neurogenic bladder dysfunction, oxybutynin for, 251
long-term antibiotic prophylaxis, adverse reactions of nitrofurantoin, trimethoprim, and sulfamethoxazole, 240
pelvic floor relaxation therapy for pelvic floor spasms, 248
urinary tract infections, follow-up urine cultures and fever in, 238
vesicoureteral reflux
modified subureteral transurethral injection procedure for, 244
timing of follow-up of voiding cystourethrogram in, 243
Chlamydial infections
prevalence in young adults in the United States, 87
Circumcision
neonatal, cost-utility analysis, 274
Clomipramine
for on-demand treatment of premature ejaculation, 234
Colpopexy
abdominal sacral with autologous fascia lata, 67
Computed tomographic angiography (CTA)
vs. digital subtraction angiography for diagnosis of renal artery stenosis, 17
Computed tomography (CT)
angiography (*see* Computed tomographic angiography)
helical, for identification of urinary stone composition using attenuation values, 15

multiphase helical, in planning surgical treatment of pelvi-uretric junction obstruction, 16
Cooled thermotherapy
for benign prostatic hyperplasia, 115
Coronary heart disease
in kidney transplant recipients, nontraditional risk factors, 51
Cryoablation
laparoscopic, for solid renal masses, 37
Cryptorchidism
difference in prevalence in infants between two Nordic countries, 279
intra-abdominal, long-term outcome of Fowler-Stephens orchiopexy for, 280
CT (*see* Computed tomography)
CTA (*see* Computed tomographic angiography)
CYP1B1 gene
polymorphisms as risk factors for renal cell carcinoma, 137
Cystectomy (*see* Urothelial cancer)
Cystitis
interstitial, botulinum-A toxin for, 62
Cytomegalovirus disease
valganciclovir for, in kidney transplant recipients, 47

D

daVinci robotic system
for laparoscopic partial nephrectomy, 37
Detrusor
contractility, noninvasive assessment in men, 95, 96
correlation between collagen content and urinary symptoms in symptomatic benign prostatic hyperplasia, 97
hyperreflexia secondary to neurogenic bladder dysfunction in children, oxybutynin for, 251
underactivity, influence on long-term outcome of TURP, 121
Dihydrotestosterone
levels in prostatic tissue before and after androgen deprivation therapy for prostate cancer, 211
DNA hypermethylation
of multiple genes in renal cancer, 138
Docetaxel
plus estramustine vs. mitoxantrone plus prednisone for advanced refractory prostate cancer, 199
plus prednisone vs. mitoxantrone plus prednisone for advanced prostate cancer, 200
Donor insemination
adolescent offspring with open-identity, 222
Donor-specific transfusion
in inducing tolerance in transplantation, 43
Doxazosin
(*see also* Alpha-blockers)
with or without tolterodine in men with bladder outlet obstruction and an overactive bladder, 109
Dutasteride
for benign prostatic hyperplasia, long-term efficacy and safety, 107

E

Ejaculation
frequency and subsequent risk of prostate cancer, 168
premature (*see* Premature ejaculation)
Enuresis
nocturnal, persisting into adulthood, urodynamics in treatment of, 249
Erectile dysfunction
after a long-distance cycling event, associations with bicycle characteristics, 231
bicycle riding and, 232
sildenafil for, long-term safety of, 233
Escherichia coli
pyelonephritis, purified PapDG protein as vaccine for, 85
Estramustine
plus docetaxel vs. mitoxantrone and prednisone for advanced refractory prostate cancer, 199
Ethanol ablation
transurethral, for benign prostatic hyperplasia, 110, 112
Evidence-based medicine
pretest probability estimates and, 1
Extracorporeal shock wave lithotripsy
risk factors for subcapsular hematoma formation after, 22
vs. uteroscopy/laser lithotripsy for proximal ureteral stones, 23

F

Fascia lata, autologous
in abdominal sacral colpopexy for vaginal prolapse, 67
in sling cystourethropexy for stress incontinence, 66

Fetus (*see* Prenatal diagnosis)
Finasteride
  vs. alpha-blockers for benign prostatic hyperplasia, 106
5α-reductase inhibitors (*see* Dutasteride; Finasteride)
FK778
  as immunosuppressive agent in kidney transplantation, 48
Fractures
  risk with androgen-deprivation therapy for prostate cancer, 208, 209
Frequency-volume charts
  in adults without voiding complaints, reference values and variables, 93
  vs. voiding symptom questionnaire, accuracy for nocturic episodes, 92

G

Genital ambiguity
  genetic males with severe phallic inadequacy assigned female, 7-year experience, 277
Gonococcal infections
  prevalence in young adults in the United States, 87
GreenLight laser prostatectomy
  for benign prostatic hyperplasia, 117
GSTP1 methylation levels
  correlation with Gleason grade and tumor volume in prostate needle biopsies, 186

H

Hematoma
  perinephric, after extracorporeal shock wave lithotripsy, 22
Heminephroureterectomy
  ureterectomy for symptomatic refluxing distal ureteral stumps after, 267
Hip fracture
  risk with androgen-deprivation therapy for prostate cancer, 208
Holmium laser prostatectomy
  vs. TURP, 119
Hormone ablation (*see* Androgen suppression)
Hospital costs
  for surgical complications, 10
Hypermethylation
  in tumor, urine, and serum DNA of patients with renal cancer, 138
Hypertension
  in living kidney donors, 50
Hypospadias
  buccal onlay graft reconstruction for, long-term results, 273
  island tube and island onlay repair, 271
  sexual behavior and sexual function of adults after, 274
  staged buccal graft urethroplasty after failed initial repair, 272
  tubularized incised plate urethroplasty for repair, 269

I

Immunosuppression
  FK778 for, in kidney transplantation, 48
Incontinence, urinary (*see* Urinary incontinence)
Infants
  (*see also* Children)
  cost-utility analysis of neonatal circumcision, 274
  febrile urinary tract infections, renal ultrasonography for, 237
  mild prenatal pyelectasis
    2-year outcomes, 257
    neonatal ultrasound as screening tool for significant nephrouropathies, 255
    thresholds of renal pelvic diameter associated with normal postnatal renal function, 256
  prenatally detected ureteroceles associated with multicystic dysplasia, outcome analysis, 258
Infertility, male
  (*see also* Azoospermia)
  adolescent varicocele repair and, 283
  association of meiotic arrest with lack of *BOULE* protein expression in, 219
  with defective spermatogenesis and hypotestosteronemia in male mice lacking the androgen receptor in Sertoli cells, 225
  deletion of the *Parkin* coregulated gene as cause in the *quaking*^{viable} mouse mutant, 226
  impaired Leydig cell function in, 218
Internet
  full-text journal article availability, 2
Interstitial cystitis
  botulinum-A toxin for, 62
Island onlay repair
  for hypospadias, 271
Island tube repair
  for hypospadias, 271

K

Kidney cancer (*see* Renal cell carcinoma)
Kidney masses
  laparoscopic cryoablation for, 37
Kidney stones (*see* Urolithiasis)
Kidney transplantation (*see* Renal transplantation)

L

Laparoscopy
  for cryoablation of solid renal masses, 37
  en bloc stapling of renal hilum during nephrectomy or nephroureterectomy, 33
  intraoperative local anesthesia for decreased postoperative opioid requirements, 34
  pancreatic injuries during, 41
  for partial nephrectomy
    complications, 38
    daVinci robotic system for, 36
    long-term oncological outcome, 35
  practice patterns in the Midwest, 30
  for radical nephrectomy
    retroperitoneoscopic, vena cava transection during, 32
    transperitoneal laparoscopic vs. retroperitoneoscopic, 31
  for radical prostatectomy
    body mass index and, 29
    extraperitoneal vs. transperitoneal approach, early oncologic results, 28
    vs. open, cost comparison, 28
  thoracic complications, 40
  tumor seeding in, 39
Laser prostatectomy
  GreenLight, for benign prostatic hyperplasia, 117
  holmium, vs. TURP, 119
Leydig cells
  impaired function in infertile men, 218
Living donors
  hypertension in, 50
Local anesthesia
  intraoperative, for decreased postoperative opioid requirements after transperitoneal laparoscopic renal and adrenal surgery, 34
Lower urinary tract
  obstruction in fetus, diagnosis and outcome, 258
  reconstruction for nonfunctioning renal moieties associated with obstructing ureteroceles, 266
  symptoms (*see also* Benign prostatic hyperplasia)
    in black American men, longitudinal changes, 89
    botulinum toxin for (*see* Botulinum toxin)
    correlation with detrusor collagen content, 97
    doxazosin with or without tolterodine in men with bladder outlet obstruction and overactive bladder, 109
    intermittent tamsulosin therapy for, 105
    male sexual function and, 229
    natural history in men, 121

M

Macrophage inhibitor cytokine-1 (MIC-1) gene
  down-regulation of, association with prostatic inflammation in benign prostatic hyperplasia, 99
Magnetic resonance angiography (MRA)
  vs. digital subtraction angiography for diagnosis of renal artery stenosis, 17
Male germline stem cells
  regeneration by spermatogonial dedifferentiation in vivo, 215
  transgenic modification before fertilization by retroviral infection of cultured sperm in the zebrafish, 227
Malone antegrade continence enema (MACE)
  for neuropathic bowel dysfunction, 262
Medical education
  urology graduate, trends in, 5 (*see also* Urology residents)
  validated instrument to measure medical student learning in clinical urology, 6
Medicare
  effect of changes in reimbursement rates on urology practice, 9
MEDLINE
  full-text journal article availability, 2
Megaureter
  primary obstructive, Starr placation for, 265
MET proto-oncogene
  missense mutations in tyrosine kinase domain in early onset hereditary papillary renal carcinoma, 136

Methylation analysis
  for molecular profiling of renal cell carcinoma, 138, 139
MIC-1 (macrophage inhibitor cytokine-1) gene
  down-regulation of, association with prostatic inflammation in benign prostatic hyperplasia, 99
Microwave feedback thermotherapy
  transurethral, vs. TURP for benign prostatic hyperplasia, 113
Microwave heating
  for catheters reused for clean intermittent catheterization, 241
Mitoxantrone
  plus prednisone vs. docetaxel plus estramustine for advanced refractory prostate cancer, 199
  plus prednisone vs. docetaxel plus prednisone for advanced prostate cancer, 200
Molecular profiling
  of benign prostatic hyperplasia, using a large scale real-time reverse transcriptase-polymerase chain reaction approach, 101
  of renal cell carcinoma, by quantitative methylation analysis, 139
MRA (magnetic resonance angiography)
  vs. digital subtraction angiography for diagnosis of renal artery stenosis, 17

N

NASH/dx copolymer insertion
  using Implacer device, for stress incontinence, 81
National Surgical Quality Improvement Program (NSQIP)
  reduced morbidity costs as offset of costs of participation, 10
Nephrectomy
  laparoscopic
    en bloc stapling of renal hilum during, 33
    partial
      complications, 38
      daVinci robotic system for, 36
      long-term oncological outcome, 35
    radical
      retroperitoneoscopic, vena cava transection during, 32
      transperitoneal vs. retroperitoneoscopic, 31
  nephron-sparing, frozen section analysis in, 143
Nephrolithotomy
  percutaneous
    vs. open surgery for complete staghorn stones, 24
    predictions of length of stay, 25
Nephroureterectomy
  ureterectomy for symptomatic refluxing distal ureteral stumps after, 267
Neurogenic bladder
  with bowel dysfunction, in situ Malone antegrade continence enema for, 262
  detrusor hyperreflexia secondary to, in children, oxybutynin for, 251
  reconstruction
    non-cycled artificial urinary sphincter for, 263
    stomal complications in children with cutaneous catheterizable continent stomas, 261
  transitional cell carcinoma following augmentation cystoplasty for, 252
Nitrofurantoin
  prophylactic long-term use in children, adverse reactions, 240
  prophylactic use after surgery for pelvic organ prolapse and/or stress incontinence with suprapubic catheterization, 82
NMP22
  proteomic urine assay for detection of bladder cancer, 145
Nocturia
  questionnaire vs. frequency-volume charts for assessment, 92
Nocturnal enuresis
  persisting into adulthood, urodynamics in treatment of, 249
Nonsteroidal anti-inflammatory drugs (NSAIDs)
  vs. opioids for treatment of acute renal colic, 21
NSQIP (National Surgical Quality Improvement Program)
  reduced morbidity costs as offset of costs of participation, 10

O

Obesity
  laparoscopic radical prostatectomy and, 29
  PSA levels and, 183
  as risk factor for kidney stones, 20
  as risk factor for renal cell carcinoma, 125

Opioids
vs. NSAIDs for treatment of acute renal colic, 21
postoperative requirements after intraoperative local anesthesia during transperitoneal laparoscopic renal and adrenal surgery, 34
Orchiectomy
(*see also* Androgen suppression)
spermatic cord anesthesia block for, 213
Orchiopexy
Fowler-Stephens, long-term outcome in prune-belly syndrome, 280
Orthoptic urinary diversion
urethral recurrence of transitional cell carcinoma following, 158
Osteoporosis
in men on androgen deprivation therapy
diagnosis and treatment, 208
fracture risk and, 209
hip fracture and, 208
Overactive bladder
botulinum-A toxin for, 62
costs in the United States, 55
solifenacin succinate for, 58
Oxybutynin
in children with detrusor hyperreflexia secondary to neurogenic bladder dysfunction, efficacy and safety, 251

P

Pancreas
injuries during urologic laparoscopy, 41
PapDG protein
as vaccine for *E. coli*-mediated pyelonephritis, 85
Parkin coregulated gene
deletion as cause of male sterility in the *quaking*^{viable} mouse mutant, 226
Paroxetine
for on-demand treatment of premature ejaculation, 234
Pelvi-uretric junction obstruction
multiphase helical CT in planning surgical treatment, 16
Pelvic floor muscle training
for pelvic floor spasms in children, 248
for stress incontinence, patient characteristics predictive of outcome, 60
Pelvic organ descent
in young nulligravid women, 78
Pelvic organ prolapse
abdominal sacral colpopexy for, with autologous fascia lata, 67
sexual function before and after surgery for, 83
with stress incontinence, tension-free vaginal tape vs. endopelvic fascia plication for, 70
Penile compression release
for noninvasive assessment of bladder contractility in men, 95, 96
Percutaneous nephrolithotomy
vs. open surgery for complete staghorn stones, 24
predictions of length of stay, 25
Perineal magnetic stimulation
for urinary incontinence, 64
Perineal sling
for stress incontinence in men, 123
Permixon (*see Serenoa repens*)
Photoselective vaporization of the prostate
for benign prostatic hyperplasia, 117
Postoperative complications (*see* Surgical complications)
Practice management (*see* Urology practice)
Prednisone
plus mitoxantrone vs. docetaxel plus estramustine for advanced refractory prostate cancer, 199
Premature ejaculation
AUA guidelines on pharmacologic management, 230
on-demand treatment with clomipramine vs. paroxetine, 234
Prenatal diagnosis
lower urinary tract obstruction, prognosis and management, 258
pyelectasis (*see* Pyelectasis)
ureteroceles associated with multicystic dysplasia, outcome analysis, 258
Pretest probability estimates
in evidence-based medicine, 1
ProstaLund microwave feedback
vs. TURP for benign prostatic hyperplasia, 113
Prostate biopsy
factors predicting cancer detection in extended needle, 185
nomogram for prediction of positive repeat, 184
validity of primary care patient self-report of abnormal results, 188
Prostate cancer
advanced
docetaxel and estramustine vs. mitoxantrone and prednisone for, 199
docetaxel plus prednisone vs. mitoxantrone vs. prednisone for, 200

intermediate endpoint for mortality following salvage hormonal therapy, 203
assay for humoral response to α-methylacyl-CoA racemase as supplement to PSA screening, 201
bicalutamide in addition to standard care for localized or locally advanced
efficacy and tolerability, 204
lymph node status and, 204
comorbidity as independent predictor of mortality in older patients, 164
correlation of *GSTP1* methylation levels with Gleason grade and tumor volume in needle biopsies, 186
ejaculation frequency and subsequent risk of, 168
geographic variation in treatment, 167
immediate vs. deferred hormone treatment for patients not undergoing for curative local treatment, 171
impact of percentage of positive prostate cores on mortality, 169
impact of surgical delay on long-term control for clinically localized, 165
incidence and survival in a population that is not screened, 162
natural history of early localized, 161
preoperative PSA velocity and risk of death after radical prostatectomy, 205
prognostic significance of high grade prostatic intraepithelial neoplasia and atypical small acinar proliferation, 170
prostate specific antigen and (*see* Prostate specific antigen)
prostatectomy for (*see* Prostatectomy)
salvage radiotherapy for recurrent, 197
testosterone replacement therapy after radical prostatectomy for, 174
Prostate specific antigen (PSA)
levels
body mass index and, 183
changes in relationship to cancer parameters over last 20 years, 177
clinical utility of proPSA and "benign" PSA when percent free PSA is less than 15%, 182
preoperative velocity and risk of death after radical prostatectomy, 205
prevalence of prostate cancer among men with a level 4.0 ng/mL or less, 175
relationship between initial level and subsequent prostate cancer detection in a longitudinal study, 178
screening
biennial, 176
ecologic study of screening and prostate cancer mortality in nine geographic areas of the United States, 180
Prostatectomy
in lymph node positive prostate cancer, prognosis and long-term survival, 192
radical
frequency of positive surgical margins in patients with extraprostatic extension in the region of the neurovascular bundle, 189
Hispanic race as predictor of treatment failure, 193
impact of unilateral interposition sural nerve grafting on recovery of urinary function after, 194
laparoscopic
body mass index and, 29
extraperitoneal vs. transperitoneal approach, early oncologic results, 28
vs. open, cost comparison, 27
vs. radiotherapy, five-year quality-of-life outcomes, 173
residual benign prostatic glands at the urethrovesical anastomosis, prediction and impact on disease outcome, 190
"vanishing" prostate cancer in specimens, incidence and long-term follow-up, 191
Proteomic assay
of urine, for detection of bladder cancer, 145
Proteosome inhibitors (*see* Bortezomib)
Prune-belly syndrome
long-term outcome of Fowler-Stephens orchiopexy for, 280
PSA (*see* Prostate specific antigen)
Pubovaginal sling
with bone anchor fixation, complications after, 79, 80
persistent stress incontinence after, excessively proximal position and, 74
vs. tension-free vaginal tape for urodynamic stress incontinence, 71
Pyelectasis, mild prenatal
2-year outcomes, 257

neonatal ultrasound as screening tool for significant nephrouropathies, 256
thresholds of associated with normal postnatal renal function, 255
Pyelonephritis
in children, correlation of renal ultrasonography with inflammatory volume from dimercaptosuccinic acid renal scans, 239
E. coli-mediated, purified PapDG protein vaccination for, 85

R

Radical nephrectomy (*see* Nephrectomy)
Radical prostatectomy (*see* Prostatectomy)
Radiotherapy, for prostate cancer
for disease recurrence after radical prostatectomy, 197
vs. prostatectomy, five-year quality-of-life outcomes, 173
with and without androgen suppression for clinically localized, 195
Renal artery stenosis
computed tomographic angiography and magnetic resonance angiography vs. digital subtraction angiography for diagnosis, 17
Renal cell carcinoma
height, body mass, and physical activity as risk factors, 125
hereditary papillary, germline missense mutations in the tyrosine kinase domain of the *MET* proto-oncogene in the early onset form, 136
hypermethylation of multiple genes in tumor, urine, and serum DNA, 138
locally advanced, autologous renal tumor cell vaccine and tumor progression after radical nephrectomy in, 141
metastatic, bortezomib for, 140
molecular profiling and classification by quantitative methylation analysis, 139
natural history, 126
nephron-sparing surgery for, frozen section analysis in, 143
polymorphisms of the *CYP1B1* gene as risk factors for, 137
postoperative nomogram for prediction of recurrence, 130
pT2 classification, subcategories for improved prognostic accuracy, 131
relationship between renal tumor size and metastases in von Hippel-Lindau disease, 128
surveillance guidelines based on patterns of relapse after nephrectomy, 127
unilateral sporadic multifocal, long-term survival according to histologic subtype compared to patients with solitary tumors, 135
University of California Integrated Staging System for prediction of survival, 131
venous thrombus extension in
prognostic significance of renal vein vs. inferior vena cava involvement, 133
prognostic significance of tumor thrombus level, 132
Renal colic
nonsteroidal anti-inflammatory drugs vs. opioids for, 21
Renal masses
laparoscopic cryoablation for, 37
Renal transplantation
coronary heart disease in recipients, nontraditional risk factors, 51
immunosuppression in
alemtuzumab for, 53
FK778 for, 48
living donors, hypertension in, 50
restricted paired list exchange program, 44
valganciclovir for cytomegalovirus disease in recipients, 47
Research
impact of full-text in MEDLINE on visibility of, 2
Residents
urology (*see* Urology residents)

S

Scrotal procedures
spermatic cord anesthesia block for, 213
Semen studies
selection bias due to self-selection of volunteer donors, 221
Serenoa repens
for benign prostatic hyperplasia, 103
Sexual function
female, before and after surgery for pelvic organ prolapse and/or stress incontinence, 83
male (*see also* Erectile dysfunction; Premature ejaculation)
of adults after hypospadias surgery, 274

lower urinary tract symptoms and, 229
Sexual identity
genetic males with severe phallic inadequacy assigned female, 7-year experience, 277
Sildenafil
for erectile dysfunction, long-term safety of, 233
Sling surgery
autologous fascia lata, efficacy and morbidity, 66
delayed treatment of bladder outlet obstruction after, 68
minimally invasive polypropylene (*see* Tension-free vaginal tape; Transobturator tape)
Snodgrass repair
for hypospadias, 269
Solifenacin succinate
for overactive bladder, 58
Sperm donors
open-identity, adolescent offspring of, 222
volunteers for semen studies, selection bias and, 221
Spermatogenesis
defective, in male mice with androgen receptor deleted using a Cre-Lox conditional knockout strategy, 225
male germline stem cells regeneration by spermatogonial dedifferentiation in vivo, 215
Sertoli cell-selective knockout of the androgen receptor and meiotic arrest in, 223
Spermatogonial cells
dedifferentiation in vivo, 215
Starr plication
for primary obstructive megaureters, 265
STING (subureteral transurethral injection)
modified, for vesicoureteral reflux in children, 244
Stress incontinence
(*see also* Urinary incontinence)
in men, perineal sling for, 123
in women
with bladder outlet obstruction, 59
effect of previous treatment experience and incontinence severity on placebo response, 56
NASH/dx copolymer insertion using Implacer device for, 81
pelvic floor muscle training for, patient characteristics predictive of outcome, 60
persistent after pubovaginal sling, excessively proximal sling position and, 74
sexual function before and after surgery for, 83
sling cystourethropexy with autologous fascia lata for, efficacy and morbidity, 66
tension-free vaginal tape for (*see* Tension-free vaginal tape)
transobturator tape for (*see* Transobturator tape)
Subureteral transurethral injection (STING)
modified, for vesicoureteral reflux in children, 244
Sulfamethoxazole
prophylactic long-term use in children, adverse reactions, 240
Suprapubic catheterization
after surgery for pelvic organ prolapse and/or stress incontinence, prophylactic use of nitrofurantoin monohydrate macrocrystals for, 82
Sural nerve graft
impact on recovery of urinary function after radical prostatectomy, 194
Surgical complications
changes in prognosis after, 12
hospital costs associated with, 10
during laparoscopic partial nephrectomy, 38
pancreatic injuries during urologic laparoscopy, 41
thoracic, during urologic laparoscopy, 40

T

Tamsulosin
(*see also* Alpha-blockers)
intermittent therapy for lower urinary tract symptoms, 105
TARGIS cooled thermotherapy
for benign prostatic hyperplasia, 115
TEAP (transurethral ethanol ablation of the prostate)
for benign prostatic hyperplasia, 110
Tension-free vaginal tape
for stress incontinence
vs. endopelvic fascia plication for genital prolapse and, 70
with low Valsalva leak point pressure, 72
position and mobility, correlation with postoperative symptoms of bladder dysfunction, 74
vs. pubovaginal sling, 71

tape-related complications, 75
vs. transobturator tape, 69
Valsalva leak point pressure for prediction of outcome, 73
Testicular sperm extraction
microdissection for idiopathic nonobstructive azoospermia, prediction of successful outcome, 216
Testicular stem cells
regeneration by spermatogonial dedifferentiation in vivo, 215
Testis
prepubertal tumors, prevalence rates of histological types, 285
Testosterone replacement therapy
after radical prostatectomy for prostate cancer, 174
Thermotherapy
for benign prostatic hyperplasia
cooled, 115
microwave feedback vs. TURP, 113
TIP (tubularized incised plate) urethroplasty
for hypospadias repair, 269
Transgenic modification
by retroviral infection of cultured sperm before fertilization in the zebrafish, 227
Transobturator tape
for stress incontinence
bladder injury during procedure, 77
short-term results, 76
vs. tension-free vaginal tape, 69
Transplantation
kidney (*see* Renal transplantation)
mechanism of action of donor-specific transfusion in inducing tolerance, 43
Transurethral ethanol ablation of the prostate (TEAP)
for benign prostatic hyperplasia, 110, 112
Transurethral needle ablation (TUNA) of the prostate
vs. TURP, 5-year results, 116
Transurethral resection of the bladder (TURB)
vs. immediate cystectomy in primary T1G3 bladder cancer, 149
immediate postoperative instillation of chemotherapy in superficial bladder cancer, 156
Transurethral resection of the prostate (TURP)
vs. feedback microwave thermotherapy, 113
vs. holmium laser prostatectomy, 119
long-term outcome, influence of detrusor underactivity on, 121
quantitative morphometric analysis of specimens using immunohistochemical staining and color-image analysis, 100
vs. TUNA, 5-year results, 116
Transvaginal bone anchor fixation
complications after, 79, 80
Trimethoprim
prophylactic long-term use in children, adverse reactions, 240
Tubularized incised plate (TIP) urethroplasty
for hypospadias repair, 269
Tumor seeding
in urologic laparoscopy, 39
TUNA (transurethral needle ablation) of the prostate
vs. TURP, 5-year results, 116
TURB (*see* Transurethral resection of the bladder)
TURP (*see* Transurethral resection of the prostate)

U

Ultrasonography, renal
correlation with inflammatory volume from dimercaptosuccinic acid renal scans in children with acute pyelonephritis, 239
for febrile urinary tract infections in infants, 237
University of California Integrated Staging System (UISS)
for prediction of survival in renal cell carcinoma, 131
Upper tract transitional cell carcinoma
bladder cancer as prognostic factor for, 148
Ureterectomy
for symptomatic refluxing distal ureteral stumps after nephroureterectomy and heminephroureterectomy, 267
Ureteroceles
associated with multicystic dysplasia, outcome analysis of prenatally detected, 258
Urethral stricture
self-expanding wallstent for, long-term results, 236
urethrotomy and dilation followed by urethroplasty for, 235
Urethroplasty
buccal onlay graft, for hypospadias repair, long-term results, 273

staged buccal graft, for hypospadias reoperation, 272
tubularized incised plate for hypospadias repair, 269
Urge incontinence (*see* Urinary incontinence)
Urinary incontinence
costs in the United States, 55
in men, perineal bone-anchored sling for, 123
in women
perineal magnetic stimulation for, 64
stress (*see* Stress incontinence)
unblinding in randomized controlled drug trials, implications for assessing outcomes, 56
urge, botulinum-A toxin for, 61
Urinary retention
in benign prostatic hyperplasia, alfuzosin once daily for, 104
Urinary sphincter
non-cycled artificial, 269
Urinary stones (*see* Urolithiasis)
Urinary tract infections
in children, follow-up urine cultures and fever in, 238
febrile in infants, renal ultrasound in, 273
Urolithiasis
dietary risk factors, 19
extracorporeal shock wave lithotripsy vs. uteroscopy/laser lithotripsy for proximal ureteral stones, 23
helical CT for identification of stone composition using attenuation values, 15
obesity and weight gain as risk factors, 20
percutaneous nephrolithotomy for
vs. open surgery, for complete staghorn stones, 24
predictions of length of stay, 25
Urology practice
effects of changes in Medicare reimbursement rates, 9
laparoscopic practice patterns in the Midwest, 30
Urology residents
trends in training programs, 5
Urothelial cancer
arylamine exposure as risk factor in nonsmokers, 146
intravesical instillation of chemotherapy immediately after transurethral resection, 156
invasive, neoadjuvant platinum-based combination chemotherapy for, 155
microscopic and gross extravesical extension in pathologic staging of, 150
nodal involvement in cases treated with radical cystectomy, 151
partial cystectomy for, patient selection recommendations, 153
primary T1G3, organ-preserving approach vs. immediate cystectomy, 149
as prognostic factor for upper tract transitional cell carcinoma, 148
proteomic urine assay for detection of, 145
surgical factors in prediction of outcome, 152
transitional cell, following augmentation cystoplasty for neuropathic bladder, 252
urethral recurrence following radical cystectomy
diagnosis, management, and outcome, 159
with ileal bladder substitution, transurethral bacillus Calmette-Guerin treatment, 157
with orthoptic urinary diversion, 158
Uteroceles
obstructing, lower urinary tract reconstruction for nonfunctioning renal moieties associated with, 266
Uteroscopy
with laser lithotripsy vs. extracorporeal shock wave lithotripsy for proximal ureteral stones, 23

V

Vaginal prolapse (*see* Pelvic organ prolapse)
Valganciclovir
for cytomegalovirus disease in kidney transplant recipients, 47
Valsalva leak point pressure
low, tension-free vaginal tape for stress incontinence with, 72
for prediction of outcome after distal urethral polypropylene sling, 73
Varicocele
in adolescents
fertility following repair of, 283
progression in grade and volume, 284
Venous thrombus
in renal cell carcinoma
prognostic significance of renal vein vs. inferior vena cava involvement, 132

prognostic significance of tumor thrombus level, 132
Vesicoureteral reflux
modified subureteral transurethral injection procedure for, 244
timing of follow-up of voiding cystourethrogram in children, 243
Voiding cystourethrogram
follow-up, timing in children with vesicoureteral reflux, 243
Voiding symptom questionnaire
vs. frequency-volume charts, accuracy for nocturic episodes, 92
Von Hippel-Lindau disease
relationship between renal tumor size and metastases in, 128

W

Wallstent
self-expanding, for urethral stricture, 236

Author Index

A

Abdel-Fattah M, 71
Abdel-Latif M, 151
Abol-Enein H, 151
Abou-El-Ghar M, 16
Abreu SC, 40
Adolfsson J, 208
Agarwal PK, 174
Ahyai S, 119
Albertsen PC, 232
Al-Kohlany KM, 24
Allaf ME, 35, 41
Almeida FG, 64
Al-Zahrani H, 31
Amundsen CL, 61
Andersson A-M, 218
Andersson S-O, 161
Andrén O, 161
Andrich DE, 235
Angeloni D, 136
Antenor JAV, 178
Anumba DO, 258
Arunkalaivanan AS, 71
Åström K, 208
Atala A, 284
Auchincloss H Jr, 43
Auethavekiat P, 2
Auger J, 221
Aus G, 162, 176
Austin JC, 265
Austin PF, 258

B

Babel N, 47
Bae DC, 208
Baillargeon J, 183
Baker H, 6
Barkin J, 107
Barqawi A, 261
Barrington JW, 71
Barry MJ, 188
Bartlett E, 121
Baskin G, 85
Bassel YS, 213
Begum S, 138
Belville W, 116
Bentkover JD, 55
Bhayani SB, 27, 32, 35, 41
Bishop CE, 226
Bjørge T, 125
Blaivas JG, 65
Blockeel C, 60
Blute ML, 36, 130
Bochner BH, 153
Bogaert GA, 241
Boisen KA, 279
Borkowski A, 62
Boshier A, 233
Bostwick DG, 191
Bostwick KC, 191
Boudewijn G, 17
Bove P, 39
Boyle P, 106
Bradley CS, 59
Bratslavsky G, 237
Brawley C, 215
Broderick GA, 230
Brotzman M, 115
Brown JA, 29, 67
Bruschini H, 64
Bruskewitz R, 116
Bubanj TB, 274
Bump RC, 56
Burgess SM, 227
Burkhard FC, 157

C

Cabrol D, 221
Cadeddu JA, 9
Cain MP, 252, 262
Caldwell M, 177
Cammu H, 60
Cannon A, 121
Cardozo L, 58
Carey JM, 79
Carroll PR, 203
Casale P, 267
Castle C, 235
Caubet J-F, 188
Celia A, 39
Cestari A, 37
Chalopin J-M, 51
Chan DW, 182
Chang C, 225
Chang JH, 123
Chen M-H, 205
Chen M-J, 239
Chen SL, 10
Chen Y-T, 225
Chene L, 101
Cheng EY, 266
Chetner MP, 127
Chiu N-T, 239
Chow GK, 36
Choyke PL, 128
Clark PE, 150, 159
Conn IG, 63
Cookson MS, 158
Cooper CS, 265
Coplen DE, 258
Costa P, 76
Cote K, 169
Cummings P, 231
Curhan GC, 19, 20
Currie ML, 238

D

D'Amico AV, 169, 195, 203, 205
Daneshmand S, 192
Darrow A, 83
Davies BJ, 68
Davis WW, 172
de Almeida F, 73
Debruyne F, 107
Deffieux X, 69
De Gendt K, 223
De La Rochebrochard E, 221
Dell'Acqua V, 37
de Ridder D, 241
Desai M, 193
Desai MM, 38
deTayrac R, 69
Dettori JR, 231
de Valdenebro M, 261
Dhar NB, 22
Diamond DA, 284
Dickman PW, 208
Dietz HP, 74, 78
Dikranian AH, 123
DiMarco DS, 135
Dimick JB, 10
Djavan B, 90
Dogan I, 217
Dorey F, 73
Drinnan MJ, 95, 96
Driscoll N, 50
Droupy S, 69, 76
Drucker B, 140
Dubeau CE, 56
Ducloux D, 51
Duffey BG, 128
Duffy PG, 280
Duvdevani M, 143

E

El-Baz M, 151
Eldridge A, 78
Eliçevik M, 269
Ellis G, 74
Elmore J, 272

El-Nahas AR, 16
Elovitz M, 255
Engeland A, 125
Epstein JI, 165, 189
Erasmie U, 257
Escribano-Burgos M, 103
Etzioni R, 180
Eustache F, 221

F

Farré AL, 103
Faulkner JR, 152
Fernandez LA, 53
Fialkow MF, 80
Fichtner J, 273
Filipas D, 273
Fisch M, 273
Flisser AJ, 65
Flynn MK, 61
Fong YK, 90
Ford CA, 87
Fouad MN, 164
Franco I, 251
Frank I, 130
Frederick RW, 23, 79
Freeman JL, 209
Freschi M, 185
Fretz PC, 265
Fromont G, 101
Frydelund-Larsen L, 218
Fung CH, 167
Funkhouser EM, 164
Furness PD III, 261

G

Gabdrakhmanova L, 47
Gago-Dominguez, 146
Gan J, 146
Gerber GS, 33
Gettman MT, 36
Gilling P, 119
Giorgi LJ Jr, 237
Glassberg KI, 283
Glavind K, 83
Glenn G, 128
Goeman L, 241
Goktas S, 105
Golijanin D, 148
Gonen M, 184
Gonzalgo ML, 139
Goodman PJ, 175
Goya N, 110
Grace M, 78
Grady R, 251
Grady RW, 267
Gran CD, 266
Greenwell TJ, 235, 236
Griffiths CJ, 95
Grise P, 76, 112
Groshen SG, 159
Grossman HB, 145, 152
Guazzoni G, 37

H

Habib FK, 100
Han K-R, 133
Han M, 178
Hanselmann S, 171
Harding CK, 96
Harik M, 90
Harkaway R, 106
Hashimoto Y, 211
Hassan JM, 158
Hauri D, 171
Heldeweg EA, 93
Hernandez DJ, 189
Herndon CDA, 262, 263
Herr HW, 152
Hill B, 116
Hodges SJ, 25
Hoebeke P, 248
Hoffman RM, 172
Hoffmann L, 141
Holdgate A, 21
Holzbeierlein JM, 153
Hong SK, 92
Hoppmann M, 190
Hoque MO, 138
Horowitz M, 251
Hoznek A, 28
Hsiao K, 213
Hu T-W, 55
Hugosson J, 176
Hussain M, 236
Hussain MHA, 199
Hussain Z, 229

I

Imbimbo C, 97
Ishikawa M, 99
Ishikawa N, 110
Ismaili K, 256
Issa MM, 213
Ito F, 110
Iversen P, 206

J

Jacobsen SJ, 89
Jarow J, 230
Jeschke S, 31
Jeurgensen J-S, 47
Jocham D, 141
Johansson J-E, 161
Johnston C, 229
Jørgensen N, 218
Justice MJ, 226

K

Kaack MB, 85
Kaleva M, 279
Kammerer-Doak D, 82, 83
Kao T-C, 232
Kapadia H, 257
Karafa MT, 22
Karakiewicz P, 194
Karikehalli S, 170
Karpman E, 240
Kastin A, 143
Kato M, 126
Kattan MW, 130
Katz EE, 62
Kaunders PTK, 223
Kazory A, 51
Kennett K, 119
Kerfoot BP, 6
Kessler O, 75
Khaira HS, 34
Khan MA, 165, 182
Khullar V, 56
Kibar Y, 105
Kiemeney LALM, 125
Kim HH, 92
Kim HL, 131, 133
Kim HW, 109
Kirsch AJ, 244
Kishimoto K, 43
Klinger M, 48
Klutke C, 77
Knechtle SJ, 53
Koepsell TD, 231
Kogan BA, 237
Kondagunta GV, 140
Kreder KJ, 66, 67
Kristal AR, 183
Kropp BP, 266, 277
Ku JH, 72, 92
Kukul E, 249
Kuntz RM, 119
Kuo Y-F, 209
Kurita K, 227
Kurzrock EA, 240
Kutlu O, 249

L

Labbé-Declèves C, 221
Lahdes-Vasama TT, 247

Lam JS, 131, 193
Larsson G, 81
Latil A, 101
Latini JM, 66, 67
Laufer M, 143
Laxman B, 201
Leach GE, 79
Lee B, 29
Lee JY, 109
Lee RS, 267
Lee SJ, 109
Lehrich K, 119
Leibovich BC, 130
Leipzig, 141
Leitzmann MF, 168
Leng WW, 68
Lentz GM, 80
Lerman SE, 247
Levitt MA, 1
Libertino JA, 132
Lidefelt K-J, 257
Lilja H, 176
Link RE, 27
Lisec M, 58
Loffredo M, 195
Lohse CM, 135
Lopez-Corona E, 153
Lorenzetti D, 226
Lotan Y, 9
Lucioni A, 62
Luetjens CM, 219
Lux MM, 66

M

Main KM, 279
Malloy TR, 117
Mangold LA, 165
Manola J, 195
Markwalder R, 149
Matlaga BR, 25
Matsumiya K, 216
Matunis E, 215
Mayo CP, 164
McAllister M, 32
McAteer JA, 15
McIntosh SL, 95
McLaughlin JC, 89
McLeod DG, 204
McNaughton-Collins M, 188
McNeal JE, 177
McNeill A, 100
McNeill SA, 104
Meschia M, 70
Messing E, 145
Metcalf PD, 285
Micali S, 39
Milicevic RM, 274
Millard R, 58
Miller DC, 5
Miller EA, 80
Miller WC, 87
Minaglia S, 77
Mirone V, 97
Misseri R, 252
Mitz L, 238
Miyagawa Y, 216
Mogutin B, 75
Moinzadeh A, 132
Montague DK, 230
Moore CK, 170
Morris M, 87
Mosbah A, 24
Moul JW, 203
Mouritsen L, 74
Muller A, 221
Mullerad M, 148
Murali HR, 2
Murali NS, 2

N

Nambirajan T, 31
Nazeer T, 170
Newling DW, 93
Nguyen MT, 269
Nickerson ML, 136
Nishiyama T, 211
Nordling J, 113

O

Odibo AO, 255
Oefelein MG, 174
Okino ST, 137
Olivier B, 234
Olsen A, 82
Ong A, 32
Onur R, 123
Oosterlinck W, 156
Orvieto MA, 33
Özel B, 77

P

Paick J-S, 72
Palmer J, 112
Parker BD, 23
Patard J-J, 131
Patel RP, 271
Patil KK, 280
Paul R, 190
Pauler DK, 175
Pera RAR, 219
Perez-Brayfield M, 244
Perovic SV, 274
Petrylak DP, 199
Phelps MA, 1
Phipps S, 100
Pifarotti P, 70
Pirsch JD, 53
Plant ND, 258
Plante M, 112
Platz EA, 168
Pohl HG, 285
Pollock BH, 183
Pollock T, 21
Poon C, 74
Potosky AL, 172

Q

Quek ML, 150, 192

R

Raab E, 255
Raasch CS, 238
Radziszewski P, 62
Rajkumar GN, 63
Rajpurkar A, 123
Ramani AP, 38, 40
Rapp DE, 33, 62
Reilly TP, 23
Reiner WG, 277
Renshaw AA, 169
Renson C, 248
Rhee EY, 123
Rhodes DR, 201
Richter A, 141
Rink RC, 262, 263
Riordan M, 222
Roberts HA, 85
Robson W, 96
Rodin DM, 29
Rodríguez LV, 73
Roehl KA, 178, 205
Roehrborn C, 106
Roehrborn CG, 9
Rogers C, 35
Rogers RG, 82, 83
Roscigno M, 185
Rosenbaum PR, 12
Ross LF, 44
Rourke K, 127
Rovner ES, 59
Rubin S, 222
Ruiz L, 28
Russo P, 148

S

Sak SC, 229
Sakai N, 227
Salomon L, 28
Salzhauer EW, 285
Samli MM, 217
Sander S, 269
Sarma AV, 89
Sasaki M, 137
Scardino PT, 184
Scattoni V, 185
Scheib JE, 222
Schelin S, 113
Schmidt LS, 136
Schouten LJ, 125
Schwartz L, 140
Sclar JD, 193
Scott JE, 258
See WA, 204
Sessa G, 97
Shah J, 236
Shah OD, 25
Shahin O, 149
Shahinian VB, 209
Shakir SAW, 233
Shariat SF, 194, 197
Sharma V, 243
Sharp DS, 40
Shaw MBK, 263
Shaw PA, 180
Shin JW, 72
Shokeir AA, 24
Shoma AM, 16
Shukla AR, 271
Sidransky D, 186
Silber JH, 12
Simon SD, 243
Singh H, 194
Singla A, 123
Skipper PL, 146
Smith CP, 62
Smith EA, 244
Smith JA Jr, 158
Snodgrass W, 272
Snodgrass WT, 269
Snyder HM III, 271
Snyder ME, 130
Soergel TM, 252
Sokol A, 283
Sokoll LJ, 182
Soloway M, 145
Sorbellini M, 130
Spencer BA, 167
Spennacchio M, 70
Sreekumar A, 201
Srougi M, 64
Stamey TA, 177
Stampfer MJ, 19, 20, 168
Stein BS, 117, 208
Stein JP, 150, 159, 192
Steinberg AP, 38
Stephenson AJ, 127, 197
Studer UE, 171
Su L-M, 27
Suzuki T, 126
Suzuki Y, 126
Swinnen JV, 223
Sylvester RJ, 156

T

Taheri PA, 10
Takahashi K, 211
Taler SJ, 50
Tanaka Y, 137
Tangen CM, 199
Tann M, 15
Tannock IF, 200
Taoka R, 99
Tarin T, 68
Tash JA, 65
Taylor EN, 19, 20
Taylor JA III, 232
Te AE, 117
ter Meulen F, 81
Tetsche MS, 83
Textor SC, 50
Thalmann GN, 149, 157
Thomas AW, 121
Thompson IM, 175
Thompson M, 243
Thornton J, 22
Tireli G, 269
Tokumaru Y, 186
Topaloglu O, 138
Tretil S, 125
Trock BJ, 115, 189
Trudeau ME, 12
Tsivian A, 75
Tsujimura A, 216
Tsukuda F, 99

U

Utz WJ, 115

V

Vale C, 155
van der Meijden APM, 156
van Dijk BAC, 125
van Erps P, 107
van Haarst EP, 93
van Hooff JP, 48
Van Howe RS, 274
van Kerrebroeck P, 81
Van Laecke E, 248
Van Nylen M, 60
van Randenborgh H, 190
Vanrenterghem Y, 48
Varkarakis IM, 41
Varol C, 157
Vela-Navarrete R, 103
Versi E, 56
Volkan K, 6

W

Wagner TH, 55
Wagrell L, 113
Wahl EF, 247
Waldinger MD, 234
Wang DS, 30
Wang M, 167
Wang Y-T, 239
Webster GD, 61
Westenberg A, 119
Wilton LV, 233
Winfield HN, 30
Wirth MP, 204
Wolf JS Jr, 34
Woodhouse CRJ, 280

X

Xu EY, 219

Y

Yalcin I, 56
Yan G, 139
Yanardag H, 105
Yanke BV, 184
Yegnasubramanian S, 139
Yeh S-D, 225
Yuan X, 43
Yucel S, 249

Z

Zarse CA, 15
Zelefsky MJ, 197
Zeliadt SB, 180
Zenios S, 44
Zhou M, 186
Zimmern P, 74
Zincke H, 135
Zisman A, 133
Zurakowski D, 284
Zwinderman AH, 234